HMONG WOMEN AND REPRODUCTION

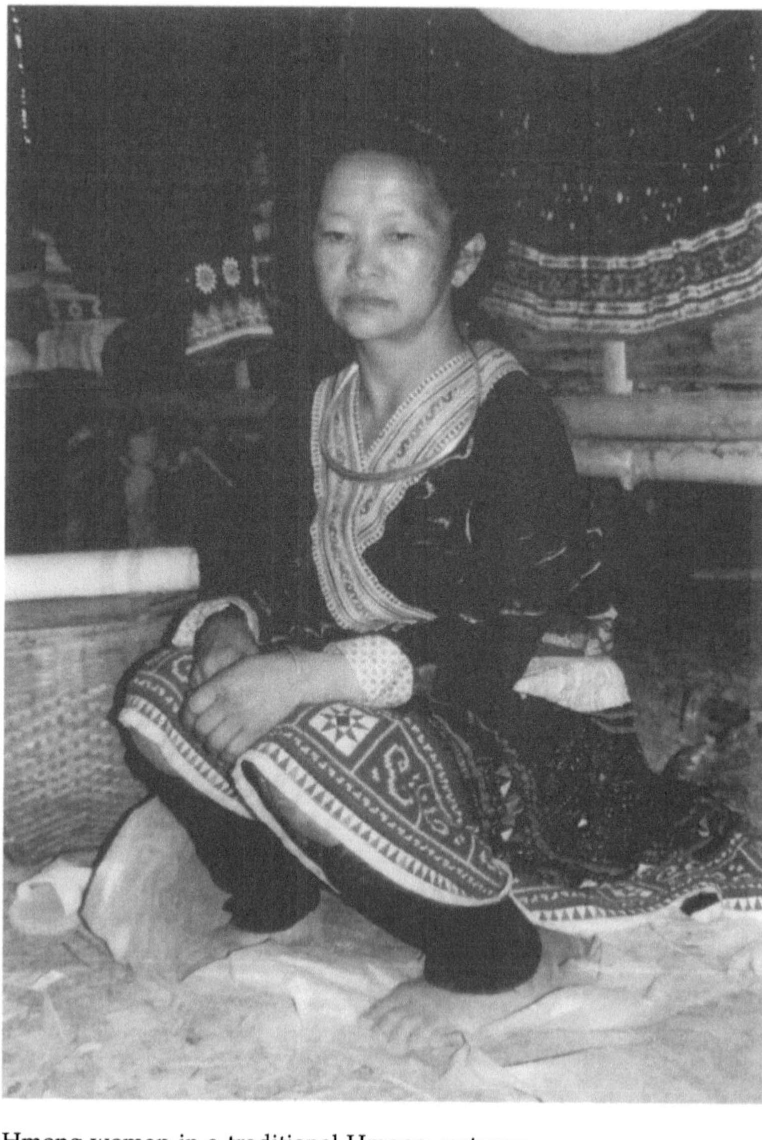

Hmong woman in a traditional Hmong costume.

HMONG WOMEN AND REPRODUCTION

Pranee Liamputtong Rice

Bergin & Garvey
Westport, Connecticut • London

Library of Congress Cataloging-in-Publication Data

Rice, Pranee Liamputtong, 1955–
Hmong women and reproduction / Pranee Liamputtong Rice.
p. cm.
Includes bibliographical references and index.
ISBN 0–89789–679–3 (alk. paper)
1. Women, Hmong—Social life and customs. 2. Birth customs—Cross-cultural studies. 3. Child rearing—Cross-cultural studies. 4. Women, Hmong—Australia—Melbourne (Vic.) 5. Maternal and child welfare—Australia—Melbourne (Vic.) I. Title.
DS509.5.H66R53 2000
305.48'895942—dc21 99–055890

British Library Cataloguing in Publication Data is available.

Library of Congress Catalog Card Number: 99–055890
ISBN: 0–89789–679–3

First published in 2000

Bergin & Garvey, 88 Post Road West, Westport, CT 06881
An imprint of Greenwood Publishing Group, Inc.
www.greenwood.com

Printed in the United States of America

The paper used in this book complies with the Permanent Paper Standard issued by the National Information Standards Organization (Z39.48–1984).

10 9 8 7 6 5 4 3 2 1

Copyright Acknowledgments

The author and the publisher gratefully acknowledge permission for use of the following material:

Excerpts from P. V. Symonds, "Cosmology and the Cycle of Life: Hmong Views of Birth, Death and Gender in a Mountain Village in Northern Thailand," Ph.D. dissertation, Department of Anthropology at Brown University, Providence, RI, 1991. Reprinted with permission of the author.

Excerpts from Megan McNamer, "Musical Change and Change in Music: Implications for Hmong Identity." In *The Hmong World 1*, edited by B. Johns and D. Strecker, 137–163. New Haven, CT: Yale Southeast Asia Studies. Reprinted with permission of Yale University, Council of Southeast Asia Studies.

Excerpts from Pranee Liamputtong Rice, Blia Ly and Judith Lumley, "Childbirth and Soul Loss: The Case of a Hmong Woman," *MJA* 1994; 160: 577–578. © Copyright 1994. *The Medical Journal of Australia*, reproduced with permission.

Chapter 10 is based on P. L. Rice, "Childhood Health and Illness: Cultural Beliefs and Practices among the Hmong in Victoria," in *Australian Journal of Primary Health–Interchange*, Vol. 4, No. 4, 44–59, 1998, reprinted with permission.

Excerpts from P. L. Rice, "When Baby Falls!: The Cultural Construction of Miscarriage among Hmong Women in Australia." *Women & Health*. Vol. 3 (1), 87–109, 1999. Reprinted with permission.

Reprinted from *Midwifery*, Vol. 16, No. 1, P. L. Rice, "Nyo Dya Hli—Thirty Days Confinement: Traditions and Changed Childbearing Beliefs and Practices among Hmong Women in Australia," pp. 22–34, 2000, by permission of the publisher Churchill Livingstone.

Excerpts from P. L. Rice, "Traditional and Changed Childrearing Beliefs and Practices and Child Health among the Hmong in Australia: Implications for Health Services," *International Journal of Health Services*, reprinted with permission of International Journal of Health Services.

Every reasonable effort has been made to trace the owners of copyright materials in this book, but in some instances this has proven impossible. The author and publisher will be glad to receive information leading to more complete acknowledgments in subsequent printings of the book and in the meantime extend their apologies for any omissions.

To all Hmong women
Who have taught me to see the world in a more meaningful way.

And
To my mother
Yindee Liamputtong
Who taught me to be a mother.

Contents

Part Three. Women and Child Rearing

Part Four. Women and Reproductive Health

Illustrations

MAPS

FIGURE

PHOTOGRAPHS

Preface

In the past decade or so, a number of publications have brought together ethnographic accounts of birth and reproduction. Brigitte Jordan's work, written relatively recently (1978), was one of the first comprehensive comparative studies to draw attention to the diverse ways of managing birth and nurturing the new mother in different social and cultural settings—the Yucatan, Sweden, the United States and the Netherlands. Subsequent books by Kay (1982), MacCormack (1982), Michaelson (1988) and Jeffery et al. (1988), among others, have highlighted women's experiences of pregnancy, childbirth, the postpartum and the days of early mothering, and draw attention to the roles played by others—kinswomen, husbands, children, traditional birth attendants—in the management and care of the new mother and the unborn/newborn child. Works such as this are valuable because they highlight the importance to women of reproduction in terms of their personal identity and social status as well as the ways in which their lives have centered on biological events. However, they do not adequately address the issues of reproduction of women from minority groups who have settled in Western societies. This book intends to fill this gap.

The focus of this book is the process of reproduction of one particular group of women from Southeast Asia—Hmong women who are now living in Australia. How Hmong women perceive, achieve, maintain and deal with reproduction is the main focus of this book, which also examines how women try to adapt to changes—social, economical and political—that affect their reproduction and their reproductive health. Data presented in this book are derived from my ethnographic research concerning the Hmong in Melbourne, Australia.

Since 1975, large numbers of Hmong people have settled in Australia, France and the United States. In the United States in particular, there are more than 200,000 Hmong scattered across many states. In Australia and France, the numbers are less, but significant enough to be taken into account by health and welfare services. In their countries of origin in Southeast Asia and China, Hmong people still live in significant numbers. Despite this, their voices are generally not heard. This is particularly true for Hmong women. Yet, in all countries—particularly in the West, where the Hmong have settled—health and welfare professionals complain of the lack of available knowledge about their lives, their history, their health needs and their reproduction. My experience in the area of reproduction among Hmong women has enabled me to fill some of these gaps in knowledge. When I published articles or chapters in books about the Hmong (Rice et al., 1994; Rice, 1993, 1994, 1995, 1997), they became important resources for professionals working with Hmong people. However, there has been no comprehensive collection concerning the Hmong and reproduction.

This book will also be useful to those who wish to better understand the lives of migrant women; for example, to those involved in Feminist Studies, Women's Health Studies, Ethnic Health Studies, Sociology and Anthropology and Social Work.

I hope this book will add to the reader's knowledge of Hmong women and reproduction and help overcome ethnocentric views about the Hmong and Hmong women. This will, hopefully, lead to more sensitive and culturally appropriate health care for Hmong women wherever they may be living.

Ua Tsaug: Acknowledgments

This book would never have been written without the help of many people: first and foremost, I thank all Hmong women and key male informants who participated in the study, who passed on to me a wealth of knowledge about the Hmong way and who helped me to better understand the Hmong world. This book is dedicated to all *Poj niam Hmoob*; Hmong women.

I thank Blia Ly and her family. Blia's endless tasks as a bicultural researcher and her wealth of knowledge and enthusiasm are indeed appreciated. I also thank Aunt Va Lee, who has become a key informant and who fed me on so many occasions.

I thank Hua Yang and his family, who invited me into their home many times so that I could participate in Hmong traditions more fully. I also thank him for his knowledge of the Hmong way, which he freely passed on to me. Aunt Xao Lee, a Hmong woman shaman who treated me like her daughter and passed on so much knowledge about shamanic ritual and herbal medicines, I also thank. The assistance of Chai Vue, who shared his knowledge on the Hmong way and Lee Vang, who reported what I have written to the community leaders, is greatly appreciated.

I sincerely thank my dear friends: Dia Cha of the University of Colorado at Boulder, who read the manuscript to check on whether I have used the wrong Hmong words or misunderstood the Hmong way, and who welcomed me into her warm home when I visited Denver; and Professor Lenore Manderson and Michael Esler, who read the entire manuscript before submission.

My sincere thanks extend to many friends and colleagues who at one time or another read and made comments on different chapters. These include Jason Ayre, Dr. Gary Yia Lee, Rhonda Small, Lyn Watson, Dr. Rosalie Cooper, Fiona Brushima, Associate Professor Heather Gardner, Dr. Simon Baraclough and Dr. Christopher Peterson.

I also wish to thank James Moua, who assisted me with the map of the United States I have included in this book; and Mao Saykeo in Australia and Maykou Vang in the United States for their assistance in various ways. My thanks also extend to Jane Garry, my editor and publisher, who saw the importance of this book and who endlessly worked with me to bring it to life.

I cannot leave this section without saying thank you to my own children, Zoe Sanipreeya Rice and Emma Inturatana Rice, who share with me so many ideas about motherhood and mothering, who always admire my work and tolerate the demands of writing. Lastly, my gratitude goes to my own mother, Yindee Liamputtong, who shares so much in common with the Hmong in so many ways. When Hmong women talked about childbearing and childrearing, I shed a tear on many occasions because they were so close to the experiences of my mother. This book is also dedicated to her.

Ua tsaug ntau to you all.

Introduction: Why Hmong Women and Reproduction?

> Woman to primitive man is . . . at once weak and magical, oppressed, yet feared. She is charged with powers of childbearing denied to man, powers only half-understood . . . forces that all over the world seem to fill him with terror. The attitude of man to woman, and, though perhaps in a lesser degree, of woman to man, is still today essentially magical.
>
> (Jane Harrison, cited in Rich, 1992: 84)

WHY DO WOMEN GIVE BIRTH?

A long time ago Hmong men used to give birth to the babies of the lineage. It was difficult and painful for men to do as they only had a small hole for the child to come out of. This caused them to labor for seven days and seven nights. One day a man delivered a child as small as a grasshopper. The man killed and ate a cow in order to replenish his strength and, because he was too lazy to carry the infant on his back, he tied it to his chin. Then, he went off to the field to join his wife who was already working there. As he walked along, he came upon a chicken. The chicken saw the baby and pecked if off the man's chin and ate it. The man started to cry and continued to do so until he reached the field where his wife was working. "Why are you crying?" his wife asked. "Because the chicken ate my baby after I laboured painfully for seven days and seven nights," he answered. "Stop crying," said his wife, "from now on why don't I have the babies? The hole I have is bigger and if I open my legs the child would be

> as big as a small stool we sit on. Then the chicken will not be able to eat it. But, if I do this you must kill me a chicken to eat every day for a month after I give birth and I must stay at home eating chicken that you have prepared for me, regaining my blood and strength." The man agreed and from then on women gave birth and men killed chickens for them to eat and cared for them for a month after the birth of each child. (Symonds, 1996: 111)

CROSSING PATHS

When I was a young child growing up in Thailand, I always heard people talking about the Hmong in a negative manner. Other hill tribes did not escape such negative attitudes, either. Very often, people judged the Hmong based on ethnocentric views that disregarded Hmong culture and traditions. Now that I am older and living in Australia, I find that negative sentiment toward the Hmong continues. "They [Hmong women] breed like rabbits" (Julian, 1994), was one comment insensitive health care providers in Australian hospitals made in reference to Hmong women. "Why are they having so many children? I don't understand it when they are so poor already," I was once asked. And a comment like: "Oh! They always want to have children, you can't stop them," is very common when people begin to talk about Hmong women in Melbourne. In addition, to outsiders, Hmong women appear to tend to be passive and submit themselves to their men, and hence have no power at all in their culture.

But do Hmong women want to "breed like rabbits"? Is it really true that Hmong women do not want to stop giving birth? And is it true that they do not care about their children? Are Hmong women altogether powerless? Would these questions be asked if Hmong women were looked at from their own perspective or within the context of Hmong culture? One may well find that Hmong women have good reasons for behaving as they do. This book will help to clarify many myths about the Hmong in general and Hmong women in particular.

Why do we need to know more about Hmong women and their reproduction? Perhaps this can be answered with the following case study.

MAI

Mai is 34 years old. She is married and has six children. Four children were born in a refugee camp in Thailand and two in Australia. Five of her children were born naturally. However, when Mai had her last child she was advised that she needed a caesarean operation, since the fetus was in a transverse lie. Mai refused the caesarean operation and insisted that she could give birth naturally. She was told that if she attempted a vaginal birth the fetus might not survive. Because of the concern about the survival of her fetus, Mai agreed to a caesarean operation. However, the caesarean operation was done under a general anesthetic and she was alone in the operating room, as her husband was not allowed to stay with her. Since the birth of her last child, Mai has been physically unwell. She has seen a number of specialists about her health, but they have not been able to find anything wrong with her.

Mai believes that while she was unconscious under the general anesthetic, one of her souls, which takes care of her well-being, left her body and was unable to re-enter. Because she was moved out of the operating room and regained consciousness in a recovery room, she believes that her soul was left in the operating room. She strongly believes that the departure of this soul is the main cause of her ill health, because during the last ten months she has frequently been awakened by bad dreams. The dreams occur two or three times a week. Each time, after the dream, she feels very ill and has bad pains. Her dream is that she is wandering to faraway places. She does not know where she is going, because she has never seen these places before. It is as if she just has to keep walking and there is no end. Mai believes this is the sign that her lost soul wanders in another world.

In order to regain her health, she must undergo a soul-calling ceremony and this must be performed at the room in which the caesarean was done, where the soul is still waiting to be called back. We asked her if she ever considered a soul-calling ceremony in the operating room in the hospital where she had the caesarean operation. Her quick response was that this would not be possible; the hospital staff would not understand her customs and would refuse the request, since the ceremony involves a live chicken and the burning of an incense stick. Her husband commented that it was hard enough to accompany his wife into an operating room, and that it would have been impossible to perform a ceremony there that is alien to western health care providers. Being unable to perform a soul-calling ceremony in the operating room, Mai's family believes that the soul has transformed into another living thing because it has left her body for a lengthy period of time. Thus, as a consequence, her health is deteriorating.

Concerned about the well-being of Mai, I promptly met with my superior and discussed the possibility of taking Mai back to the hospital to perform a soul-calling. My superior immediately contacted one of the hospital staff. Through this person, the Deputy Chief Executive Officer of the hospital agreed to the request. Her positive response was that "the hospital is more than happy to do anything for the woman if this can help her." She then left the name of a person to contact for making the arrangements.

I contacted the operating room manager to arrange the soul-calling ceremony. I was told the operating room was quite busy during the week, so I suggested to Mai that she have it done on the weekend. Because the date was not important, Mai agreed to have the ceremony performed on Sunday morning. At 8:00 A.M. one Sunday morning, Mai, her husband and a shaman met us at the ground floor of the hospital with the essential ingredients, which included a live chicken in a cardboard box. When we reached the operating room, the charge nurses were expecting us. They were very helpful and supportive, showing Mai where she was anesthetized and where she regained consciousness. They even showed Mai the path along which she was carried to the operating room, because they wanted to ensure that the ceremony was performed appropriately. At 8.30 A.M., the shaman performed a soul-calling ritual in the operating room. It took him about twenty minutes there to persuade Mai's soul to come home with her. However, to ensure that the soul would return to the "right body," the shaman also performed the same ritual at the spot where Mai regained consciousness in the recovery room. This took him only ten minutes after which we all went back to Mai's house to perform another ceremony. This was to welcome the soul back to its home.

Could this situation have been prevented? I believe so, if the cultural beliefs and practices of the Hmong women had been taken into account. There is no doubt that a caesarean operation was essential for the survival of the infant in this particular case. However, it could have been managed differently. For example, an epidural anesthetic could have been used, and Mai's husband should have been with her in the operating room to be able to call her soul into the recovery room for her.

The agreement of the hospital to allow Mai and her family to perform a soul-calling ceremony in the operating room, as well as concerns about her well-being by the hospital staff, were positive responses. They illustrate how mainstream health services can provide culturally sensitive care to consumers from different cultural backgrounds if informed of these cultural beliefs and practices.

Within multicultural societies such as the United States and Australia, different cultural sensibilities need to be understood not only as a matter of cultural tolerance but because they may have a direct effect upon the health and well-being of a mother and her newborn as well as her use of health services. A knowledge of existing patterns of childbirth beliefs and practices among Hmong women needs to be a prime concern when establishing maternal health programs. This knowledge can improve our understanding of women's acceptance or rejection of certain practices and health resources. When misunderstanding and mismanagement are eliminated, there will be better health care delivery for consumers from different cultural backgrounds. This is particularly important for the

Hmong, since the majority of Hmong women are of childbearing age. Because the Hmong put a high value on having many children, they will be major users of mainstream health services. This means that health care providers will have more contacts with Hmong women. And this is precisely the reason this book was written.

POINT OF DEPARTURE

When I had my first child 11 years ago, I gave birth in a public maternity hospital that had a good reputation for quality maternity care. My experience in the hospital, however, was not as good as I had expected. My personal experience prompted me to look at the childbirth experiences of other women. But which group of women should I study? I decided that because there are so many myths and misunderstandings about the Hmong, and because they are refugees and often recent arrivals, I should talk with Hmong women first. I approached Fitzroy Community Health Centre, where most Hmong people seek help with health issues. It is close to the Housing Commission flats, where the majority of Hmong people live. By talking with a female health care worker who, I was told, had a good relationship with Hmong women, I was able to contact a Hmong woman, Blia Ly, who later became my research assistant, assisting me during fieldwork.

During the course of my fieldwork with Hmong women in Melbourne, I had the opportunity to be introduced to another medical anthropologist, Dr. Patricia Symonds, who worked on similar issues with Hmong women in Thailand. Through her, I learned that Hmong women in America face similar problems. I heard many stories about the dilemmas of Hmong women in the United States concerning giving birth, their children's health, or some other aspect of reproductive health. All of these incidents prompted me to write this book in the hope that Hmong women might become better understood and as respected as any women in any other culture.

THE STUDY

This book is based on research in Australia among Hmong women who are refugees from Laos and have migrated to Australia since 1975. I conducted ethnographic interviews covering a number of issues concerning childbearing and child rearing with 27 Hmong women in Melbourne, Victoria.

The majority of the women had experienced childbirth while living in a refugee camp in Thailand or in hospitals in Melbourne. Older women were asked to participate so that I could obtain more information about

Hmong cultural beliefs and practices. In addition, I interviewed several Hmong traditional healers (shamans, medicine women and a magic man) in order to obtain more in-depth details of traditional healing methods.

The women were initially recruited through a community center they and their families frequently visited and from the personal network of Blia Ly, the bi-cultural researcher who is a native-born Hmong woman. She has worked for and represented the Hmong community in Melbourne for more than ten years and is well known and accepted by most Hmong here. A "snow ball" sampling technique (Minichiello et al., 1995; Yodumnern-Attig et al., 1993) was also used to recruit the women in the study; that is, the women were asked to nominate or contact friends or relatives who would be interested in participating in the study.

Entry into the community was sought from community leaders. Prior to entering the Hmong community for my fieldwork, I attended one of the community's fortnightly meetings and sought permission from the community leaders. The Hmong community was aware and informed of my presence and of my research purpose.

Women were contacted by telephone. An agreement to participate in the study was gained after information about the research and the nature of the woman's participation were explained. Each woman was also notified about the time needed for the interview. The date of the interview was then arranged to suit the woman. The women were then individually interviewed in their own homes after an informed consent was obtained. All interviews were conducted in the Hmong language by the author with the assistance of a bi-cultural research assistant. Each interview was tape-recorded. The length of the interviews varied, depending on the women's responses. In general, each interview took between two and three hours. Most women were interviewed once. There were, however, a number of occasions when I needed to obtain more information, and those respondents were visited a second time and in some cases, a third.

In addition, a participant observation method was used to allow me to observe and record the Hmong cultural beliefs and practices and their experiences in Australia more fully. I attended a number of Hmong ceremonies and participated in Hmong activities. The main interviews and participant observations were conducted between May 1993 and July 1994. However, since the initial fieldwork, I have made several more visits to the community to obtain more up-to-date information as well as to keep in contact with my key informants. My most recent participant observation was conducted in late March 1998, when I joined a soul-calling ceremony for the newborn baby of one of my key informants.

REFLECTIONS ON FIELDWORK

Morse (1992: xi, emphasis added) writes:

> To be immersed in qualitative research inquiry is *fun and exciting*. Although the process may be filled with many traps that trip the unwary researcher, the rewards are immense. Researchers get to know the participants in their studies as real people, become part of their lives and often make lifelong friends in the process.

As Morse says, immersion in fieldwork helps one better understand the Hmong, despite certain unique experiences one may have during the period. The following incident is one example of my experience while immersed in the Hmong culture.

> When I participated in a *hu plig* (soul-calling) ceremony for a newborn infant in one family, I was invited to sit at the table with the Hmong men. It is usual in Hmong culture for the men to sit at the table while the women are in the kitchen or other parts of the house, but not sitting at the table with the men. Therefore, it was rather unusual to have me at the table. I was told that because I had been known within the Hmong community and because I was highly educated, I could legitimately sit at the table with the men.
>
> Before the eating started, the family members and junior men (younger men who did not sit at the table) said "thank you" to the senior members who had helped them in general and with the *hu plig* ceremony and asked the senior members to accept their thanks. They then bowed low on the floor three times. The senior members stood up and said they accepted the thanks, and let the party begin. The alcohol tray was handed out to a man at the top of the table. He poured beer into two glasses (in full) and then handed them to the man next to him. The man drank two glasses of beer, continously (so quickly to me). I asked the man next to me why he had to drink two glasses at one time. "There is always a pair in Hmong culture, like marriage which needs a pair of woman and a man, father and mother and so on," he said. The man who had drunk the beer then poured two more glasses of beer and handed out to the next person. By now, I started to realize what was going to happen to me. I would have to drink two glasses of beer at once like the men at the table. Oh, dear! I started to panic since I cannot have alcohol. Every time I touch alcohol I become unconscious. "What do I do?" I kept wondering. I decided to ask the man with whom I had been talking about a solution. I explained to him that I understood that this was the Hmong tradition and I indeed respected it, but I could not drink any kind of alcohol. He looked at me with funny eyes, and then he smiled and said, "I will do my best to help you out."
>
> Then it was my turn. The beer was passed to me. I looked desperately at the man at the top of the table who was in charge of this drinking round. The man next to me whispered to me that I should seek permission from

> the in-charge man. I stood up and told him about my problem. Everyone laughed. The man in charge stood up and said that he accepted my problem and he knew that as a woman I should not drink alcohol anyway. He then poured two glasses of Coke and passed them to me. What a relief! I thanked everyone at the table and then drank the Coke as quickly as I could.

What followed my initial fieldwork was extended contact between the Hmong community and myself. My role now is seen not so much as a researcher who wants to find out about their lives, but rather as a friend. I have been invited to family functions. For example, Mai has asked me for advice on matters including health and family. Mai also gives me her advice on health issues. For example, during the fieldwork I accidentally burned my little girl with hot coffee. I talked with Mai about my concern about the burn. She quickly advised me to bring my daughter to see the Hmong magic man, who had a reputation for curing burn tissue with magic. She instructed me on what to bring to honor the healer and how to go about asking for help within the Hmong culture. I followed her advice. Unfortunately, he was not home and after a lengthy wait, I had to bring my girl home without receiving his healing power.

I had contact not only with Mai, but with others in the community. One Hmong man, Hua, has become like a brother. My research assistant, Blia Ly, has become like a little sister. Her mother-in-law has fed me whenever I turned up at her house, giving me fresh vegetables if she had come back from a farm. There were many times, too, that the women would make comments about my life as a migrant mother and other aspects of my life. Because I have only two daughters, some would tell me to have more children, particularly boys. They also promised that if I had another child, they would make me a baby carrier so that I could carry my baby like they do. When I first met Aunt Xao Lee, a woman shaman, she said I looked just like her mother who had passed away a long time ago in Laos. After that, whenever I saw her she would give me a big cuddle and kiss. It felt very special and moving.

This does not mean that I am totally accepted and trusted by the community. I had to seek permission before commencing my fieldwork, as indicated in the study section. There are certain aspects of Hmong life that I was told not to write about, as to do so could harm the community. Consequently, I am reluctant to write in depth on certain issues. This may be obvious to those who are familiar with Hmong culture, and some topics may be seen as lacking in detail. This is my ethical dilemma.

Many times, the Hmong would comment that they were happy to tell me about Hmong culture and customs, but that they did not expect me to help them improve their lives in their new homeland. I believe they appreciate my limitations as a researcher and as an academic who might not be able to perform the tasks of a social worker.

Morse (1992: xi) says that "researchers' lives are enriched as participants share their stories, their suffering, and their lives" when one engages in qualitative methodology. I have found this to be particularly true in my study, on which the information in this book has been based.

Part One

The History and the Culture

Chapter 1

The Hmong

THE ORIGIN OF THE HMONG: HMONG LEGEND

The Great Flood and Children of Incest

Once upon a time, the whole universe turned upside down, and the whole world was flooded with water. All living beings were killed, except one brother and sister, who were safe by staying in a wooden boat. Later the flood stop and the land dried up, and the brother and sister started to plant seeds and looked after their fields. The brother asked his older sister to marry him but she refused. He persisted. After being tricked, his sister eventually agreed to marry him. Soon she became pregnant and gave birth to a formless infant, which shaped like an egg. The parents cut it open, believing the infant was inside. However, when each piece of the infant's flesh touched the ground it transformed into a normal child. The parents cut more pieces in order to turn them into as many babies as possible. This created the Hmong population in the world. Since the parents threw the infant's flesh in different directions, it landed in different places and created many Hmong clans. (Adapted from Johnson and Yang, 1992; Quincy, 1995)

Why the Hmong Live on Mountains

The very first king of the Hmong was a child who had remained in his mother's womb for three years. Because he was such a special child, he

> grew up to be king. He then lived in a palace of pure gold. One day, the Hmong and their neighbors had a dispute over ownership of land. The king ordered both parties to depart at nightfall and to return before sunrise. He decreed that each would be the owner of the land they had traveled over during the night. The party that did not return on time would have to remain at the place where the rising sun caught them travelling. At daybreak, the Hmong found themselves on a high mountain, and since that time the Hmong have lived on mountains. (Livo and Cha, 1991:57)

These are only two of the Hmong legends about the creation and the location of the Hmong. These stories are only part of many Hmong oral histories told as myths or legends.[1] However, in real history, how the Hmong came to be as we know them today is another story.

HISTORY OF THE HMONG

The Hmong do not have their own written history, but rely on oral history passed down by older generations.[2] Consequently, most of what we know about the Hmong has been written by outsiders, very often with "prejudiced observations" (Cooper et al., 1995: 5). However, what seems to be consistent is the fact that the Hmong living in Laos, Thailand, Vietnam and several countries of resettlement migrated from the mountainous areas of southern China (see Map 1.1).

In China, the Hmong are referred to as "Miao," meaning "barbarians," the term the Chinese use to refer to all minority groups who have different beliefs and practices from their own. The Hmong do not accept this. Hence, they call themselves "Hmong," which some take to mean "free people," a term that I believe best portrays the Hmong wherever they live. Trueba et al. (1990: 21) have this to say about the Hmong:

> Oral traditions and recorded personal histories depict the Hmong as a fierce, independent and invincible people who took to the mountains rather than submit to the domination of lowlanders. Their quest for autonomy led them from the forest of southern China to the fertile mountains of Burma, Laos, Vietnam and Thailand.

In early times, the Hmong were said to live in lowland valleys. Early Chinese history described the Hmong as "an ancient people who occupied the fertile Yellow River basin long before the Chinese themselves migrated into the area" (Quincy, 1995: 17). Because of wars, suppression and the demand for assimilation from the Chinese, the Hmong retreated into the mountains where "the freedom to live as they pleased became the prime consolation" of their life (Quincy, 1995: 33). From the late sixteenth century, there were many wars between the Chinese and the

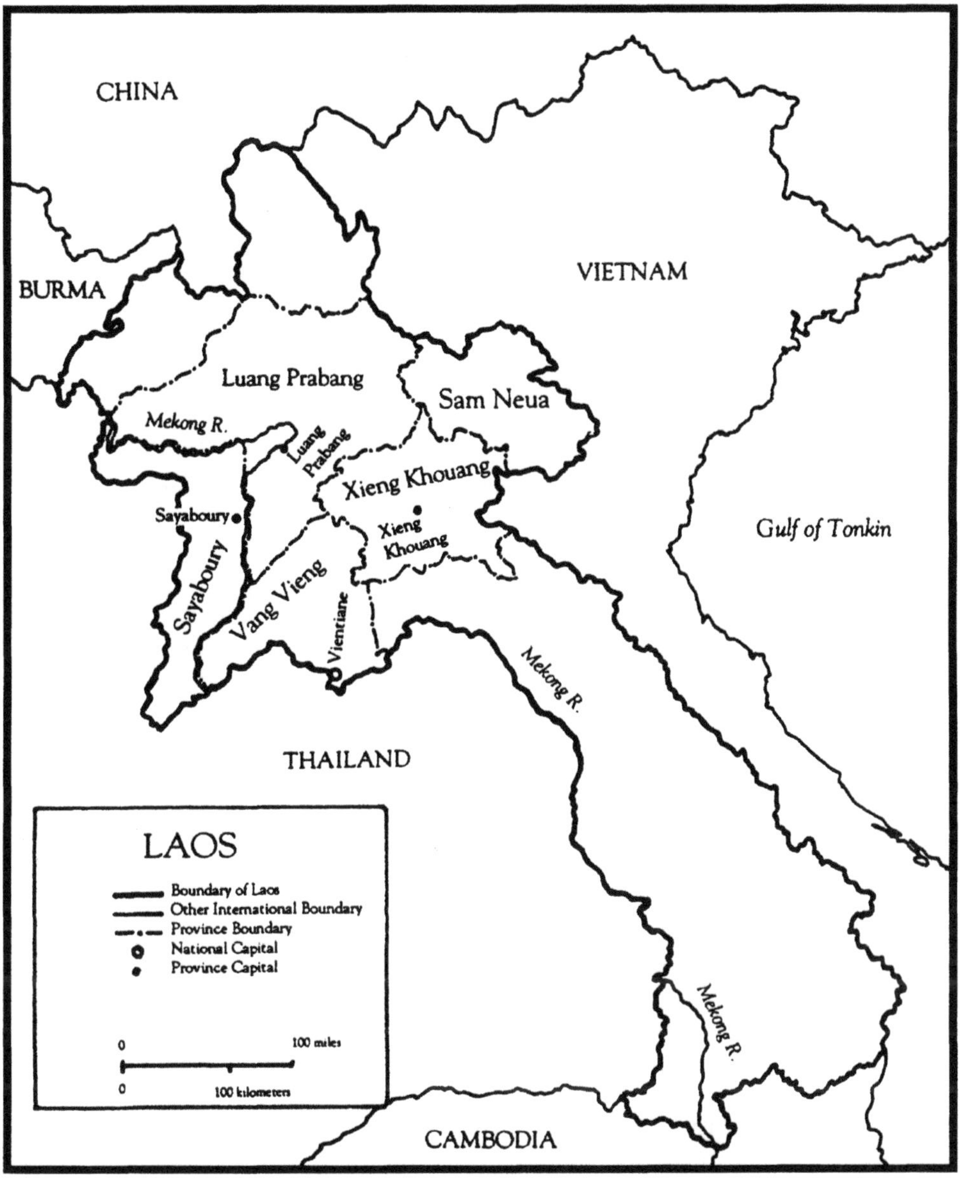

Map 1.1 Laos. *Source*: Adapted by N. D. Donnelly, 1994. *Changing Lives of Refugee Hmong Women*. Seattle: University of Washington Press. From original by Dr. Joel Halpern. Reprinted by permission of the University of Washington Press.

Hmong, but the bloodiest wars occurred between 1855 and 1881, forcing many Hmong to migrate southwards into Southeast Asia (Trueba and Zou, 1994).

It is said that the Hmong began to move into Laos somewhere between 1815 and 1818 (Quincy, 1995). They settled in the mountainous areas, where there was no competition with those who occupied the land earlier. Later on, they moved into Xieng Khouang province in eastern Laos, where there were plenty of lush and uninhabited mountains.[3] In their early years of settlement in Laos, the Hmong lived in a relatively peaceful environment. However, they rebelled against the French when the French imposed a tax on them in 1918, and the rebellion ended in 1921. The bloodiest war, which decimated many Hmong lives and changed their way of living, was the civil war in Laos between 1949 and 1975.

The Hmong began their migration into Thailand around 1855. Most Hmong in Thailand live in mountainous areas in the north, including Chiang Mai, Chiang Rai and Mae Hong Son. Cooper et al. (1995) state that by 1929 there were Hmong in Tak province, a town located at the southern tip of the mountain range stretching north into the southern provinces of China, where most Hmong still live today. Compared to their lives in China and Laos, the Hmong in Thailand live relatively peacefully, since they have not been involved in any civil war such as in Laos, or suppressions as in China, except for the so-called "Red Meo War," a rebellion that resulted in the destruction of many Hmong villages and the resettlement of many Hmong in the lowlands or flight into the jungles (Mottin, 1980; Lee, 1986).[4]

HMONG AS REFUGEES

Because of their reputation as fierce fighters and their familiarity with mountains, Hmong were recruited by the Central Intelligence Agency (CIA) to become secret guerrillas and help American pilots shot down over mountains during the Vietnam War. From 1961 to 1973, thousands of Hmong were involved in a "secret war," and it was said that Hmong casualties were ten times higher than those of the American soldiers fighting in Vietnam (Fadiman, 1997; Cerquone, 1986). Hmong civilians lost their homes and became displaced persons living in refugee camps in Laos.[5]

When the American forces withdrew from Indochina and the Lao coalition government fell in May 1975, the Pathet Lao began a plan to "exterminate" all Hmong. On May 9, 1975, the Pathet Lao newspaper published the party's intention: "It is necessary to extirpate, down to earth, the 'Hmong' minority" (Quincy, 1995: 208). We then saw another sad episode of Hmong migrations, beginning with a long march towards the Thai borders, crossing the Mekong River, and long stays in refugee camps in Thailand. Those who stayed were executed or died from the deadly effects of the "red" and "yellow" rain. Many were sent to re-education camps, where starvation took many lives, and many were forced into agricultural communes in the lowlands, where they were stricken with tropical diseases. As Quincy (1995: 210) poignantly puts it: "After thirty years of more or less continuous fighting and the loss of approximately one third of their population, the Laotian Hmong found themselves back where they had started three generations earlier: poor, repressed, and longing for freedom."

Many Hmong have been able to resettle in Western countries as refugees. The majority have been accepted into the United States because of their involvement with the CIA. There are a small number of Hmong in other countries, including Canada, France (including French Guiana), Argentina and Australia. The most recent estimation indicates there are 220,000 Hmong in the United States and Canada, 11,500 in France, and 1,800 in Australia (Yang, 1992; Adler, 1995; Moua, 1996; Stone, 1998; Lee, 1999; Cha, personal communication, 1999). Those in refugee camps in Thailand number about 50,000.

THE HMONG IN AMERICA

Since the end of the Vietnam War in 1975, about 220,000 Hmong have resettled in the United States (Cha, personal communication, 1999). A large number settled in three main states: California, Minnesota and Wisconsin (Moua, 1996). However, since the early 1980s there have been secondary migrations among the Hmong, mainly into areas where the climate is similar to their homeland and where they can farm. A secondary migration took place into the Central Valley of California. At present, California has the largest Hmong population in the United States. The Census of the Population and Housing of California State in 1990 indicated that 46,892 Hmong live in California, with the largest concentration located in Fresno (Moua, 1996). The Hmong spread across other states in the United States, as shown in Map 1.2. Recent estimation (Cha, personal communication, 1999) indicates that there are about 50,000 Hmong in California, 45,000 in Minnesota, and 30,000 in Wisconsin. Colorado, Michigan, North Carolina and Georgia have more than 5,000 Hmong. Other states have less than 2,000 Hmong.

The Hmong in the United States face many difficulties in adjusting to their new society. The toughest adjustment has been economic (Quincy, 1995). Unemployment among the Hmong in the United States is relatively high. In Fresno, for example, the rate is as high as 90%. Rates in North Carolina and Texas are lower (Yang, 1992). A large number of Hmong rely on welfare for survival. Quincy (1995) points out that in 1987, nearly 63% were on welfare and in some Californian communities

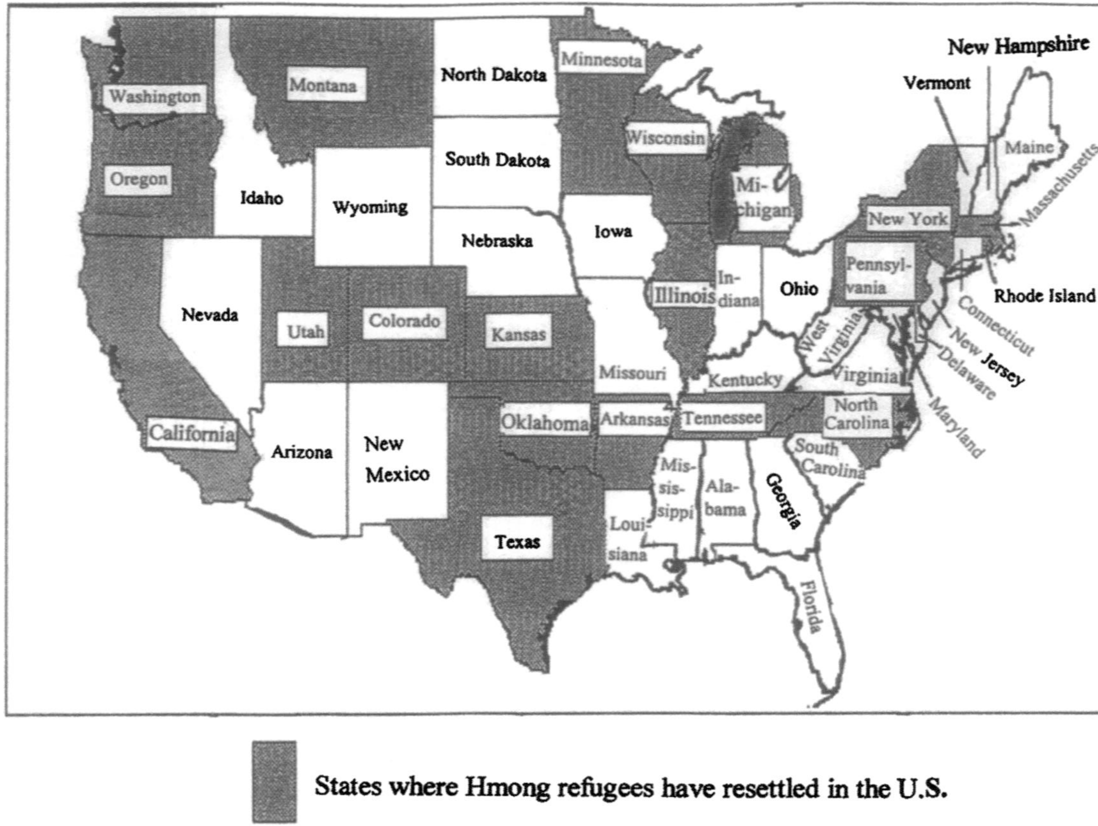

Map 1.2 Hmong refugee resettlement in the United States. *Source*: J. L. Moua, 1996. "The Uses of Herbal Medicine in Health Care Practices of Hmong Refugees, and Policy Implications in Merced County, California." Masters thesis, California State University, Stanislaus. Reprinted with permission.

the welfare rate was over 80%. However, many younger Hmong are doing well with their educations (Yang, 1992; Quincy, 1995). At present, many Hmong have graduated with Bachelor, Masters and Doctoral degrees, and the number of highly educated Hmong continues to rise.[6] Quincy (1995) points out that because of their academic achievements, Hmong children are likely to be successful in gaining skilled employment. Some Hmong have already worked as engineers, social workers, computer programmers and university professors.

For the Hmong in the United States, religion and culture have been affected by resettlement. Many Hmong in the United States have been converted to Christianity, and this has a great effect on beliefs and practices concerning health and illness as well as on the relationships between Christian and non-Christian Hmong. This is particularly true regarding shamanic beliefs, which have no place in Christian theology (Quincy, 1995). Some traditional practices, such as marriage by abduction, have caused some Hmong men to be jailed or subjected to heavy fines. Cultural interpretations of health and illness have also led to accusations of child neglect or abuse, and children have been taken from their parents' homes (e.g., Fadiman, 1997; Chan, 1994). Such interpretations have also led to interference from government officials, such as court orders for medical procedures (e.g., Lusetich, 1994; Murphy and Chamberlin, 1994).

THE HMONG IN AUSTRALIA

Like the Hmong in America, the Hmong in Australia are refugees from Laos.[7] By and large, they left their country in the same period as their counterparts in the United States. However, their resettlement in Australia has been slower. The Hmong first settled as refugees in Australia in 1976 (Lee, 1999), mostly in New South Wales. Between 1980 and 1991 a small number of Hmong migrated to Australia under the Family Reunion Program and the Community Refugee Settlement Scheme (Lee, 1999).

In Australia, the number of Hmong is far less than in the United States. It is estimated that there are about 1,500 to 1,800 Hmong in Australia (Stone, 1998; Lee, personal communication, 1999). This number is based on an estimation by Hmong community leaders in Melbourne, as there are no official statistics collected on the Hmong *per se*. Officially, the Hmong in Australia are included under "people born in Laos."

According to Lee (1999), in 1986 there were 384 Hmong living in Sydney, Melbourne, Hobart, Adelaide and Canberra. However, the 1996 Australian census indicated 1,420 "Hmong-speakers" in Australia: 603 in Queensland, 384 in Victoria, 272 in Tasmania, 126 in New South Wales, 29 in the ACT, 3 in South Australia, and 3 in Western Australia. However, for those who defined themselves as having "Hmong ethnicity," the number is 1,603. These include: 748 in Queensland, 397 in Victoria, 257 in Tasmania, 161 in New South Wales, 28 in the Australian Capital Territory, 7 in Western Australia, and 5 in South Australia (Map 1.3). In the last eight years, we have seen a secondary migration among the Hmong from the southeastern states to the far north of Queensland, mainly for economic reasons. This is the only area where they can do farming, and as Lee (1999) argues, the region's rain forests "remind them of their old home in the highlands of Laos."

In Victoria, where the study was undertaken, the Hmong live in close-knit groups, mainly in high-rise public housing in an inner suburb and one outer suburb in the state capital, Melbourne. With new children being born into families, the number of Hmong in Melbourne, estimated in 1998 (Hmong Australia Society Inc., 1998), was 497. These included 98 males and 96 females over age 18 and 153 males and 150 females under age 18.

Although more Hmong are unemployed in comparison with other Southeast Asian refugees in Australia, it is estimated that 35% of Hmong households now engage in small businesses. In addition, many Hmong now either have their own banana farms or work as hired labor for banana growers in northern Queensland around Cairns and Innisfail (Lee, 1999).

Most Hmong in Australia have not been converted to Christianity, as have their counterparts in the United States.[8] Although we have seen changes in Hmong life because of the need to adapt to a new environment, their culture has not altered greatly. Quincy (1995) states that Hmong children in the United States speak little Hmong, and more and more Hmong women exercise greater independence in the family. According to my observations, the same trend is not reflected among the Hmong in Australia, except for a few families that have done better than most, or those who have been resettled for a longer period of time.

By and large, the Hmong in Australia—particularly the first generation—try to maintain their cultural heritage. They live relatively quiet lives, as most small minorities do. Health and illness are still interpreted within their cultural framework, but they have no hesitation in seeking Western health care if need be (Wang, 1998). They still strive for freedom and resist being absorbed or assimilated into the host society. This has always been the case historically, but is more pronounced in Australia, with its multicultural approach to migrant settlement. This will be seen clearly in the chapters that follow.

HMONG SOCIAL STRUCTURE

The Hmong are not homogeneous, but are divided into different subgroups. The most well-known groups are White Hmong (*Hmoob Dawb*)

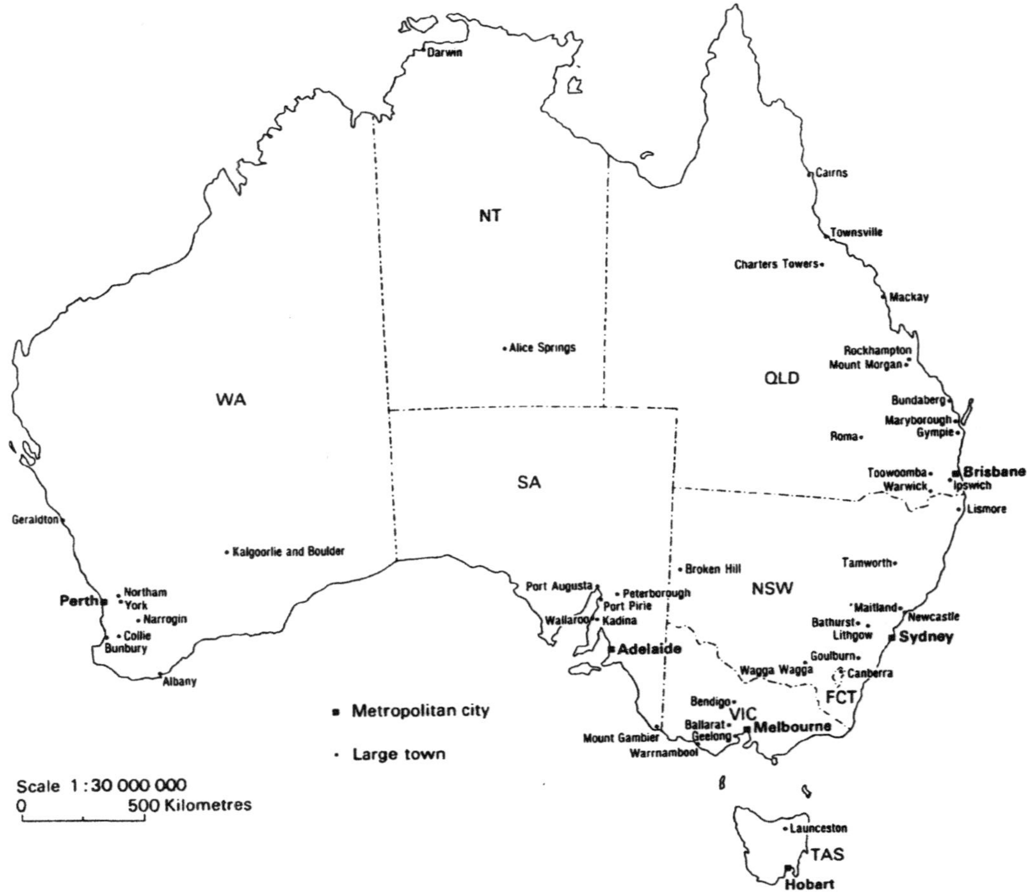

Map 1.3 Australia. *Source*: Reprinted from J.C.R. Camm and J. McQuilton (eds.), "Australians: A Historical Atlas," Fairfax, Syme and Weldon Associates (1987) by kind permission of The Macquarie Library Pty Ltd.

and Green Hmong (*Hmoob Ntsuab*). There are also other Hmong subgroups known as Striped Hmong and Flowery Hmong; they are differentiated by women's costumes. Green Hmong women wear a blue skirt that is batiked, embroidered and pleated. White Hmong women wear black trousers, but they also wear a plain white skirt, particularly at New Year's time and as a burial costume. Striped Hmong women dress like White Hmong but have striped decorations on the sleeves of their jackets.[9]

Although there are differences in their identity and differences in dialect, many similarities exist, and these are the main identity of the Hmong. As Cooper et al. (1995: 25) point out, "The similarities uniting the various components of Hmong identity certainly outweigh the significance of cultural-linguistic distinctions. As every coin must have two sides, so Green and White identities make up a single Hmong identity."

Hmong society is patrilineal. Family names follow the clan system (*xeem*). The original clans are said to number about 20 (Lee, 1981; Bliatout 1982; Cooper et al., 1995; Moua, 1996). These include: Cha/Chang (*Tsaab/Tsab*), Chai (*Cai*), Chee (*Tshib*), Cheng (*Tsheej*), Chue (*Tswb*), Fang (*Faaj/Faj*), Hang (*Haam/Ham*), Her (*Hawj*), Khang (*Khaab*), Kong (*Koo*), Kue (*Kwm*), Lao/Lor (*Lauj*), Lee/Ly (*Lis*), Moua/Mua (*Muas*), Phang (*Phaab/Phab*), Plua (*Plua*), Tang (*Taj*), Thao/Thor (*Thoj*), Vang (*Vaaj/Vaj*), Vue (*Vwj*), Xiong (*Xyooj*), and Yang (*Yaaj/Yaj*) (Bliatout, 1982: 5; Moua, 1996: 30). In Laos and Thailand there are only 18 clans (Cooper et al., 1995). In Australia in 1984 there were only 8 clans, but by 1996 there were 12 clans (Lee, 1999). In Melbourne, however, there are only 8 clans, including Hang, Lee, Lor, Moua, Thao, Vang, Vue, and Yang[10] (Hmong Australia Society Inc., 1998).

Within a clan, the Hmong observe a lineage system. Lineage is a "cluster of brothers" (*ib cuab kwv tij*) or a group of people who can trace their descent through a male line from a common ancestor (Lee, 1981; Symonds, 1991; Cooper et al., 1995). The eldest male of the lineage, usually the father, is the spiritual leader who organizes rituals and other important matters. Lineage members should be invited to important social and religious occasions such as weddings and funerals. Lee (1981: 670) refers to the lineage as "one ceremonial household" because "it is in this household that specific mortuary rituals take place and into which a member is ideally born and dies" (Symonds, 1991: 31).

The practice of clan system means the prohibition of incest taboo. A clan name prohibits a Hmong man from having sexual relations with or marrying a woman who has the same clan name as himself. However, sexual relations or marriage are permitted between people of the same clan names who are not related by blood ties, especially among the Vang and Xiong clans in Laos and Thailand (Lee, 1981). Ideally, a son should marry his mother's brother's daughter or his first cousin on his mother's side (Cooper et al., 1995).

Hmong residence is patrivirilocal. Women, when married, move into their husband's household. Upon their marriage they are accepted into their husband's clan. This means that they follow the customs of their husband's clan, not their natal families. Women therefore define themselves in relation to the household in which they reside. However, women do not change their clan name upon marriage (Moua, 1996).[11]

The Hmong, traditionally, practice polygyny. It has been argued that this practice was originally born out of economic necessity, because more wives meant more children to help in farming. However, the practice was later adapted because many Hmong men perished quickly during the war, leaving many widows without men to protect them (Moua, 1996; Scott, 1986). Therefore, a Hmong man may have as many wives as he can afford. In reality, however, only a wealthy man can do so because of the substantial bride price that must be paid to the woman's family.[12]

The Hmong also practice levirate; that is, a widow may marry her husband's younger brother after his death (Symonds, 1991). This takes place only if the widow's family wishes to remain within the extended family and gain its economic support. She can otherwise marry other men outside the family (Moua, 1996). The brother may have already had a wife or several wives. Hence, polygyny, in this case, acts as a form of social security for the widow.

From this discussion, it becomes clear that Hmong value the group more than the individual. Yang (1993: 22) puts this succinctly: "The Hmong mentality has, through the ages, been profoundly steeped in the concept of group. What counts is most often the group—the family, the clan—rather than the individual, whose sojourn on earth is a brief one."

HMONG COSMOLOGY

The Hmong are animistic and practice ancestral worship. They believe in reincarnation; the rebirth cycle. This has led to belief in a great variety of deities, spirits and other supernatural beings in the Hmong cosmos.

The Hmong Universe

Symonds (1991: 43) states that the Hmong divide the universe into two worlds. One is the "World of Light" (*Yaj ceeb*), the world of the living. Another is the "World of Darkness" (*Yeeb ceeb*), the metaphysical world of spirits. According to Symonds (1991: 43), everything that lives in the World of Light is interconnected. Hence, the living, such as people, animals and plants, are connected with the supernatural beings, such as wild spirits and caring spirits.

The worlds of light and darkness are also connected.

> All of these animated beings are connected to the dark land of the ancestors, supernatural spirits, and gods—the land where souls (*tus plig*) come from when they are called to enter the body of a new born infant and where souls return after they leave the mortal body of a dead person. These souls return again when called to a new body in a continuous and never-ending cycle of rebirth. (Symonds, 1991: 44)

This interconnection of the two worlds is clearly shown in Hmong beliefs and rituals, which will be discussed in the following sections and throughout this book.

Hmong Deities

In Hmong cosmology, benevolent deities govern the world of darkness. The creator and ruler of the world is *Huab Tais Ntuj*. Although he creates human beings, *Huab Tais Ntuj* has no interest in their affairs. He can see what humans are doing in the world below him, but he does not interfere with them.[13] A shaman told me that *Huab Tais Ntuj* is the king of heaven and his children are the Hmong, since he gave his permission for the Hmong to become human beings. *Huab Tais Ntuj*, or God, also governs all living beings including humans and animals in the mundane world. He explained "Every one on earth is under the rulership of *Huab Tais Ntuj*; whether it be an animal or human, they are all the same. *Huab Tais Ntuj* made humans to live on earth so he must make some animals to feed the humans. If they only made humans then what will they eat? This is why humans have the right to eat animals, and eating them will not curse them in any way."

It is, however, one of his lieutenants, *Saub*, who has compassion for human beings (Quincy, 1995). *Saub* is known as a kindly deity to whom humans can appeal in times of need. *Saub* is associated with fertility and reproduction. According to Hmong folklore: "It was *Saub* who supplied the first seeds and *Saub* who caused the first hen to lay eggs. It was *Saub* who, after the mighty floods, receded from the Earth, and told the surviving brother and sister to carve up the shapeless flesh or their incestuous child. From the pieces of flesh grew the 12 original Hmong clans" (Cooper et al., 1995: 54). According to Symond's Hmong informants in Thailand (1991), *Saub* has wives. Hence, sometimes people may refer to *Saub* as *Puj* and *Yawm Saub* (Grandmother and Grandfather *Saub*). *Puj* and *Yawm Saub* live in heaven and do not interact too often with humans.

Another important deity is *Siv Yis*, who was "given the power to cure illness and disease" and became the first shaman. He is the master that all other shamans look to in healing rituals. *Siv Yis* lives in a cave in the Otherworld. When a shaman dies, his spirit helpers (*neeb*) will return to this cave. When another person is called to become a shaman, it is *Siv*

Yis who will send spirit helpers to assist the shaman in healing. *Siv Yis* does not make any distinctions between male and female; this is why both men and women are able to become shamans if he or she is chosen to help other human beings.[14]

In my interviews with the Hmong in Melbourne I came across another deity couple who have not been much mentioned in previous literature.[15] This couple is *Txoov Kab Yeeb*, the "Spirit Parents" who bring the soul of the newborn to earth and who assist in fertility (Symonds, 1991).[16] It is said that *Txoov Kab Yeeb* are able, through a shaman, to give children to women who are infertile. The Hmong believe that if a woman is unable to conceive, she did not bring "a piece of paper" (mandate of life) from heaven when she was born indicating that she would have children. This piece of paper is written and given out by *Txoov Kab Yeeb*. If the paper does not indicate that a woman can have children, she becomes childless. Hmong women understand that to be able to conceive, a woman must have a husband or at least a man involved in the affair. However, pregnancy cannot happen solely by having a husband. It is determined by *Txoov Kab Yeeb*. A child can be born only when *Txoov Kab Yeeb* give permission. Only they can direct the child to be born to the woman they have stated is to do so on her "piece of paper," written before her own birth.

On the third day after birth, parents must hold a *hu plig* (soul-calling and naming) ceremony to thank the spirit parents for bringing the child into the world of men and to the family, lineage and clan. It is believed that the spirit parents have an interest in the well-being of the child, and they may take the child back if the child is not properly looked after by his or her human parents.[17]

Lords of the Otherworld

In the World of Darkness there are two Lords of the Otherworld who are "wicked and cruel" and greatly feared by the Hmong. One is *Ntxwj Nyug*, and another *Nyuj Vaj Tuam Teem*, who together control birth and death. *Ntxwj Nyug* resides at the top of a great mountain. The souls of the dead must pass his many gates before joining their ancestors. "It is to him one must present one's papers, to show the correct rituals were performed; he is the judge who gives souls permission to be reborn and in what form" (Symonds, 1991: 52). *Ntxwj Nyug* is assisted by *Nyuj Vaj Tuam Teem*, who sits on a mighty throne behind a great writing desk and gives out licenses for rebirth (Cooper et al., 1995; Symonds, 1991). These two Lords of the Otherworld are more commonly known by the Hmong as those who give out a "mandate of life," which will indicate the length of a person's existence and his or her fate in the mundane world. When the person becomes ill and dies, the Hmong say that it is because his or her death was due (Thao, 1986).

Plig (Soul) and Life

In Hmong belief, souls play a major role in a human's health and well-being. Hmong say that each person has three souls (*plig*).[18] Each soul has its own duty. One soul looks after the body when a person is still living. This soul travels to the other world and awaits the opportunity for re-birth. A second soul stays to look after the grave of the person after his or her death and it is not reincarnated. A third soul travels to live with their ancestors in the other world when the person dies (Lee, 1981; Symonds, 1991; Bliatout, 1991).[19]

If all souls reside in the body, a person will be well and healthy. A soul is able to wander off occasionally and is usually able to return to its body. However, ill health occurs when a soul leaves the body because it is frightened away for any reason and is unable to find its way home. The causes of soul loss are many; among them are injury and wounds, a great fall, a loud noise, being alone in darkness, being unconscious, or feeling sad and lonely (Symonds, 1991; Thao, 1984; Chindasri, 1976). To restore a person to wellness, a soul-calling ceremony (*hu plig*) must be performed at the place at which the soul has left the body. The soul-calling ceremony is often performed by a shaman, who will "travel to the other world" to bring the soul back. However, I was told that the ceremony could also be performed by an older person who has knowledge of the soul-calling ritual.[20]

Chindasri (1976) found that the Hmong in his study perceived that souls were related to human strength. They believed that a human body is held up by his or her souls like strings, connecting the body to the sky. If one or more strings are cut, the person will then be sickly and less strongly held up. But Symonds (1991:46) points us to the significance of souls in the Hmong cosmos:

> The souls are also perceived as being transferred from one social order to another. This soul transference occurs at birth, when one of the souls travels from the world of darkness to the world of light to be incorporated into the family, lineage, and the clan. It also occurs at marriage, when a woman's souls change their allegiance and residence from one family, lineage and clan to another. Finally, souls are transferred at death, when they leave the body and travel back to the land of darkness, one soul to be incorporated into the community of ancestors and one to await the opportunity for rebirth.

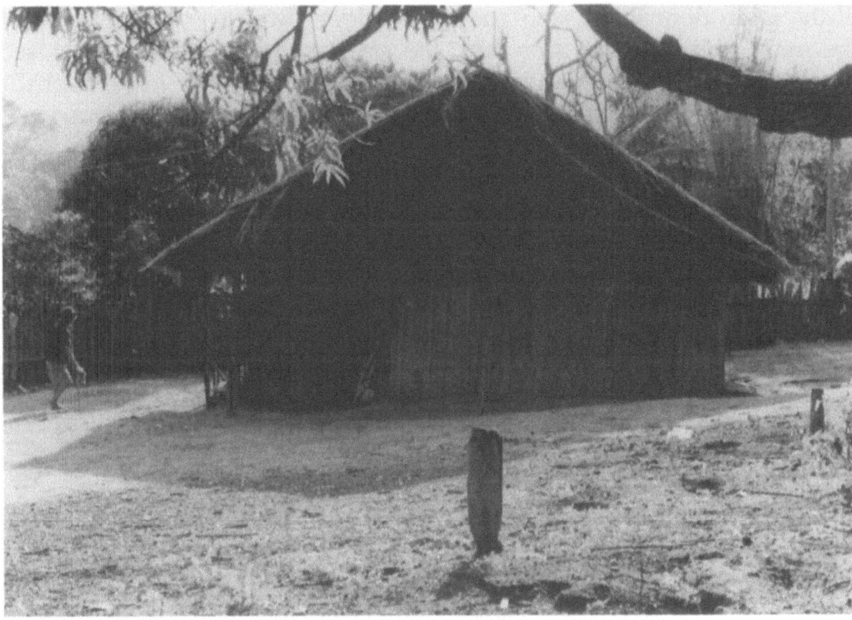

Photo 1.1 A typical Hmong house in northern Thailand.

Dab (Spirits)

Hmong call spirits *dab*. It is believed that the Hmong world is inhabited by many *dab*. The *dab* are divided into two main groups: the *dab nyeg* and the *dab qus*. *Dab nyeg*, include *dab qhuas*, the house spirits who are benevolent. The *dab qus*, however, are those wild or evil spirits who reside in specific areas and roam around waiting for an opportunity to strike people or capture their souls (Cooper et al., 1995).

A Hmong house is built simply. The house has three major posts, the most important being the middle. The other two posts support the roof. A Green Hmong house usually has only one door and no windows. White Hmong houses, however, have another side door, which family members may use instead of the front door.[21] Despite its structural simplicity, a Hmong house is a symbol of the Hmong cosmos. Cooper et al. (1995: 56) state that "the roof and rafters of the house represent the vault of heaven, the earthen floor represents the world of nature, and between heaven and earth is the world of men [*and women*]" [italics added] (see Photo 1.1).

It is believed that many spirits reside in the house and that these spirits protect the house and its members. They must be treated with respect, however. Cooper et al. (1995: 14) identify seven house spirits as follows: *Dab xwm kab*, the spirit of wealth and prosperity; *dab txhij meej*, the spirit of the main door lintel who guards the door; *dab qhov cub*, the spirit of the main fireplace; *dab qhov txos*, the spirit of the secondary enclosed hearth; *dab roog*, who guards the bedroom door and who looks after the fertility of the animals; *dab ncej cuab*,[22] the spirit of the central housepost; and *dab nthab*, guardian of the loft. Offerings must be made to these spirits and all Hmong taboos must be observed so as not to offend them. Failure to do so results in disaster, including poverty, illness and death.[23]

These spirits are greatly feared by the Hmong as they believe these spirits "set their sights on the household." They may strike at any time. They must also be exorcised occasionally so that they will not cause bad health or death (Cooper et al., 1995).

Hmong also believe in the power of traditional healing methods, including herbal medicines (*tshuaj Hmoob* or *tshuaj ntsuab*), shamanism (*ua neeb*) and magic healing (*ua khawv koob*). Each healing ritual is believed to be assisted by specific *dab*. These will be discussed in detail in Chapter 3.

The Ancestors

The Hmong believe that all the remembered dead are still interested in the living. It is said that if ancestors are looked after well, all family members will be well. However, if they are neglected, they will be angry and may cause illness and misfortune to befall their negligent children (Symonds, 1991). Therefore, ancestral spirits must be fed and honored frequently. At certain rituals, the ancestors will be invited to partake of the meals. Ideally, those left behind must always remember them. In reality, however, only four generations may be remembered because of the Hmong's reliance on memorizing names, having no means of writing them down. The distant ancestors will be called collectively by generational terms (Chindasri, 1976). Within a Hmong house, ancestral spirits live in the pillars where most rituals, including the sacrifice of animals to patrilineal ancestors, take place (Symonds, 1991: 53).

HMONG CALENDAR

The calendar in the Hmong cosmos plays a major role in the well-being, health and fortune of the people. The Hmong calendar comprises 30-day cycles. The first day of the first quarter of the moon is counted as the first day of the month, whereas the last day of the full dark moon is the last day of the month (Chindasri, 1976). Certain animals represent days in the Hmong calendar. There are 12 days in a cycle; hence, in one lunar month there will be two completed cycles and part of a third cycle. My Hmong informants mentioned that these days are counted in the same way as the years in Chinese cosmology, as follows:

1	day of the chicken
2	day of the dog
3	day of the pig
4	day of the rat
5	day of the ox
6	day of the tiger
7	day of the rabbit
8	day of the big snake or dragon
9	day of the small snake
10	day of the horse
11	day of the goat
12	day of the monkey

These 12 days continue until the 30th day of the month. Then the first day (day of the chicken) starts the cycle again.

Each animal day has its influence on the personality of the person. This is very similar to the way the Chinese interpret their years. Within the 12 days, the day of the dragon or big snake is the best day for birth and other matters. The worst days will be the day of the chicken, because chickens are often killed and used in sacrifice.

The time of the day also plays an important role in a human's health and well-being (Figure 1.1). According to this chart, the day commences on the far-left corner and proceeds to the right hand side, from the first to the fifth day. The sixth day will be counted from the beginning again. This continues until the 30th day. Times of the day are divided into five times: morning, late morning, afternoon, evening and night. These times start from the bottom left hand and go upward from morning to night. Dots, crosses and empty spots on the chart represent good and bad times of the day. It is said that the best times are where the empty and the "four dots" spots occur. The worst times are where the crosses land, since it means that a person is "being cut" by others all the time. Time represented by a "four dots" spot is a good time, as is "two dots." But time with a "one dot" spot is seen as a bad time. According to the chart, if, for example, a baby is born at night time on the first day, he or she will have bad health and misfortune. Similarly, if the person is setting off to war and leaves home in late morning on the first day, he is likely to be involved in fighting and may be killed. If a baby is born on the third day, at night time, he or she will be good, will not often become sick, and later in life may go anywhere and nothing bad will happen. If a baby is born in the morning on the third day, he or she brings prosperity and enters into a large family with wealth. If a person is setting off to perform a certain task in the morning on the second day, it is likely that

Night	O	OO		X	OO OO
Late Afternoon	OO		X	OO OO	O
Afternoon		X	OO OO	O	OO
Late Morning	X	OO OO	O	OO	
Morning	OO OO	O	OO		X
Days	One	Two	Three	Four	Five

Figure 1.1 Hmong calendar

he or she will not be successful and will suffer a loss. It is seen as a "time for loss." Lastly, if a woman gives birth to a baby in the morning on the fifth day, the birth will be a difficult one and the baby may not survive.[24]

HMONG CONCEPTS OF HEALTH AND ILLNESS

The Hmong have a legend of how illness and disease originated in their world.

> The wife of a wicked god named Nyong laid an egg as large as a pig house. For three years, the egg did not hatch. Nyong's father chanted to the egg and, in response, heard the jabbering voices of many evil dabs inside. He ordered Nyong to burn the egg, but Nyong refused. So the egg burst, and out swarmed the dabs. The first thing they did was to eat Nyong's wife, down to the last bone, hair, and eyelash. Then, still hungry, they came after Nyong. Nyong opened the door that led from the sky, where he lived, to the earth. Through it flew the dabs, as big as a water buffalo and as red as fire, with showers of sparks in their wake. Nyong was safe, but from that day on, the people of the earth have known illness and death. (Fadiman, 1997:278)

As illustrated earlier, the Hmong have a number of beliefs concerning supernatural beings who can cause illness and death to humans. Although they believe the primary cause of such misfortune is the loss of soul, they also see that some illnesses are due to natural or organic factors (Thao, 1986; Bliatout, 1991). This also will be illustrated in the chapters that follow.

According to Thao (1986), the Hmong are conscious of the influence of natural forces on a person's good health or illness. When a woman has just given birth, her body is believed to be in a state of disequilibrium with nature. She therefore is prohibited from participating in daily work for 30 days. During this period she needs to rest and be mindful of "cold" and "wrong" food. Hot food, mainly chicken cooked with herbal medicines, is consumed for the entire period of 30 days. Failure to do this will result in ill health later in life.[25]

Thao (1986) also points out that in the Hmong worldview, many illnesses have organic causes. These include stomach ache, chicken pox, nose bleeding and leprosy. A weak body is believed to be the result of a lack of certain elements in the body. For example, if a person eats well but does not gain proper weight, it is because the person does not carry enough fat and blood to feed his or her body. In order to recover from organically caused illnesses, a variety of healing methods is used. To produce more fat and blood, for example, herbal medicines are used in conjunction with chicken to nourish the body. Stomachache can be remedied by massage as well as by herbal medicines. Ill health associated with childbearing and reproduction is often treated in similar ways.

CONCLUSION

The Hmong have a long history of migration; from beyond China to Southeast Asia and now into far-Western societies. As Quincy (1995:224) points out, "It is nothing new for the Hmong to be driven from their homeland and to be forced to start life anew in a foreign country." They have endured an inordinate number of oppressions and hardships throughout history. Despite this, the Hmong survive. Evidence has shown that it is the nature of the Hmong to strive for freedom. Savina (cited in Fadiman, 1997: 19) says it all in his writing of the Hmong's history:

> Though they are but a small people, the Hmong still prove to be great men. What particularly strikes me is to see how this small race has always managed . . . to survive though they often had to face more powerful nations. . . . The Hmong . . . have never possessed a country of their own, they have never got a king worthy of this name, and yet they have passed through the ages remaining what they have always wished to be, that is to say: *free men with a right to live in this world as Hmong.* (italics added)

However, their nature is not only characterized by their strong desire to live as free men and women. I believe that the Hmong social structure, particularly their clan and lineage systems, also plays a significant role in their endurance and survival. What is more, the Hmong social structure and cosmology, particularly their beliefs in deities, souls and spirits, form Hmong perceptions of well-being, which again help them to endure hardship and cope with difficulties. The roles of Hmong social structure and cosmology concerning women and reproduction are no exception. These will be illustrated throughout the chapters that follow.

NOTES

1. See also Vang and Lewis, 1990; Livo and Cha, 1991; Johnson and Yang, 1992; and Quincy 1995 for further details of Hmong legends and folklore.

2. The Hmong have only had a written language since 1959, when Shong Lue Yang, a messianic Hmong leader who was previously illiterate, devised alphabetic writing systems for the Hmong language and Khmu' language of his mother. He is known among the Hmong as "Mother of Writing" (Vang et al., 1990). See also Smalley et al., 1990 and Lee and Smalley, 1991 for more details about Hmong writing. See also Cooper et al., 1995 about Hmong language folklore.

3. Quincy (1995: 61) points out that the Hmong moved to Xieng Khouang province because of the persuasion of a Chinese opium merchant named Ton Ma. He told the Hmong about "the lush, uninhabited mountains of Xieng Khouang in eastern Laos where the Hmong could grow better opium." He even guided them there.

4. But this does not mean that their lives are easy. In the past the Hmong were treated badly because they were powerless and uneducated. Today, the Hmong are better treated by the Thai people and government, largely because of the influence of the Thai king, who has initiated many development projects to improve the lives of all Thai people regardless of their social or cultural backgrounds.

5. See Quincy (1995) for his account of Hmong civilians who became refugees and lived around the Plain of Jars in Xieng Khouang province, because Pathet Lao regularly invaded their villages, killed the village chiefs and burned their houses down.

6. My personal observation confirms this. I have attended Hmong National Conferences in the United States since 1995 and noticed that each year there have been more and more young educated Hmong people who organized, attended and presented their papers.

7. Except for several Hmong who came to Australia as Columbo Plan students and their families; beginning with the arrival of Dr. Gar Jia Lee, who was the first and only Hmong to receive a Doctorate degree in Australia in 1965.

8. According to Dr. Gar Yia Lee (1999), only four families were Christian, but they were converted before coming to Australia.

9. In this study, most women are Green Hmong, but there are also White and Striped Hmong.

10. There is another Hmong family name known as Saykao in Melbourne. Saykao is not a traditional Hmong clan name; it is a family lineal name. Many Hmong have recently (since the 1970s) adapted the Lao custom of changing one's last (clan) name to the middle name and adding one's well-known father, grandfather or great-grandfather's name as the last name. Saykao is one example. Their clan name is Thao. This reflects one of the many adaptations that the Hmong have made as they attempt to become acculturated to whatever dominant cultural groups they find themselves in (Cha, personal communication, 1999).

11. This is in great contrast to other women in Southeast Asia, such as Lao and Thai women, who will use their husbands' family names after marriage. Some Hmong women in the West have started to adopt this practice as well, to make things easier when dealing with service providers.

12. See also Chapter 3 in this volume for more details on brideprice in Hmong society.

13. See also Chindasri (1976) Kunstadter et al. (1987); Quincy (1995); and Cooper et al. (1995) for further detail on Hmong deities.

14. See also Chapter 3 on the first shaman and *neeb* spirits in Hmong shamanism.

15. There is a mention in Chindasri (1976) and in Symonds (1991).

16. *Txoov Kab Yeeb* is also called *nkawm niam txiv Kab Yeeb* or *nkawm niam txiv dab pog* by other different regional Hmong groups. See also Chapter 10 in this volume.

17. See also Chapters 9 and 11 in this volume for further discussions on the influence of *Txoov Kab Yeeb* on women's fertility and the rearing of young children.

18. It is difficult to pinpoint exactly how many souls reside in an individual's body, as different numbers are given by different people. In most writings, three souls are specified (Lee, 1981; Kunstadter et al., 1987; Symonds, 1991; Bliatout, 1991). However, as Symonds (1991: 45) points out, even though the number of souls is uncertain, "the theme behind the concept of soul and soul loss is similar." Chindasri (1976: 30) also mentions that the Hmong are not so much concerned about the number or nature of the souls as in their well-being, which affects the body and life. In my interviews, most lay Hmong said that there were three souls, but some shamans specified seven and others, 12. For simplicity and consistency, I will refer here to only the three common souls.

19. Kunstadter et al. (1987: 61) point out that the three souls include, first, *plig duab* (shadow of soul), who will remain to watch over the burial place when the person dies. A second soul is *plig qaib* (chicken soul), who will be reborn. A third soul is *plig nyuj* (ox spirit), who will go to the spirit land after the person dies.

20. See also Chapter 9 in this volume for more details on a soul-calling ceremony.

21. Kunstadter et al. (1987) argue that a major difference between Green and White Hmong houses are the doors. White Hmong houses usually have two doors but Green Hmong have only one. However, the most important door is located at the front of the house and is of similar importance to both groups.

22. This *dab* is also called *dab ncej tag* or *tas* by different regional Hmong groups.

23. Of these house spirits, my informants spoke mainly of *dab xwm kab* and *dab txhij meej*, who play major roles in childbirth and infant feeding practices. See also Chapters 9 and 10 in this volume.

24. It is noted that knowledge of the Hmong calendar belongs mainly to shamans and elders. The average Hmong do not know or believe in this. This is perceived as astrology or fortune telling.

25. See also Chapter 6 in this volume for greater details about Hmong confinement practices.

Chapter 2

Hmong Women in Hmong Society

> Nine fireplaces are not as warm as the sun;
> Nine daughters do not equal one son.
>
> Hmong proverb (Vang and Lewis, 1990: 66)

INTRODUCTION

> The sun is the constant and reliable source of light and heat, but the moon is changeable.... The darkness falls at the setting of the sun. Surely the moon should then rise and give us light throughout the dark hours, but she is not to be relied on.... In these unaccountable qualities of the moon, man has seen a symbol of woman's nature which to him appears erratic, changeable... not to be relied on. (Harding, 1973: 78–79)

Hmong understanding of gender differentiates sharply between girls and boys. Hmong girls are perceived as "other people's daughters," since upon marriage they must move into their husbands' household. However, girls are valued because they are the ones who bring a bride price into their family. The bride price is paid to the woman's family as compensation for her parents' "milk and care" in raising their daughter. Depending on the girl's status and the relationships of her parents with the groom's family, the level of the bride price paid will vary.

When a Hmong girl is at an eligible age for courting, she is referred to as *hluas nkauj* (a young, single, courting girl); a "ball game" held at Hmong New Year marks the occasion when Hmong adolescents start to court and, perhaps, subsequently wed. Parents encourage their marriageable daughters to join the ball game so that they may find a husband. Young women are encouraged to marry and bear children as soon as possible, although they may have their own view of whom they wish to choose to marry and when they want to be married. Upon marriage, a Hmong woman is placed under the authority of her mother-in-law, who will ensure that she is trained to be a good wife and a good mother. The shift in a young woman's status can be seen upon her marriage, when she becomes *tus poj niam* (a woman), and particularly when she is able to produce a first child, as this proves her ability to procreate and thus ensure the continuity of her husband's lineage.

This chapter focuses on female status, courtship, marriage and motherhood among young Hmong adults. It also examines the Hmong's perceptions and practices in the context of a new environment; the results of social and cultural changes that have occurred since settling in Australia.

GENDER AND THE STATUS OF HMONG GIRLS

The Hmong believe that men are more important than women. Women hold no place in rituals concerning the patriline. Only men are allowed to perform spiritual ceremonies such as ancestral worship and clan or family lineal rituals known as *dab qhuas*; only men carry on the family's clan name, which ensures the continuity of family lineage; and men, not women, look after aged parents. The status of men is therefore higher than that of women. In writing about the Hmong in Thailand, Symonds (1991: 29) states: "The ideology of Hmong society states that men are more important. Men are the 'skeleton of the society' upon which all else is built. If the skeleton breaks down . . . there is no Hmong society left." Doua Hang (1986: 33–34), a Hmong man now living in the United States, writes:

> The important part of a Hmong family from one generation to the next is the men. This is because the clan name is handed down through men, and the sons carry the family traditions from their fathers to their own sons from each generation down to the next. . . . Women are important, but women change. When they grow up they leave their family and go to their husband's family.

Similarly, Tapp (1985) points out that the Hmong see daughters as worthless, since daughters leave the family upon marriage and, hence, will not be able to contribute to the household. This may explain why women are metaphorically compared with the leaves and flowers,

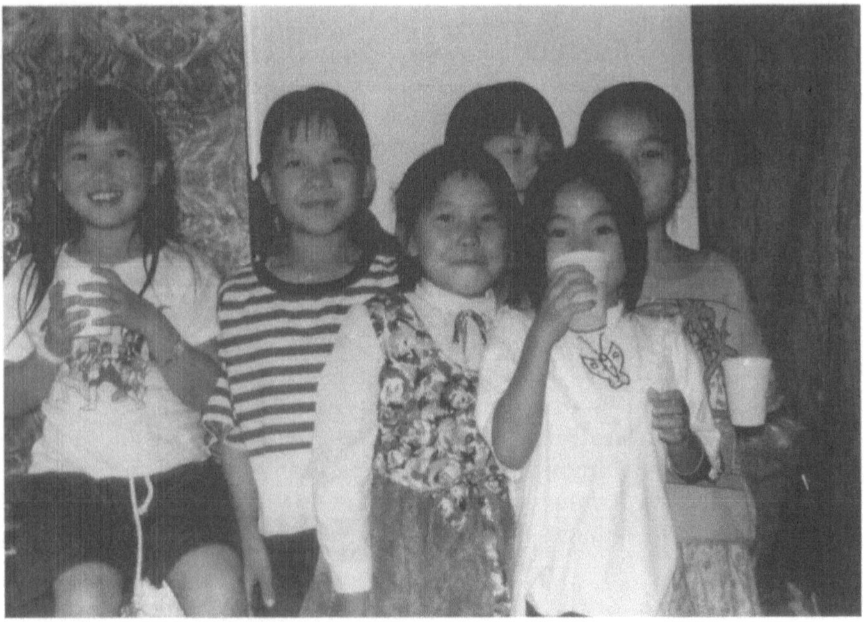

Photo 2.1 Hmong girls at home.

whereas men are compared with the trunk and roots of the tree, as Hang (1986: 34) writes: "always strong and never changing."[1]

When I asked Hmong women how girls are perceived in Hmong culture, a mother told me that "Girls are not as valuable as boys. If you were to sell the boys, you would sell them at a more expensive price, as boys are more important than girls." Gender inequality begins at birth with the burial of the placenta. The boys' placentas are buried at the most important part of the house, near the middle post where the spirit of the clan resides. The girls' placentas are buried under the birth bed, signifying the inferior status of women in Hmong culture (Symonds, 1991; Donnelly, 1994; Rice, 1994). The Hmong see girls as "other people's daughters" (Photo 2.1).

Despite their inferiority, women play an important part in the Hmong universe. The Hmong have a story about "why men rule the world," in which a king and a queen were competing over who should rule the world. The king was assigned by *Yawm Saub* (a beneficent deity of Hmong people) to cut off the heads of his seven wives. He then went to his home:

> He saw his wives all sitting together in the house breastfeeding his children. He thought about the test and he knew he could not do as he had been told. He went back to *Yawm Saub* and said, "*Saub,* I cannot do as you

> ask. My wives are feeding our children milk. If I kill them and bring their heads to you, my children will have no food and they will die." (Symonds, 1991: 107)

However, when the queen was asked to cut off the heads of her husbands, she did. And so *Yawm Saub* said, "The king shall rule the world for he knows the meaning of life" (Symonds, 1991: 107).

Although the moral of this story is that men's judgment is superior to women's, it also indicates the importance of women, their procreative power and their ability to maintain lives. Without women, there can be no children to continue the family's line. Women, therefore, have their place in the society and they hold status in particular areas. This is certainly recognized by both men and women, as I will discuss later in this chapter.

A GOOD HMONG GIRL

What does it mean to be a "good" girl in Hmong culture? There are several answers to this question.

Sev and Sexuality

Sev are two pieces of cloth tied around the waist with a belt over a girl's trousers, with one piece hanging over the front to cover her genitals, and another piece hanging over the back to cover her buttocks. If a girl wears a skirt then there is only one piece of *sev* covering the front.

Sev are symbolic of womanhood and sexuality. Symonds (1991: 127) argues that "women wear them to cover their sexuality and to protect themselves . . . wearing of the *sev* for Hmong women constitutes the most visible act of modest deference." Girls start wearing *sev* when they are old enough to go to the farm (around five or six years of age). Their mothers continue to encourage them to wear *sev*. Prior to puberty, a young Hmong girl is taught that sexuality is secret and she must keep her genital area covered by wearing *sev*. Girls wear *sev* at home and in public. They are taught that to leave home without *sev* is to make oneself shameful, since people, particularly men, will see the outline of their genitals.

Hmong women in Melbourne gave me the following reasons for girls to wear *sev*:

> With the Hmong, from generation to generation we always have the *sev*; that is *the way it is*. . . . Ever since I was a girl I have been wearing it. . . . For men you don't have to, but a woman she has to wear it for the rest of her life.

And another one remarked:

> *It is the Hmong way, it is the way it is.* If you don't wear them you look strange, and you look different. People will look at you and say that you look very funny because all Hmong girls have to wear these all the time.

When I asked what the reaction of Hmong men would be if they were to see a woman without *sev*, a Hmong woman said:

> They will laugh at you and would not want to look at you. When you wear *sev*, you also wear the belt—sometimes just pieces of red and green cloths tied around your waist. Without these, people will not want to look at you, and will say that you do not dress properly according to the Hmong way, and they will laugh at you too.

For some women, a woman who does not wear *sev* is shamed because she is not modestly dressed.[2] Women in Melbourne primarily associated *sev* with cultural tradition—"the Hmong way" (see Photo 2.2). In addition, however, *sev* becomes a symbol of fertility when girls start courting. Hmong girls do not fully participate in courting until the onset of menstruation. Once they reach puberty, young women wear the most decorative and colorful *sev* for courting at the New Year celebration. The beautiful *sev* signifies the girl's readiness for courtship, marriage and motherhood. The decorated *sev* therefore identifies to young men those young women now considered ready to be married.

Women continue wearing *sev* once they are married and when they become elderly (see Photo 2.3). Aged women make several new *sev* in preparation for their death and upon death the *sev* are buried with them. The Hmong in Melbourne wear *sev* whenever they dress in Hmong costumes, and young girls continue to wear colorful and decorated *sev* if their parents can afford them. Women of all ages agree that to be a good Hmong woman, a woman must wear *sev* whenever she puts on Hmong clothes. However, the Hmong in Melbourne, both young and old, predominantly wear Western clothes—trousers, mainly, for warmth in cold weather—and they refer to these trousers as *soua*, "Chinese pants." With this type of clothing, *sev* are not regarded as necessary despite the fact that trousers do outline buttocks, which reveal women's sexuality.

Paj Ntaub: Needlework and Flower Cloths

Needlework refers here to pieces of embroidery or reverse appliqué, which are used to decorate Hmong clothing; hence the term flower cloths. Embroidered *paj ntaub* are also used as a form of tapestry that

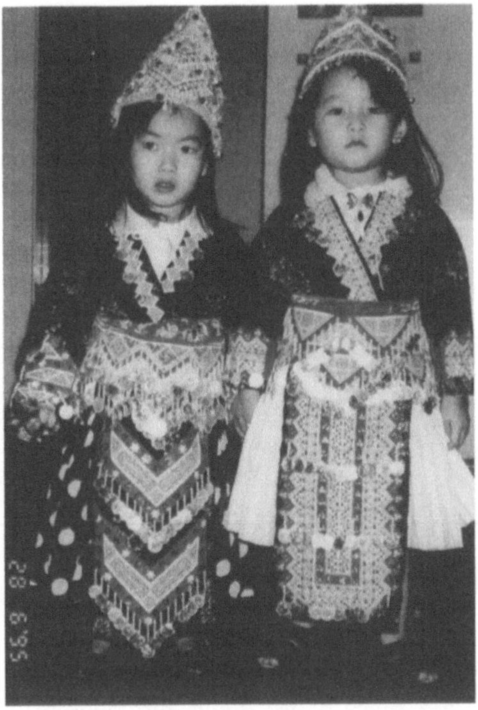

Photo 2.2 Hmong girls in their costumes at Hmong New Year.

may include patterns of traditional Hmong lives, images of wildlife and plants, and illustrations of folk stories.[3]

Hmong girls begin to learn needlework as early as six to seven years of age. However, it is not until ages 10 or 12 that most Hmong girls are able to do their own pieces of needlework. Hmong women say that some girls can look at *paj ntaub* and know how to do it, so they just go ahead and sew it. If a girl is unable to do needlework by herself, then she needs lessons from older women, and it is mainly her grandmother, aunts and older sisters who give her lessons until she is competent.

A good Hmong girl must be good at needlework. Some girls are quick to learn and, hence, enjoy the praise of their mother or grandmother. Young women are respected if they are good at needlework. Girls use the pieces of appliqué for everyday wear. However, when they begin courting they produce special pieces to wear at New Year celebrations to attract the attention of the boys. When a young woman is of marriageable age, people begin to look at her needlework. The Hmong believe that the needlework a young woman produces can tell a lot about whether she will be a good woman and wife. A Hmong mother told me,

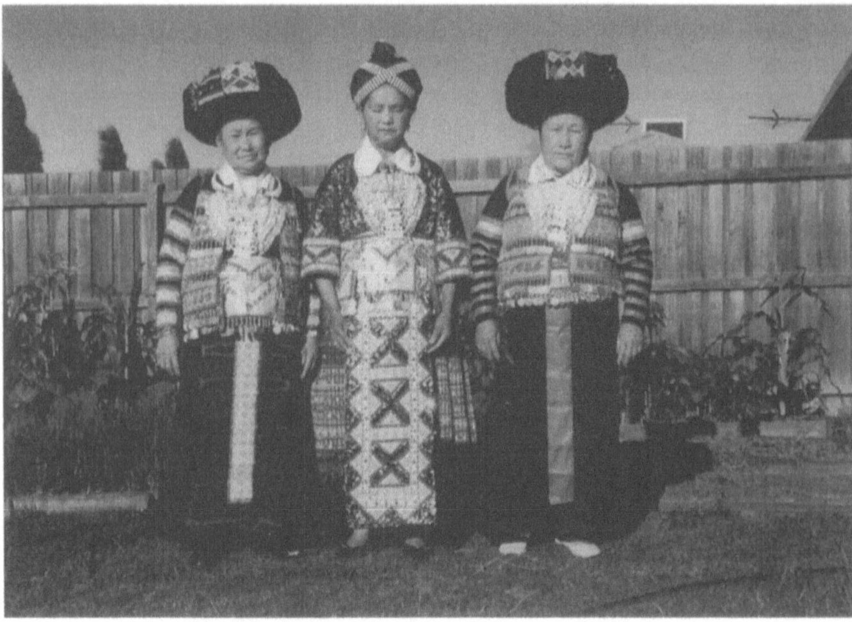

Photo 2.3 Hmong elderly in Melbourne in their costumes at Hmong New Year.

"When you make a piece of *paj ntaub* and people look at your work, they can tell from your needlework whether or not you will be a good wife and a good mother."

However, a good Hmong girl needs to have other qualities as well in order to attract a man. As one grandmother explained, "If you can do *paj ntaub* and you are educated, then people will say that you are very good, and a man will want to marry you; it will make you highly sought after as a wife." As young girls become more mature, they are expected to produce more intricate and more colorful work and be able to make *paj ntaub* that is based on traditional stories and myths and their own imagination.

This emphasis on needlework skills reflects the importance women place on familiarity with Hmong tradition. However, to some women needlework is only essential if the girl is not educated, as indicated by the following conversation:

Pranee: Why is it that girls and women have to learn to make *paj ntaub?*

Va: You must learn it so that when you are older and you have children, you can make them for your children.

Pranee: But, do all Hmong girls have to learn this?

Va: If you study then you don't need to learn it, but if you do not study then yes, you need to learn it. If you are a woman and you do not have education then you have to make your own clothes.

These remarks are certainly borne out in the Hmong community in Melbourne, where several young women have studied and do not know how to do *paj ntaub* or know very little. My bicultural research assistant, for example, says that she cannot do as nice a piece of *paj ntaub* as can her mother-in-law. When I asked her why that was so, she explained that she did not work on *paj ntaub* from an early age as other Hmong girls did, and she studied until she married. There was no opportunity for her to learn *paj ntaub*.

Several mothers in my study commented that education is extremely important for their children today, because it is the way in which employment may be obtained. Consequently, the family may have the opportunity to secure better income and live in better conditions. Many mothers, therefore, do not really insist on their daughters doing as good a job on *paj ntaub* as in the past.

However, most Hmong girls and women do not leave any opportunity to work on their *paj ntaub* despite other tasks to be done in the house. When I visited women at their homes to interview them during my field work, all of them would sit down on a small stool in front of a warm heater and work on their *paj ntaub* as we talked. They would answer my questions and engage in any conversation, but their heads would be bent down and their hands would keep moving, threading the needle up and down on the piece of *paj ntaub*. Although women were very engaged in our conversation—as they are engaged in everything—they remained committed to acting in a conventional and appropriate fashion, ensuring that they made good use of their time, as they are expected to do in their culture.

When young women become mothers, they continue to work on *paj ntaub* for their children. In one of the houses I visited, as a Hmong mother and I sat and talked, her eldest daughter (12 years of age) came to sit near us and listened. But she also kept working on her *paj ntaub*. At that time she was making a piece of *paj ntaub* for her *sev*, to be worn at the coming New Year celebration.

Many Hmong women and girls in Australia also make pieces of *paj ntaub* for sale, to earn money. In Melbourne, there is a Hmong craft market in Fitzroy where women can sell their pieces. Similarly, in Hobart, at the Salamanca Place market, the center of arts and crafts in this city, there are many pieces made by Hmong women for sale as well. Women act similarly wherever they are located.

BRIDE PRICE: MILK AND FOOD MONEY

Girls are also regarded as an asset to the family because they bring in a bride price, which in turn helps the family bring in daughters-in-law. When marriage is proposed, the bride price must be negotiated. The bride price is paid to the bride's family as compensation for her mother's milk and the care she has given her daughter to bring her to maturity: "The bride price is for your mother's milk and the price of looking after you."

In the Hmong language, the bride price itself refers to "a head price," but its meaning is "milk and food" (*nqe mis nqe hno*) of the mother. Traditionally, it must be paid in silver, the most precious metal in Hmong homelands. The Bride price is therefore not a commercial trade by which women can be bought and sold, but, as Geddes (1976: 58) argues, is symbolic of the importance of women:

> The main utility of bride-price . . . is the symbolisation it gives to a new creative act in the Miao [i.e., Hmong] social universe. The symbolisation is both general and particular. There is probably significance in the fact that the price should be paid in silver and not in ordinary money, thus setting it apart from a commercial transaction and relating it directly to the traditions of . . . [Hmong] culture. The most precious metal, the material of ornamentation as well as wealth, symbolises the most important occasion and celebrates the worth of the woman.

Thao (1986: 80) states that for Hmong people, the bride price represents two things: "It is a symbolic recognition of the hardship of raising the girl, and it is a consideration for a promise to love." During the marriage negotiation, the girl's parents will ask the man's family if they promise to love the girl. The girl's family will request a monetary value as a security upon that promise. If the promise is broken, the bride price will be forfeited.[4]

Thao's second point is reflected in the variation in bride prices that the bride's parents demand. Prices are normally measured by the welfare of other girls of the family who have been married out to members of the groom's family. Hmong women refer to this measurement as either "a difficult case" or "an easy case," as illustrated in the following conversation:

Pranee: How much is the bride price?

Xee: For a difficult family, it is 100 *kip*.[5]

Pranee: What does a difficult family mean?

Xee: A difficult one means that people in the groom's family have married a few girls from or other girls related to the bride's family already, and the family can see that that family does not look after the girls well or does not love the girls, but make them work hard on the farm. So they will say that for this daughter they want a high bride price, to make sure that the family will look after her well.

Pranee: What about an easy case?

Xee: For an easy case, it is only 75 *kip*.

However, upon paying the bride price, a man and his clan have the rights over a woman's labor, sexuality and children. If her husband dies, the woman and children remain with his family, and his younger brother has a right to marry her without paying a bride price. If she wishes to divorce him, the bride price has to be paid back to his family, and her children become the assets of her husband's family. Therefore, a bride price, according to Symonds (1991: 114), "ties a woman to her husband and his lineage for her lifetime."

Paying a bride price is still the norm for Hmong marriages in Melbourne. It is, however, paid in Australian dollars, because of the scarcity of silver bars. A common bride price nowadays is $2,500, whereas a few years ago it was $3,000. The decline of the bride price is mainly due to the financial difficulties many families are experiencing because of unemployment.

COURTSHIP AND SEXUALITY

Hmong girls and boys start to court as soon as they are eligible. There is some variation of opinion as to what age is suitable to begin courting. Some say that they should not be "too young."[6] Women in my study mention ages 13 to 16 as eligible ages for courtship. This age range coincides with the average age of onset of menstruation, signifying that the young woman is mature enough to court and ready to bear children. However, some say that "naughty" children may start sooner:

> Some children who are naughty and stubborn, they may start courting at a younger age like 13 or 14, but if they are obedient and they listen to their parents they will start at around 15 or 16.

When a Hmong girl is at an eligible age to court, she is referred to as *hluas nkauj* (a young, single, courting girl). Earlier ethnographies represent courting as the most popular "game" of the young (Geddes, 1976). In Laos and Thailand, courtship usually occurs at the Hmong New Year, usually around November when all harvests have been gathered and it is the twelfth lunar month of the year. At this point, a ball game is played. Young boys and girls line up opposite each other and throw soft black cloth balls to one another. On the first day of the game the throws are at random but become more selective by the second day when the young tentatively match themselves "in challenges of love in which, to conquer, the boy must prove his superior skill" (Geddes, 1976: 92). Courtship may also be initiated at other times of the year as well. One woman in my study explained:

> Courtship in the old days, back in Laos, is like this. If the boy likes the girl, he will come to the girl's house and tap on the wall and play a flute to her, and they will talk through the wall and that is all. If the boy really likes her, he will get his friends to come and catch her when they call her out of the house.

From then on, courtship may commence and develop further into love play, which is permitted among young, unmarried men and women in Hmong culture (Geddes, 1976). A girl may go off alone with a boy she likes and this may result in sexual intercourse. Geddes (1976: 81) points out that despite the fact that the Hmong ideal is that "a girl should maintain her virginity until marriage, it is also a code amongst the young that she should not resist intercourse for more than two such private meetings with the same boyfriend." The love play may precipitate marriage, since if the girl becomes pregnant the boy must marry her. If he does not wish to marry her, a fine must be paid to her parents; the father of the infant has no claim on her child.

Sexuality is thus seen as a time of freedom for young people, although their ability to interact without constraint is only permitted at certain times. Hmong girls are taught, however, not to express their sexual desire openly. They are instructed to be shy and avoid shame by not initiating and acting openly on their desires. Hmong girls may resist participation in love play unless the boy insists upon it and initiates the love play. As stated earlier, the girl will not resist sex once the boy attempts it for the second time.

When I asked women if young people could sexually experiment prior to marriage, one woman gave the following explanation:

> Some people do that, but that is for two people who really like each other. They have to sneak off so their parents do not know.

When I asked her further what would happen if their parents knew, she said:

> If the parents find out that their daughter has sneaked off with the boy and if they know that the boy is really interested in their daughter, they may not do anything to stop them. But if they know that the boy is only flirting around with her, they then can get very cross with the girl.

However, many women see premarital sex as something that only "naughty" girls will do:

> Some girls who are stubborn will have sexual intercourse while courting before they are married. They will go off with their boyfriend and have

> sex. If they fall pregnant, then there will have to be a forced marriage. It is not really acceptable in the Hmong way, but some girls will do it.

Back in Laos, wall tapping and playing of a flute were common incidences in any household that had an unmarried daughter. The girl's parents could certainly hear the sound of a soft flute tone played by the boy, and most often the dog would be barking away, but they may not have done anything to stop him. People recount this as "part of the Hmong way": a way for the young to become acquainted prior to marriage. However, wall tapping and flute playing are not practicable in Melbourne because of the changed living environment. When I asked one woman about this, she said:

> In the old days people did that, but now you can't because you won't be able to tap the wall and you won't hear it through the brick wall of the house anyway. (laugh) Nowadays you can meet at the ball game and you can meet at an outing, like a barbecue. In this country I have not seen any boy who plays a flute either.

And another woman gave the following account:

> Nowadays, because you have telephone so accessible, so you don't need that [traditional courtship] anymore. You can make a phone call and talk about it on the phone, and no one will know anyway (laugh).

In courting, a love song is usually sung to express romantic love and, sometimes, the desire for sexual intercourse, as the following love song sung by a Hmong boy indicates:

> Oh girl! Do you think of loving me?
> If so, in the evening we'll go out
> to sit by the side of the trail
> and play.
>
> Oh girl! Do you think of loving me?
> If so, in the evening we'll go out
> to sit by the side of the path
> and make love.*

Love songs are used as a means of choosing one's prospective husband or wife. Young people may be seen as more attractive if they are good at singing love songs. Young Hmong girls in my study said they would

*Song by Tova Thao in M. McNamer, "Musical Change and Change in Music: Implications for Hmong Identity," in B. Johns and D. Strecker, eds., *The Hmong World* 1, published by Yale Southeast Asian Studies, 1986: 152, reprinted by permission.

prefer a boy who knew how to sing a love song well. However, when I asked older women, the answer was somewhat different:

> What attracts the boy more is your ability to work hard. Even if you are a good singer, when they come to your house and they peep into the hole because your house is built with bamboo and has lots of holes, and they see that you have not risen by such and such hours and you are not next to the fire and kicking the coals or whatever, they will say no you are not good enough, it is no good to make you a wife. So it is your ability to work and your ability to work in the farm that attracts them more.

Conventional courtship practices such as the ball game and singing love songs have undergone a marked change in Australia. Although young Hmong still court and sexual experimentation is still practiced, traditional Hmong ways have altered. For example, although the ball game is still played at Hmong New Year, many young people do it more for fun than to look for a prospective partner, and the girls say that they can throw the ball to any man, young or old, as long as the man does not share their clan name. The ball game is also performed around Christmas time, since most people are free from work (if they have a job) and their children are not at school.

Nevertheless, the ball game at Hmong New Year still provides a good opportunity for young people to look for and meet a prospective boy or girlfriend. At this time, boys from other Australian states may travel to Melbourne to look for a prospective girlfriend. At other times, young people in Melbourne meet each other at schools, nearby playgrounds and parks. They may go to see a movie in downtown Melbourne together or, most often, go down to Richmond to have Vietnamese noodles together, since it is a much cheaper activity.

Premarital sex still takes place. There have been several cases of pregnancy before marriage in Melbourne.[7] Although there is no longer a forest into which young people may disappear, there are houses and rooms where they can experiment with sex, particularly when their parents are not at home. When this occurs and the girl becomes pregnant, a marriage is usually arranged. However, if the boy does not wish to marry the girl, he must come to pay his respects to the girl's parents, admit his mistake, and then pay a penalty. A common penalty is payment to the family of silver bars, each worth 12 *kip*. Once he pays his penalty, he is released from his responsibility. However, this practice is not really welcome, since a pregnant girl will face very costly consequences. Because abortion is not really acceptable in Hmong culture, the girl must carry her child and take full responsibility for it. Remarrying again is not in her future, because of her "bad" reputation.

MARRIAGE

According to T. C. Thao (1986: 77):

> Heaven, according to the Hmong, created man and woman to love, to care for, to share, and to help one another. Hmong believe that this is the purpose for which man and woman were created, not to be alone or to be single, but to be together in unity. That unity is marriage.

Marriage is the most important goal of all Hmong, men and women. Marriage is the means by which the clan and lineage are continued, since it is only through marriage that children are produced. Hence:

> We believe that being a Hmong woman, you have to get married and have children so you will have someone to look after you in old age. Hmong people all say that you have to farm and grow crops so you need children to help you on the farm and you need someone to look after you when you are old.

As a corollary of the belief that marriage is essential for the continuation of the clan, spinsterhood is the condition most feared by Hmong women. An unmarried woman is a disgrace to the family, since the family loses out on social relationships with other clans, which occur through marriage. The family will not receive a bride price and so will lose the money they spent in raising her as well as lose face (Symonds, 1991). Vang (1994) points out that Hmong people see a woman without a husband as "worthless"; hence, she is not respected within the community. According to Cha (personal communication, 1999), many Hmong women in this situation do eventually marry, but a woman will have a harder time finding a man she likes and may have to marry an older, divorced or widowed man. Women in my study all agreed that a Hmong girl must marry someone, unless there is something wrong with her and no man wants her.

Courtship does not lead to marriage in all cases. It is, however, likely that the young people will subsequently be wed once they are socially recognized as a couple. A marriage proposal must be made by the young man's family, and one important component in the marriage proposal is the promise to love the girl, as evidenced by the willingness to pay a bride price. Love is a precondition of marriage in people's minds and was believed to be an important aspect of marriage by the Hmong in my study.[8] When I asked the women about love and marriage, the common answer was as follows: "Yes, you have to love each other. If you don't love each other, you will end up not being married. And if the love is from one party only, it will be difficult to get married too."

Marriage in normal circumstances is arranged by *mej koob* (go-betweens): two people who the family respects (not from the same clan) act as negotiators between the bride and groom's families. The negotiation is extremely elaborate. It can last many days, depending on the relationships between the two families.[9] While this is still practiced in Melbourne, it has been altered to suit the living conditions of the community.

Since marriage is a "precondition for the formation of a new household," a father has great influence on the choice of marriage partner and in judging whether the proposed man is suitable for his daughter. According to Geddes (1976: 79), a mother has less say in the decision, since she is "expected to accept her husband's decision in household affairs." The daughter is always a junior member of the family and therefore,—theoretically—has little say in her own affairs, although she is able to exercise some influence by encouraging the attention of a young man of her choice.

Because a girl is expected to conform to the family's decision about her marriage, elopement is a common strategy when a girl wishes to avoid an unwanted marriage. A Hmong informant said:

> They [parents] can try to force you if they see that the boy is good and his parents are good. But you can always elope with somebody else at that time anyway, so you can get away by eloping.

Elopment may also occur if the young people are in love and one or both sets of parents do not consent to their wishes to marry. It also occurs when marriage negotiation is unlikely to be effective:

> For the boy and girls who are closely related, like if your parents know each other or if I have a son who is interested in my sister-in-law's daughter or another close relative's daughter, I can go to see them and arrange a go-between to arrange the marriage and there will be no problems whatsoever. But if we are not related and we don't know each other at all, it will be difficult, so it is up to the boy and girl to elope together.[10]

Eloping will then lead to a marriage negotiation, which normally follows soon after. An elopement is not regarded as a legitimate marriage until a bride price is paid.

Interestingly, young Hmong people in my study still resorted to elopment if they wished to marry each other and wanted their parents to acknowledge their wishes.[11] Although elopement occurs, in most cases the girl and boy are granted permission to marry if the girl's parents can see that the boy is diligent and responsible. As one Hmong mother said:

> Now it is totally up to the children to choose who they like. Even if you as a parent do not like the girl's chosen man you will say to her that you disapprove their marriage they will elope anyway. So you always approve your girl's partner if he is not lazy. You always say yes to them because they will elope if you do not approve their marriage.

In Laos, there is also a "marriage-by-capture" or catch-hand marriage, in which a girl may be captured by a man assisted by his friends or family members if the young couple attempts to resist parental wishes. The girl is taken to the boy's sleeping area and held capture for three days. On the second day, a negotiator is sent to the girl's family and negotiation over marriage and bride price is conducted. The "marriage-by-capture" usually results in a legitimate marriage, but not always, since the girl may not wish to be married and may escape back to her own family.[12]

Catch-hand marriage rarely occurs in Melbourne, however:

> In this country it is so accessible to the phone, so they just ring and ask, do you want to come and I will pick you up. Sometimes the boy just rings the girl up and asks her to go over to his place, so there is no catch-hand marriage any longer.

Many young women feel somewhat ambivalent about marriage. A young girl has been taught and trained to be a good woman so that she will be chosen by someone. Despite the desire to be married, young adults realize that the time has come to leave their natal kin, and this causes the girls great anxiety and distress. This is reflected in many Hmong songs, whose theme is the girl's sadness when she has to depart her own family and village.[13] A woman knows that marriage means leaving her familiar environment, losing the security, comfort and love of her clan and beginning her new life as a daughter-in-law in a new place where she will have to conform to the wishes and rules of her husband's family. Many women are anxious about their future.

Mothers also have mixed feelings about their daughters' marriages. Although they feel that it is necessary for their daughters to be married out, they also feel the pain of sending the girls away. As one mother said:

> If they are married you will be happy that they have a family of their own, they are getting on with their own family and life . . . and you have more extended family too, which is good for you. But it is like you lose something in the family. Yes, when they are married away you will have less in the family, you will cry because they are part of your blood and heart and when they go you feel lost.

Most people marry young. Yang (1993) states that in Laos most young boys are married between the ages of 18 and 20, and girls between ages 14 and 16. In Australia, most Hmong still marry when they are relatively young. Most women mention that boys and girls should be married between 15 and 18 years of age.[14] If they are too old there may not be anyone who wishes to marry them. More importantly, there may be a quick catcher who will grab the one that he or she has in his or her mind. As one woman stated:

> Hmong boys and girls are married between 15 and 18 and it is still the same here [in Australia] nowadays. Sometimes the boy may be a bit more mature than the girl and the boy thinks that if he does not marry her now, somebody might come and take her away, and it is the same for the girl. If you want to hold on to the one you like you have to do it then because it might be another girl comes in and take the man away from you. So if you really like each other you need to marry quickly.

A DAUGHTER-IN-LAW AND A MOTHER

There is a marked shift in a young woman's status upon her marriage when she becomes *tus poj niam* (a woman), and particularly when she produces a first child. Upon marriage, a woman becomes a daughter-in-law subject to the power of her mother-in-law, who will ensure that she is trained to be a good wife and a good mother: "Once the daughter-in-law moves into your home, then you need to teach them." Becoming a daughter-in-law changes the woman's status. Cultural obligations are imposed on the new bride. She has limited independence and no rights over other members of her husband's family. She has to adjust herself to her new home regardless of her social status before marriage, and she must obey the rules set in her husband's family (Thao, 1986; Donnelly, 1994). Customarily, the mark of a good daughter-in-law is as follows:

> When you are married to the son, you must understand how to run the household; you must not go out and say to everyone what happens, what goes on in the household, and gossip about your mother-in-law. You should be at home and be with other people when they are present. To be a bad daughter-in-law, you always go out and gossip about your parents [in-laws] or family and whatever goes on in your house, and be upset when everyone is around and don't want to talk to anyone in the family.

However, a woman has a right to be loved and cared for by her husband and his family. This is clarified in the wedding negotiations when the bride price is being determined. In addition, despite her obligation as a daughter-in-law to obey her mother-in-law and live harmoniously in her in-laws' home, sometimes a woman can convince her husband to leave his parents and form their own household.

As mentioned earlier, the main reason for marriage is to provide the means for bearing and raising children. A Hmong woman gains more status when she gives birth to the first child, since she has proven her ability to procreate and thus ensure the continuity of the lineage of her husband.[15] Because of this recognition, women are able to pamper themselves after giving birth. Hmong postnatal practices respect a woman's right to rest, with all household and farming tasks left to her husband and other family members for the whole lunar month (30 days). During this time she is provided with good and highly nutritious food, including food to ensure that her body regains strength lost in childbirth and that her uterus will be cleansed in readiness for the next child.[16]

During the confinement period, men cook food for women and women are nourished. Women eat meat, a prestigious food, because it is expensive and not always easily obtained. It is also food that she is not normally entitled to consume until after all the men in the family have eaten. This custom of men cooking is the opposite of the everyday routine in which women cook and nourish men, and men eat meat and eat first. A few Hmong men I interviewed said that they do this for their wives because they recognize women's procreative ability and the need to have children for the continuity of the lineage. Motherhood, in Hmong custom, is therefore an essential part of Hmong life, and women are valued for it. Hence, it is not surprising to see that most Hmong women are keen to be married and become mothers.

CONCLUSION

A Hmong woman is subject to a great deal of social control in order to meet the standards expected of a good girl, a good woman and a good mother. Women try hard to meet these expectations in a changing Australian social environment. These social controls are connected to the concept of "Hmongness." Women were not reluctant to tell me that "it is the Hmong way" whenever I questioned them about the many rules for women. The wearing of *sev*, for example, occurs because of the rules laid down for Hmong women. The love play young girls and boys are allowed to experience at courting prior to marriage, despite its unacceptability at other times, is also a Hmong custom. Elopement has always happened because it is "the Hmong way." Therefore, to be a Hmong woman, one must behave according to Hmong custom. This is the message all girls receive.

Sexuality in Hmong culture always comprises the two opposite forces: male and female. However, these two forces are not in balance. According to Cooper (1983: 175), sexual inequality exists in Hmong culture "where the position of women is generally inferior to men." Although I agree with his remark to some extent, I would argue that in certain areas Hmong women are superior and highly valued. Sexuality is the most noteworthy of these areas, because it is both feared and valued. The woman's body must be covered by wearing *sev* because it is attractive to and dangerous for men. However, it is via her sexuality that children are produced, and this enables the lineage to continue, ensuring the survival of the Hmong. This outcome can only be achieved through marriage. One might say that Hmong sexuality is expressed in terms of love and money, since one aspect of marriage is payment of a bride price. And although the Hmong may say that the bride price is to repay the mother's milk and care, it is—invariably—also the means by which to ensure that the man keeps his promise to love and care for his wife. I believe that seen from this angle, women's position within the Hmong patriarchal line appears to at least be protected.

Hmong women face changes in their new social and cultural environment in Australia, as they do in other Western countries (Vang, 1994; Donnelly, 1994). Many Hmong mothers see that their children are changing. They prefer to maintain Hmong ways in their new home as much as possible, because they believe it is the way to ensure the continuity of Hmong culture. However, most parents accept the changes, since they believe they cannot force their children to maintain "the Hmong way," even if they wish to. Some families have tried to persevere with impressing "the Hmong way" upon their children, but young people resist. This results in intergenerational conflicts between parents and their young children.

Young people, on the other hand, see that their parents are poor, backward and have no education. They want to escape their poverty and other disadvantages by trying to get away from "the Hmong way." However, they are caught between two cultures. They do not really have a good understanding of Australian ways, yet they try hard to escape "the Hmong way." This results in further conflict between old and young people.

Although I have not observed as great a change in Hmong society in Australia as has been observed in the United States (Vang, 1994; Donnelly, 1994), there is no doubt that traditional Hmong customs have been challenged by the contrasting social and political outlooks of their country of settlement. Whether Hmong women's attitudes toward sexuality will be greatly altered by these changes, as has been the case in other resettlement countries, remains to be seen.

NOTES

1. See also Tapp (1985), who provides another metaphor in which men are seen as the roots of the tree and women as the flowers.

2. See also Symonds (1991: 124).

3. Today many *paj ntaub* contain the story of refugee lives, the flights from Laos, and new life in the United States or Australia.

4. In Appell's work (1988: 97) with the Rungus of Borneo, there is emphasis on the value of the bride price, as in Hmong culture. Appell comments, "Bride-price is required, which is an expression of the cultural value of the female role. The size of a girl's bride-price is dependent primarily on the wealth of the suitor's family but also on the qualities of the girl." If she is a hard worker and good looking, her parents can expect a better price. Appell adds that bride price among the Rungus serves "to ensuring stable relationships between husband and wife. If a woman is abused by her husband, she can walk out of the marriage, and the bride-price will not be returned. The bride-price thus serves to protect the female" (p. 106).

5. *Kip* is a measurement of a silver bar in Hmong society. One *kip* is equivalent to about 300 Australian dollars.

6. But one informant in Geddes's study (1976: 91) indicated that the youngsters can begin courting at seven years of age. Geddes, however, points out that the practice does commence before adolescence.

7. See also Vang (1994: 60) and Vangay (1988: 42). Both authors find that Hmong believe that a young girl should not engage in sexual relations prior to marriage. If such an act occurs before marriage, the young girl will disgrace her family, lose her reputation and may have difficulty finding a husband. Their studies were undertaken in the United States.

8. Kunstadter (1994: 7), for example, states that most Hmong in Thailand point out that traditional forms of marriage such as bride capture, levirate and arrangement without consulting the bride and bridegroom are not favored. The young believe that "unless a marriage is based on love and understanding, and the free choice of both partners it is not likely to last." Vang (1994: 59), states that the Hmong believe that love comes after marriage. Hmong man and woman learn to love each other after they have been married; this way, the marriage will last forever.

9. For an illuminating marriage negotiation in Hmong society, see Symonds (1991).

10. In Hmong culture, a cross-cousin marriage is permitted and is the most favourable choice of marriage.

11. For more details see Thao (1986).

12. See also Vang (1994).

13. Savina (1930: 227–228, cited in Geddes, 1976: 82), for example, describes a bride in her new home singing the touching "song of the bride" to her girlhood friends before they leave her: "The song of the treacherous decoy, the poor forest bird is caught in the trap. Shut up in a cage, he looks with sorrow at his companions flying by. Such, alas, is my fate. . . . Tomorrow when you leave . . . go up the slope slowly so that I can see you the longer from the bars of my prison."

14. Vang (1994), however, points out that although some Hmong in the United States tend to get married when they are a bit older, most still practice early marriage. In her study, Hmong mothers felt that if their daughters delayed their marriages too long, they might not be able to obtain good husbands and become spinsters, since they might be too old to marry according to Hmong traditions. Nonetheless, Hmong girls in the United States feel that they must be old enough

to obtain an education and have an opportunity to do something that is meaningful for their life before becoming a married adult. In addition, those who have married young continue to pursue their educations and careers. However, as observed by Vang, this is not a trend among Hmong girls in Australia.

15. See also Symonds (1991: 35).

16. See also Chapter 6 on Hmong confinement in this volume.

Chapter 3

Hmong Healers and Hmong Medicines

INTRODUCTION

> The Hmong culture has produced a wide variety of traditional healers who have handed down their healing knowledge generation after generation through oral teaching and apprenticeship. While there was no formal health service delivery system among the Hmong in Asia, the Hmong cared for the health needs of their populations by utilizing culturally appropriate means. Many of the healing arts of the Hmong are based on the traditional religion which is a mixture of Ancestor Worship and Animism. (Bliatout, 1991: 58)

Traditional healers play a major role in health and illness in many societies. The Hmong are no exceptions. As Bliatout has pointed out, the Hmong rely heavily on their traditional healing system, which is markedly different from the Western health care system. In this chapter I discuss traditional healers and Hmong medicines relevant to reproduction and women's health as well as to the health of young children.[1] Details of the role of Hmong healers in childbearing, childrearing and women's reproductive health will be given in other chapters.

TXIV NEEB (SHAMAN)

The Hmong have a number of beliefs concerning supernatural beings, who include gods, house spirits and spirits of the forest. According to

Hmong legend, once human and supernatural entities could communicate freely, but now only the shaman retains the power to communicate with these beings (Quincy, 1995). Chindasri (1983: 187) wrote:

> The shaman is the only person who can communicate effectively with these supernatural beings, and thus plays a very important role in society. As a ritual specialist he is unique in his ability to give an "ecstatic performance," involving special chants, physical activity, and achievement of a state of trance, during which it is believed that he is in communication with supernatural beings.

According to Cooper et al. (1995: 71), "Hmong shamanism is, in effect, a psychodrama of great subtlety and power. Its ultimate aim, however, is not so much religious as medical: to heal an afflicted person, whether that affliction be physical or mental, and to restore to the patient a damaged part of his or her own self." Similarly, Lemoine (1986: 339) has pointed out that Hmong shamanism is a way of healing. This is why in every village there must be at least one shaman. Otherwise, people might not feel secure, and the village might cease to exist (Chindasri, 1983).[2]

The rituals of the Hmong shaman are often concerned with protection, curing and healing and the selection of new shamans (Chindasri, 1983). However, the most common rituals the shamans perform are to search for the lost soul and bring it back so that a person might recover from his or her illness. A Hmong shaman whom I interviewed explained that:

> The reason why we *ua neeb* (perform shamanic trance) is because we have done it for over five hundred years now and we only know according to what our ancestors tell us. If someone is sick and ask you to *ua neeb* then we have to know why they become sick, like if they have *poob plig* (soul loss) because someone frightened them and they have *poob plig*. It is like this, if the person has been heavily sick and doesn't seem to recover at all then it means that the soul has already gone to prepare a grave for them and the soul would be sleeping inside the grave and waiting for the person. Now you need to *ua neeb* to wake the soul up and out of the grave. This way the person will recover.

The shaman is also concerned with fertility and reproduction if a married couple or a male head of the family requests assistance.[3]

When seeking a shaman's assistance, the Hmong prefer to consult a shaman of the same clan, particularly a shaman who is from the same lineage (Cooper et al., 1995). This is because the shaman is well known to the family and he or she may not charge any fee. The shaman, however, usually avoids treating members of his or her own household because it is believed that the healing may not be as effective as if an outsider conducted the rituals (Chindasri, 1976).

The popularity and thus the status of a shaman is determined by the size of his or her altar and the number of pig jawbones hanging from it. Each jawbone represents one successful shamanic ritual in which the shaman has healed a patient. The number of jawbones the shaman has accumulated since the previous New Year (December) indicates the number of requests people have made. At Hmong New Year, however, these jawbones must be burnt to allow the pigs to be reborn (Cooper et al., 1995).

Siv Yis: The First Shaman

According to Hmong cosmology, evil spirits entered into the world of human beings and created terrible diseases and illnesses through a wicked and selfish god named Nyong (Fadiman, 1997; Johnson and Yang, 1992).[4] However, heaven sent a rescuer who knew "how to heal the sick, and provides protection against evil spirits" (Conquergood et al., 1989). This person was called *Siv Yis.*

Siv Yis is regarded as the first shaman in Hmong culture. When a Hmong shaman performs a shamanic trance, he or she will identify him or herself as "*Siv Yis,*" as Johnson (1985: 73) put it: "[*Siv Yis*] is the greatest of Hmong mythical magicians, and the chief or patron saint of Hmong shamans, with whom they identify themselves when performing their sacred ritual functions."

Becoming a Shaman

> I became a shaman not because it was my will
> But because it was the will of my shaman spirits
> The shaman spirits came to me
> To make me a shaman. . . .
>
> . . . .
>
> You must follow them
> They will make you sick
> Until you become a shaman.
>
> If you shake
> Then you will get better
> All Hmong know that becoming a shaman
> Does not come from your will. (Paja Thao, in Conquergood et al., 1989: 2)

This is a life history told by Paja Thao, a shaman now living in the United States. His life history describes the way a person is called to be a shaman in Hmong society. The following quote on becoming a shaman is from a Hmong shaman whom I interviewed in Melbourne:

> With our tradition of *ua neeb*, it is not that all of a sudden we want to do it because we have an idea. If the spirits come to possess anyone then he or she must do it. If all of sudden you just become a shaman because you want to be, and then I would say that all of the Hmong people would know how to do it. But it isn't like that. The spirits will say these persons are chosen, then they must do it. This is why not many people know how to *ua neeb*.

As these two quotes illustrate, a Hmong shaman cannot choose to become a shaman. He or she must be called by shaman spirits in order to become a healer. This usually occurs with a serious illness or chronic ailment (Lemoine, 1986). When this happens, an experienced shaman will be called to look into the affliction. If the shaman finds that the person's illness is a result of "the desire of a previously deceased shaman's spirit-helpers to incarnate in the afflicted person" (Conquergood et al., 1989: 48), he or she then must accept his destiny in order to be able to recover from the illness or else he or she will die. The shaman will then perform a ceremony to invite the *neeb* spirits to stay with the person in order to confirm the calling. The person usually falls into a deep trance and is then completely healed (Quincy, 1995). To accept the shaman's calling means that the person will possess a special power to enter the spirit world and dedicate his or her life to healing the sick (Quincy, 1995; Lemoine, 1986).

The following quotes are the stories of two shamans whom I interviewed, who described their initiatory sickness and how they became shamans.

Case One

> At that time, the spirits came to posses me. That year I got sick for the whole year. They made me sick, very sick and very pale and I nearly died. So we called other people to come and *ua neeb* many times. They would *ua neeb saib* and they would say that I was possessed by the *neeb* spirits. So they made the altar and put me there and then I started to shake. After I started to do this, I recovered from my sickness. And this is why I became a shaman.

Case Two

> I began to *ua neeb* because I got sick. The sickness made me very tired and lost my appetite. It made me just unable to lie down and unable to eat anything. I had fever too. But there was no medicine that was able to help me at all. *Hu plig* didn't help either. Whatever we tried didn't work. Then I had *ua neeb* but it didn't help. I was sick for one or two years but I still didn't get well. This meant that I would have to *ua neeb*. When you will become a shaman, some one will come to *ua neeb saib* and say that you

> will have to do *ua neeb* then you will be cured in a matter of a couple of days. . . . But the number of *txiv neeb* that will come to diagnose that you will *ua neeb* must be at least five. When they say that you have been given the power to cure then you will *ua neeb* and then it is not even a week when you get better. . . . My father did *ua neeb* and said that I was going to *ua neeb* but he wasn't absolutely sure so he called the second one and that one said the same thing. Then he called the third one and that one said the same thing again, and so until the fifth one who said so that we believed that this had to be done. So I became a shaman and my father was my master since he diagnosed it correctly.

But this does not mean that a shaman does not require learning and training. The shaman who diagnosed his affliction will become his or her "master shaman teacher" (Lemoine, 1986). The novice shaman usually practices with his or her master for at least three years (Lemoine, 1986). During this period the master will instruct him or her of "the sacred chants and the complex and highly elaborated techniques and procedures of the shamanic rites" as well as "the name and nature of the legion of evil spirits who bring harm and suffering to humankind" (Conquergood et al., 1989: 49).

According to Conquergood et al. (1989), the learning process is undertaken through example and imitation. The novice shaman will follow the master's words and imitate his or her actions. Instruction takes place at night or in the forest. "They would lie together on the sleeping platform and discuss the mysteries of the spirit world, the power of special chants, the intricacies of ritual technique. There are no written books or manuals. All of the learning is mnemonic, personal, and experiential" (Conquergood et al., 1989: 49).

Chindasri (1983: 188) has stated that:

> The Hmong becomes a shaman without regret. He believes firmly in the diagnosis, and in the ability of the presiding shaman. Because he is certain that if he refuses to allow the "doctor spirit" to stay he will not recover, he is also under some pressure to conform to cultural expectations and become a shaman. . . . There are other benefits in accepting the role . . . including advantage change in social position, involving material reward (meat and fees) and an opportunity to acquire increased prestige.

Occasionally there are people who try to resist becoming a shaman. As Morechand (1968: 208) has found, some have tried to escape from the prospect of having "doctor spirits" stay with them. However, none of these attempts was successful, "because the spirits were strong and persistent." I have also found this with one shaman who related a similar history (see Photo 3.1).

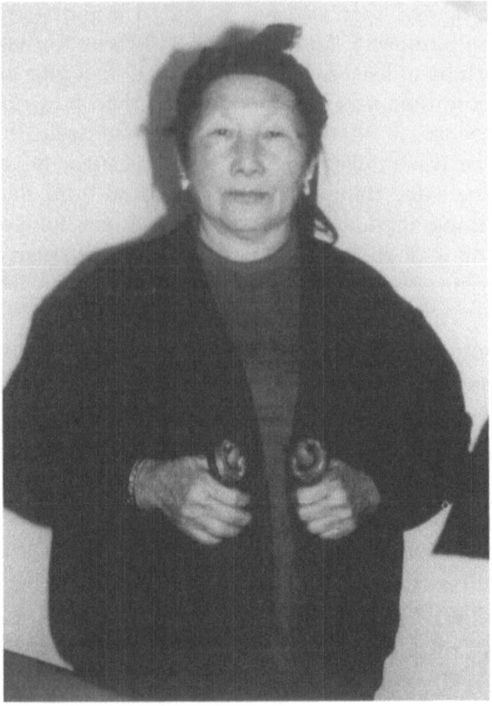

Photo 3.1 A Hmong shaman in Melbourne.

The reason why I *ua neeb* was my sickness. It started when I got sick for a long time and whoever came to *saib* would say different things. One *saib* and said "it is because your parent wants to eat a cow." So we did that but I still didn't recover. Then "it is because you have *poob plig* [lost soul,]" so *hu plig* was done but I still didn't recover. So that was why we asked my uncle to come and *ua neeb saib*. He said, "Oh! It is because you have been given a set of *neeb* and so you must *ua neeb*." I said, "Oh! I am very embarrassed I don't think that I will do it." At that time I was still very young and small. I said, "I am too young and too embarrassed." So he replied, "Even if you are embarrassed the spirits had already possessed you, you must do it." I asked him to *ua neeb* and beg the spirits to go to my husband. So I begged the spirits and when my uncle *ua neeb* my husband did not shake. Uncle spitted water on him but he still did not shake. I was sitting near a fire but I was shaking. So uncle said the spirits did not like my husband, it must be me. So he took me over to the altar and I *ua neeb*. I was very sick and couldn't move and they had to carry me to sit in front of the altar where *ua neeb* took place. When I *ua neeb* it was very powerful. I did one and I felt better. I did another one and I felt much better. I *ua neeb* twelve times then I totally recovered. And that is how I came to *ua neeb*.

Ua Neeb (Shamanic Trance): Journey into the Spirit World

In shamanic healing rituals, the shaman performs *ua neeb,* which is characterized as a trance healing process. According to Lemoine (1986: 340), trance is a particular feature of Hmong shamanism. An individual cannot become a shaman without "a predisposition to go into a trance." In *ua neeb* rituals, a shaman enters the unseen world:

> The shaman is the one who can actually cross the threshold between earth and sky, and human and spirit, and enter the side of reality that is unseen, but nonetheless real, to rescue captured or fugitive souls, battle with evil ogres, or reconcile an offended nature spirit. His or her special powers of communication with spirits are signified by out-of-body consciousness, the ecstatic trembling of trance possession. (Conquergood et al., 1989: 47)

In shamanic ritual, spirit helpers also assist in trance. There are two main spirit helpers. One is known as *Leej Nkaub,* who guides the shaman in the trance. Lemoine (1986: 341) has referred to this spirit as "the Inspiring Spirit." Another *neeb* is called *Tsheej Xeeb* who makes the shaman shake and is known as "the Spirit of the Trance." A shaman I interviewed said that these *neeb* spirits are sent down to earth to possess a shaman and help the shaman to perform *ua neeb.* These spirits also make a shaman sick in a strange way before accepting his fate. In *ua neeb* to bring a lost soul back, it is *Leej Nkaub* and *Tsheej Xeeb* who help the shaman to search for the soul. There are also other spirits who may assist in other ways. They are referred to as *tub tes tub taw* and they are seen as the shaman's "hands and feet." One shaman in my study referred to these spirits as his "soldiers" who carry his weapons in negotiating with bad spirits. He remarked:

> *Tub tes tub taw,* they are like your soldiers who carry knives and guns for you. When you call upon them they would bring the knives and guns to you and go with you. For example, the spirits are bad and do not want to negotiate, they do not listen to you who are higher than they are and have authority over them . . . then I will say to them that if they do not listen to me I will set my soldiers onto them. So if they still won't listen then I will release my soldiers to go and kill them and so they will be scared. . . . If they are willing to negotiate then I say to them, "How much money do you want?" Because they have captured your person [his or her soul] so you ask, "How much ransom do you want for the release of my person? If I give you this much and if you do not release my person then I will tell my soldiers to come and fight you." This is what happens.

Another shaman explained that there are many *neeb* who assist in trance rituals. These include *cuaj txhiab peeb zeej, yim puas peeb muas,* and *txw zeej txw koob*. However, he cited *txw zeej txw koob* as the true *neeb* spirits. In *ua neeb* rituals, he said, if we listen carefully we will always hear the shaman say "*kuv sam phiaj txw zeej xyuam phiaj txw koob*." This is the way a shaman calls upon his *neeb* spirits to assist him in the trance.

In Lemoine's (1986: 342) narration of Hmong shamanism, he explained that the shaman is never alone in trance healing. The shaman, in fact, has his or her own "task force." According to Lemoine, "His spirit helpers come to him already structured as a task force with scout spirits, engineer spirits, horsemen and foot soldiers. The Inspiring Spirit and the Spirit of the Trance, who never part from him, act as staff and liaison officers."

In shamanic trance, healing rituals take place in three sequential phases. Although in most writings on Hmong shamanism only two phases are described,[5] three Hmong shamans whom I interviewed each said that there are three ways of *ua neeb*. (1) When calling for healing, a shaman will first perform *ua neeb saib* to "see" or "divine" the seriousness and the cause of the problem. In addition, the shaman will be able to tell if the *neeb* spirits will be able to help effect a cure. (2) Once the cause of the problem is found, the shaman will perform *ua neeb cais* to "negotiate" with the spirits involved. The shaman, through his or her *neeb* (spirit helpers), will say to the spirits that they have three to five days to leave the patient alone (meaning that the patient should recover within three to five days), and—if the spirits agree to this—whether they would prefer a pig, other animals or simply spirit money in exchange for the agreement. Sometimes *ua neeb cais* is referred to as *ua neeb cais dab*, meaning to "remove" or "separate" spirits from the patient. If the spirits agree, the patient should feel better three to five days after this ritual. (3) The shaman will then perform *ua neeb kho* in order to "heal" the patient. This time an animal, as negotiated or promised, will be sacrificed as the spirits' reward for leaving the patient.

According to Cooper et al. (1995: 69), trance rituals can vary depending on the circumstances of illness and healing. However, the search for the soul is generally divided into five main parts, as follows:

> The first part is formed by the entrance of the shaman into trance and his invocation of helper-spirits. The second part is formed by the procession of the shaman and all his troops to the house of the patient to search there for his lost soul. The third part is formed by the hunt of the soul. The fourth part is formed by the return of the cavalcade, with the fugitive soul carried on the back of a female spirit (just as Hmong women carry their children) back to its home. The fifth and final part is formed by the return of the *dab neeb* to their altar and the shaman's return to normal consciousness.

Once this is done and the patient is healed, the shaman must be "paid" for his or her healing power. The payment is normally in the form of a pig's head and an attached front leg, although some may place some money on the shaman's altar to honor the *neeb* spirits. This money will not be used by the shaman. The shaman will also be invited to join the meal after the rituals are performed. However, if people come to *fiv* (beg) the shaman to perform *ua neeb* for them, they usually offer a certain amount of payment when they *fiv*. If this is the case—and only if the healing is successful—the shaman will accept the fees as promised. In addition, with difficult *ua neeb*, such as when a soul is captured by spirits, the shaman must be offered a fee. This fee is to give the shaman more "power" to negotiate and fight with the spirits. If the shaman is not paid a fee, the spirits with whom the shaman is negotiating will make him or her sick.

Quincy (1995) has pointed out that shamanism is not a profession but a vocation. Payment for healing the sick is not sufficient for the shaman to live on, as it is for health professionals in Western society. One shaman in my study remarked that "some people may give me money, but some don't. But it doesn't really matter, because *ua neeb* is not something you do for a business. It is not something that you do to get rich or wealthy. It is a means of helping people for free."

If after three or five days the patient does not recover, the shaman needs to *ua neeb cais* again in order to renegotiate with the spirits. This time a new arrangement or promise must be made. This time, it is believed, the patient should recover. However, if *ua neeb cais* fails again, the patient is allowed to seek help from another shaman. There is no loss of face in this regard, as the failure of diagnostic and healing procedures is not due to the inability of the shaman but to other circumstances, such as the *neeb* spirits being unable to help in a particular instance.

In performing a trance healing, the shaman needs his shamanic tools, which are believed to be inherited from *Siv Yis* after he returned to heaven. These include a gong (*nruas*), which is beaten by the shaman's assistant to call the *neeb* as the shaman enters the trance, during and at the end of the ritual; a rattle made of an iron hoop with several pieces of round metal, which the shaman shakes regularly throughout the trance; finger bells for his or her index fingers and a knife to put before the altar (Photos 3.2 and 3.3). The shaman also needs a wooden bench, which represents the winged horse of *Siv Yis*. He or she bounces frenziedly on this bench during the trance rituals. During the trance, the shaman also has to cover his or her face with a veil. At the shaman altar, incense sticks (usually seven sticks at one time) must also be burnt. When performing trance healing, the shaman is said to be in a trance. This is symbolized by a covering veil signifying that he or she is being cut off from the physical world. When I asked a shaman if he saw things during the trance, he answered that he did not see anything but could hear the *neeb* spirit (*Leej Nkaub*) speaking in his ears, and he followed their in-

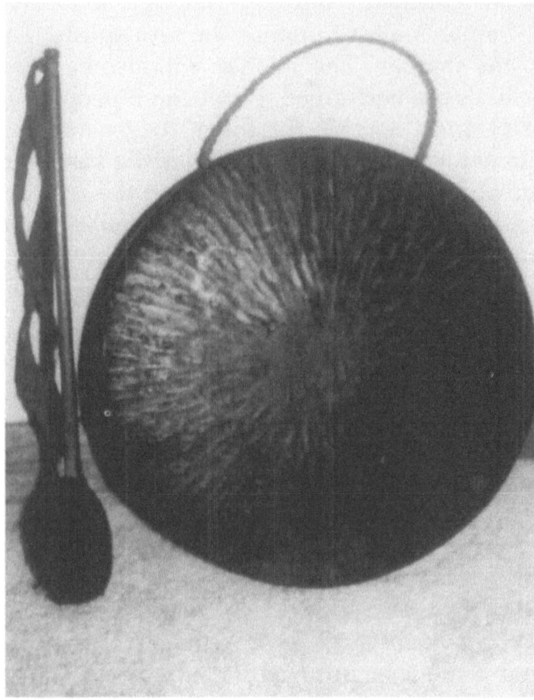

Photo 3.2 A gong used in shamanic rituals.

structions. The ritual is physically demanding and often takes a long time.

The Shaman Altar: Honoring *Dab Neeb*

A shaman keeps an altar at his house. It is usually placed on a wall near the altar of the house spirit. The altar is usually decorated with gold paper. On it, there is a bowl of water called *dej zaj* representing a dragon's pool that lies beneath the cave of *Siv Yis*. There is also a bowl of husked rice with an egg in the middle, representing the *leej nkaub*. Three incense sticks are also placed in this bowl as food-offerings to the *dab neeb*. There are three small cups containing water, tea and rice wine on the altar to offer to the spirits. Unhusked rice or maize may also be scattered on the altar as fodder for the shaman's horse. A bowl of fried raw rice or maize is always place on the altar to feed *dab neeb*. The shaman will use this at the beginning and end of his or her trance to command his or her spirit allies. A pair of divination horns (*kuam*) is also placed on the altar (Photo 3.4). On top of the altar there are three white

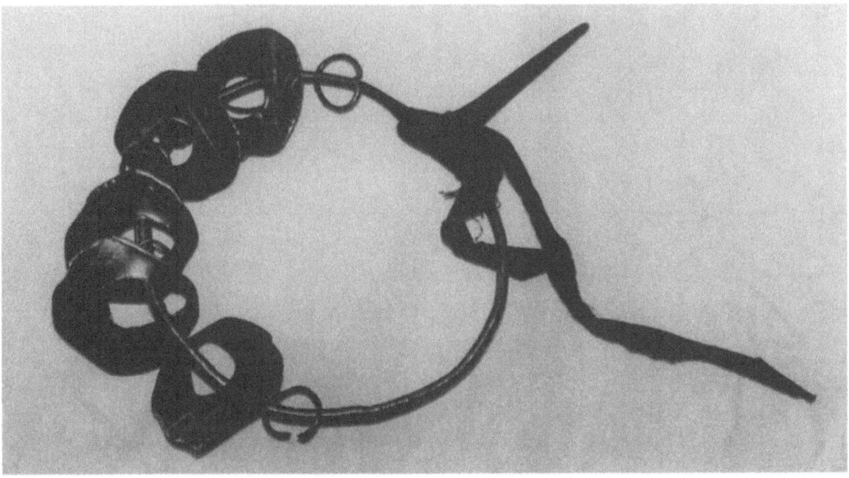

Photo 3.3 A rattle used in shamanic rituals.

strings connecting the altar to the door of the house. This set of white strings is the path the *dab neeb* travel to the altar of the shaman. Lastly, a bamboo stick is placed at the top of the altar. It represents the spear of the *neeb* king, which was thrown down to earth when shamans were created. The altar can only be removed when the shaman dies and must not be removed without a ritual for the *dab neeb*. Upon the shaman's death, the altar will be dismantled and placed in the forest, but all the tools will be carefully kept by his or her sons. Every month, usually on the ninth, fifteenth and nineteenth day, the shaman burns incense sticks on the altar and changes the water and rice wine. New raw rice must be fried to replace the old. However, these dates can be altered depending on how busy the shaman is, but they must be on odd days only.

At the Hmong New Year in December, the gold paper used to decorate the altar will be replaced. Cups and bowls will be cleaned and new food will be offered. Any food that has been offered to the spirits must be thrown away. Humans are not allowed to eat it, as it is food for the spirits. Pig jaws and chicken feet will be burnt to release the souls of these animals for their rebirth. The white strings must also be replaced. During this time, the *dab neeb* will be released to their cave in the original mountain for a period of 10 to 12 days.[6] It is said that *dab neeb* also need a period of rest. Hence, during this period, the shaman cannot perform *ua neeb* rituals. After 10 or 12 days, the shaman will summon his *dab neeb* and at that point can perform *ua neeb* again. This ritual must be undertaken on the same day each year, although each shaman may have his or her own date for releasing the *dab neeb*.[7]

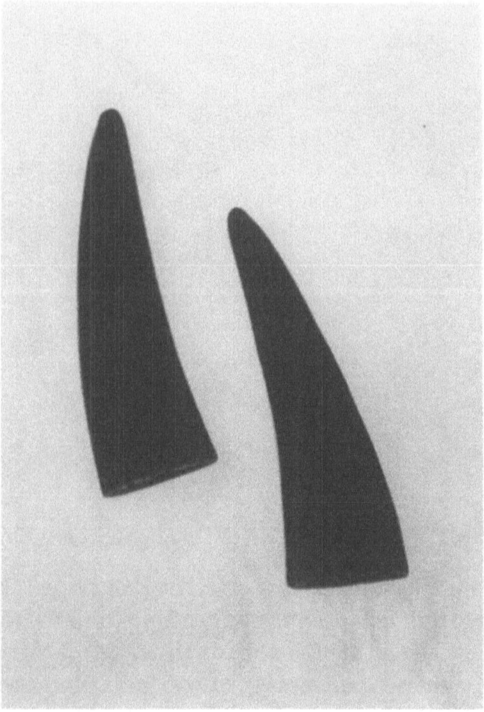

Photo 3.4 A pair of divination horns used in shamanic rituals.

A Shaman and Western Medicine: Conflicting or Complementary Approaches?

Western medicine focuses on organic disease and bases diagnosis and treatment on the physical reality of the patient. In Hmong shamanism, illness is not only a physical condition but is also the result of the interference of metaphysical realities. This leads us to the question of whether shamanism is in conflict with Western medical tradition. Conquergood et al. (1989: 60) have argued that this is not the case, as the Hmong shaman is not only concerned with the metaphysical world, but "brings physical and metaphysical realities into intimate communications."

Hmong shamans do not oppose the use of natural remedies or the physical treatments of Western medicine, as not all illnesses are caused by supernatural beings. The Hmong recognize natural causes of illness and seek help accordingly. Hence, we have seen some shamans who are also medicine women or masseurs, who treat their patients through herbal medicines and manipulation of the physical body. Lemoine (1986: 345) has also pointed out that Hmong shamans in the West do not oppose "the use of drugs or any other therapy. They are often themselves distinguished herbalists and they always welcome the use of Western drugs in conjunction with their own magic. It is not that they doubt their own power, but that they acknowledge their healing as essentially psychosomatic." Similarly Conquergood et al. (1989: 61) have stated: "It is more common than not to find shamans alternating and combining natural and supernatural healing techniques. They will try first one technique, and then another, persisting until the patient gets relief. They see the two modes of healing, natural and supernatural, as complementary rather than contradictory." Cooper et al. (1995) and Quincy (1995) have also pointed out that the Hmong are pragmatists. If they perceive that the cause of the problem is physical rather than spiritual, they will employ a physical means to cure the problem. However they also point out that although the Hmong in the United States often use Western medicine when accessible, they return to shamanism or other traditional healing methods if modern medicine fails to help them. The Hmong in Melbourne are no exception.

However, it seems that Hmong shamanism in Australia has played a lesser role in relation to women and childbirth. One shaman explained that he had helped many women with difficult births when he was in Laos and also in a refugee camp in Thailand. But he had not helped any woman in Australia, because they all went to the hospital to give birth. He had not had any opportunity to exercise his healing power on women's bodies in his new country.

KWS TSHUAJ (MEDICINE EXPERT) AND HERBAL MEDICINES

Bliatout (1991: 61) has commented that "Hmong herbalists are perhaps the most commonly used practitioners in Hmong society. For many ailments, the use of herbs is the first attempt at healing." At other times, herbs are used as shamanic healing rituals are being performed (Cooper et al., 1995). Thao (1986: 366) has pointed out that "in the Hmong community, herbal medicines rally against illness along with shamanism." Most Hmong families grow common herbs in their own gardens. These include herbs for headaches, stomachaches, morning sickness in pregnancy and herbs for confinement food (used by women in the first 30 days after giving birth).

Herbal medicines are, however, part of the women's world, since it is usually women who are knowledgeable about herbal medicines (Cooper et al., 1995).[8] As the women in Thao's study (1986: 366) claimed "We are given the gift and knowledge. Only we can make herbal medicines effective. Men are much too careless." Therefore, most herbal knowledge is held by medicine women, and they usually keep their gardens filled with herbs for all sorts of health problems. Many herbs, however, are useful for women's problems. Most medicine women are also knowledgeable about wild herbs, which are used in more serious situations such as miscarriage or abortion (see later chapters on childbirth and reproductive health). Cooper et al. (1995) commented that "wild" herbs growing in the forest are differentiated from "tame" herbs which medicine women plant secretly around the house or near the village. Some herbs must be sought in faraway fields. Moua (1996) also commented that herbs grown in the forest are considered better medicines than those grown at home, and some herbs cannot be planted domestically.[9]

Most medicine women prefer using fresh herbs, known as green herbs, rather than dried ones. Roots are most often used, but leaves and stems are used as well. They are usually boiled in chicken soup or steamed with an egg. Sometimes herbs can be boiled and drunk as tea. The usual instruction is to take the mixture for three mornings or three days. If the illness is serious and the herbs have to be prepared with chicken, the preparation must be made in secrecy and usually at night when no one is around. A medicine woman told me that if other people know that the herb is being prepared, its healing power will not be effective. Herbs prepared as tea can be prepared during the day.

Some traditional medicines are prepared from a combination of dried herbs and animal parts. This, I was told, is more common for serious health problems, such as a prolapsed uterus (Photo 3.5). The medicine is prepared with warm water as tea.[10]

Becoming a Medicine Expert

Not every woman has knowledge of and access to herbal medicines. Similar to the process of becoming a sharman, a woman will typically have an affliction on her body and a shaman will be called in to "see" her symptoms. If the spirits of medicine have caused her affliction, she will be told to try some herbs. If the herbs work, she will then become a medicine woman and have the power to cure others. The following quote is from a medicine woman whom I interviewed:

> I had pain in my hand. For no reason this hand was very sore and then the other one started to be painful too. So the *txiv neeb* came to *saib* and told me that the *tshuaj* spirit had come to possess me. . . . He said that there was nothing wrong just that the *tshuaj* spirit has come to possess me. . . . So if I had a pain anywhere I would go to get some herbs and put on the sore part then it will heal. I recovered after that. So I became a *kws tshuaj* since.

While afflicted, a medicine woman usually has a dream in which the medicine spirits show her different kinds of herbs and instruct her about

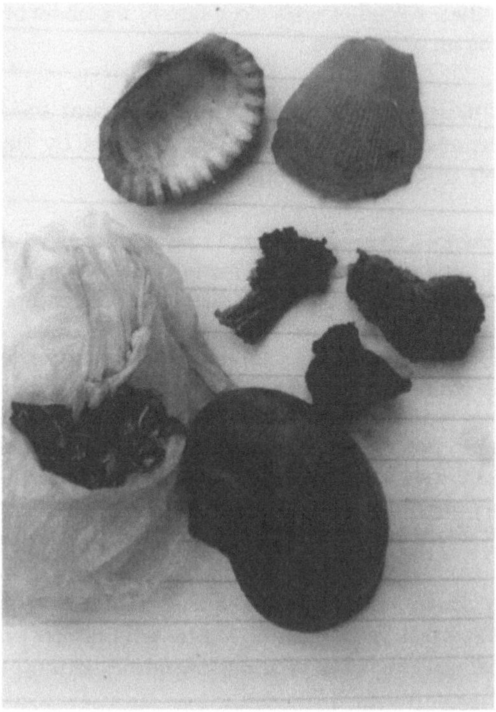

Photo 3.5 Traditional medicines used for recovering from a prolapsed uterus.

their efficacy. After waking, she will try the herbs, and they are usually as effective as in her dream.

> I would have a dream and they [spirits] would take me to show and say to me "this one is a medicine for you." I would dream because of the pain in my hand and the spirits would say to me "if you use this type of herb you will recover." The next morning when I woke up I said to myself, "since they have told me about these medicines, let me try it." If it worked then I would be able to give it to other people to take too. And it worked.

Similar to the shaman, a medicine woman must have a teacher or master who will teach her about different kinds of herbs and their healing properties. The teacher is usually an older relative or family member, such as a mother or aunt. According to Thao (1986), medicine women do not usually teach anyone unless the person is a family member, a relative or a trusted friend. Bliatout (1991: 61) has pointed out:

> Many skilled herbalists prefer to keep their remedies a secret and only give out crushed forms of their herbs to families with sick persons. They

> will only share their remedies with close family members or someone they have accepted as an apprentice.[11]

A medicine woman whom I interviewed said that she lived with some medicine women and learned the secret of herbs by begging for herbs whenever she felt unwell. She related:

> I lived with some *kws tshuaj* and when I had pain somewhere I would say to them, "Oh! I have pain here and it hurts," and the *kws tshuaj* would say that "The herb is right at your feet, the herbs for your pain is at your feet." I would then ask, "Where is it?" You have to beg them a lot and they would tell you. They would say, "Give some money." Then I would say that "I have no money, if you don't help me then I will not get better." Because they are your people [relatives] and they grow a lot of herbal medicines to help people in their garden, they would then go and pick them for you and they would tell you how to take them. They would tell you how to prepare them to be effective too. You would do this, and that is what I learnt about herbal medicines.

Women in my study also mentioned that if one is a medicine woman, one must keep the knowledge secret. If one tells others without accepting fees, one may become ill. One woman explained this to me:

> In the Hmong tradition and custom one who knows and understands the use of traditional herbal medicines cannot give out the secret of herbs. The knowledge has to be passed from parent to children or bought. The reason is because we are ancestral worshipers believing in the presence of spirits. If we give out our knowledge then we will be stricken by the illness that the medicine is supposed to cure or some other relating illness. This is believed to be caused by the medicine spirits.

There is a story of a woman who passed on her herbal knowledge to others and later became quite ill. After having several *ua neeb* she still did not recover. She later realized that she might have told someone about herbs without being paid for it. She then made a pledge to the medicine spirits: "If it was that I have been giving medicines to other people then let me get better by tomorrow." The next day she passed out some stones while urinating and she recovered.

After being requested by a novice medicine woman, the teacher will gather several kinds of herbs and place them in front of her altar. She then lights incense sticks, burns spirit paper and chants propitiatory words before her spirits of medicine (*dab tshuaj*). The herbs are then divided into two piles. Thus, as Cooper et al. (1995: 58) have written, "the spirits of medicine are symbolically divided between the two women."

The healing power of a medicine woman is believed to be assisted by medicine spirits. This power cannot easily be obtained by lay women. Bliatout (1991: 61) remarked:

> Some [Hmong] say that some of the most skilled herbalists actually utilize the power of spirits or have a healing spirit living with them. That is why herbs have a healing power when utilized by them, but will have less or no power if used by someone else.

This means that to be taught by a medicine woman, one must pay her a fee in order to honor her spirits. Without this, the learning may not be effective. A medicine woman, who was taught by her aunt who was a medicine woman, remarked:

> I had an aunt who was very experience in herbs. She took me and showed me her herbs. She told me to pay some money. I paid her *ib ki ob npib* [one dollar and twenty cents], one bunch of incense sticks, a gold paper and one chicken in order to put on her altar. Her altar was small one and I left them there. Then she showed me herbs and she taught me that "this one is good for this, that one is good for that, and so on." Since you have paid fees you should be able to remember them all. And if you give the medicine for someone, they must pay the same price and they will get better.

When I went to obtain knowledge of herbs from one medicine woman, I had to pay her a fee to honor her knowledge and skill. I was told that the amount she asked from me was similar to what she had to pay her master, and that without this fee, she might become ill.[12]

Medicine women usually keep their altars at home for *dab tshuaj* (spirits of medicine) to reside. This is set up on one side of *dab xwm kab* altar, and the spirits must be honored much as they are at the altar of the shaman. When women seek help from a medicine woman, they must bring a bunch of incense sticks tied with a piece of red material, some gold money and several silver coins. These will be put on the medicine woman's altar. The woman then can ask for help. Since leaving Laos, people have started to pay medicine women in the currency of the country they live in, such as in Thai *baht* in a refugee camp in Thailand and in Australian dollars when they are in Australia.

Hmong Herbal Medicines in a New Country

Hmong herbal medicines are still used by the Hmong despite their migratory experiences. In a refugee camp in Thailand, Pyke (1987), when working as a public health nurse at Phanat Nikhom, identified twenty medicinal plants used by Hmong herbalists. There were herbs for burns, fever, weakness, poor vision, broken bones, stomach aches, painful urination, arthritis, tuberculosis, rabies, scabies, gonorrhea, dysentery, constipation, impotence, and attacks by a *dab ntxaug* (a spirit who lives in the jungle and causes epidemics when disturbed). There were also herbs for women dealing with anemia, promoting delivery of a blood clot after birth, prolapsed uterus, and insufficient breast milk. Pyke also commented that the herbs could be used in various forms, for example, chopped, crushed, dried, shredded, powered, decocted, infused with hot or cold water, mixed with ashes, sulphur, egg or chicken.

In Merced, California, Moua (1996) conducted a study on Hmong herbs and found that the use of herbal medicines was still widespread within the Hmong communities throughout the United States. He identified many herbs which are available for all sorts of health problems. These included herbs for headache; upset stomach and loss of appetite; sore lip, gum and throat; pain due to sprained body; feeling tired and weak, with loss of appetite; constipation; bad breath; toothache and gum bleeding; indigestion and upset stomach after a meal or drink; abdominal pain; sharp chest pain; coma after eating something that does not agree with the body; high fever and cancer.

For men, there are herbs for improving fertility, lack of energy, sexual inactivity, for sexually transmitted diseases such as syphilis and for swollen penis.

For women and children, there are herbs for menstrual cramps, pain or infection in the uterus, when an unborn baby slips into a lower position because the mother stretches to reach something high above her head, relieving stomach ache after giving birth, maintaining and improving fetal health, curing fever in an unborn infant, a newborn infant who is not fully grown, chicken pox, a baby crying at night and improving weakness and energy after childbirth.

Similarly, during my fieldwork, I have observed the use of many kinds of herbs by the Hmong in Australia. There are herbs for cramps, strength, bruises, washing out bladder stones, burn, fever and stomach pain, swollen or dry limbs, skin breaks and bleeding, bladder infection, excessive coughing, fever with sore throat as well as coughing and wheezing due to smoking.

For women and children, there are herbs to stop bleeding during pregnancy and to give the baby strength to grow in the uterus, for pain in the uterus, for strength and removing childbirth blood, for a tear at birth, for heartburn during confinement, for menstruation regulation, for abortion and cleansing of the womb, for dissolving blood clots, for energy and body aches and pain, for diarrhea and for stomach pain and diarrhea in children.

Despite the fact that many herbs are grown in Australia and the United States, many more are not available to the Hmong in their new country. This is particularly true of wild herbs. Therefore, many Hmong use dried herbs ordered from Thailand or Laos, or they buy similar dried herbs from Chinese herbalists. The Hmong also modify their herb intake. For example, there are 12 or 13 kinds of herbs traditionally used in the chicken soup consumed during the confinement period. Today, Hmong women only use three or four herbs. Many herbs that can be grown in Australia or the United States must be planted in pots and moved inside in winter. Many Hmong in Australia live in high-rise Housing Commission Flats where no land is available and, hence, cannot grow their own herbs. Some have attempted to grow herbs in pots in their flats, but they do not grow well in the limited sunlight. Nevertheless, the Hmong continue to use herbs as the first choice in the self-treatment process before seeking help from Western health care professionals.

Closely related to the medicine woman is another woman healer from whom women seek help during childbearing. This is the so-called traditional midwife, whom the Hmong refer to as "an old lady," as there is no formal term for her even though her role is the same as that of a traditional midwife in other societies. Her role will be discussed in greater detail in later chapters.[13]

KHAWV KOOB (MAGIC HEALER)

According to Bliatout (1991: 64) a *Khawv Koob* is a traditional healer who, through extensive training, learns various chants, mantras or verses to heal people with afflictions. These spoken words are believed to have a magical power. There are different types of magic healing for a wide variety of conditions such as headache, chest and stomach pain, cuts and bruises, children's common health problems such as chicken pox, sore mouth and gums, and to stop babies from crying. There are, however, four main conditions for which a magic healer offers healing; broken bones, severe cuts, burns and childbirth. To heal a person, a magic healer lights a bundle of incense sticks and then whispers magic words to the afflicted areas three times, once every day. This is usually repeated for seven days, but in cases such as broken bones it may take two weeks. Sometimes, magic words are spoken into a bowl of water and the magic water is given to the person to drink or used to blow on the afflicted parts.[14]

Moua (1996: 45) has explained the role of a magic healer in treating different types of afflictions as follows:

> For headache, chest pain, and stomach pain, the magician will suck the patient's forehead, chest, or stomach after whispering the formula each time. This is to extract an object from the patient into a small bowl of water. The object was believed to be put there by evil spirits or by other magicians. For swallowing an object, the magician will whisper and aim at a very small rice ball (*qai mov*) then give it to the patient to eat or swallow.

> This method will cause the patient to vomit to throw out the object. To treat a patient with burn or broken arm/leg, the magician will whisper, aiming at the burned or broken area three times. The magician will pour a little bit of water from a small bowl of water that was prepared for the healing to blow to the area and apply to the burned or broken area. The small bowl of water will be kept with the patient. The patient will use it to apply to burned or broken area three times a day until the water is finished. The patient will be recovered after two or three bowls of water. If the patient is injured by a car accident but received no prescription, magic healing is also used to heal the aches and pains inside the body.

A magic healer whom I interviewed explained that *khawv koob* can also be used to cure illness resulting from being struck by evil spirits. However, it is usually used when the person is extremely ill and *ua neeb* cannot help. In this case, a magic healer will use breast milk to heal the illness. In normal circumstances, adults and older children cannot drink breast milk. It is believed that in doing so they will be struck by lightning.[15] However, a magic healer can use breast milk to solve health problems, but he must conduct *ua khawv koob* before doing so. A magic healer related how he prevented a baby from being struck by the spirits:

> *Khawv koob* must be done to the breast milk and then give it to the baby to drink and also spray over his body. When you do that you have to cite verses to blame the spirits. You would say that the spirits should not come close to the baby and if they touch the breast milk then may lightning strike them.

In addition, when a person is extremely ill or when a woman is having a long and difficult labor, a magic healer may be asked to conduct *fiv yeem* (a ritual to ask for protection or insurance for the sick person's life). If the person shows signs of recovery or the woman gives birth soon afterward, animal sacrifices will be involved. Usually, a chicken, pig, cow or buffalo will be sacrificed during a second ceremony called *pauj veeb*.

Sometimes magic is used in combination with herbs and massage. A Hmong man told me that when he was in a refugee camp in Thailand, he used a knife one day to cut an object. Accidentally, the knife cut the top of his thumb so severely that it nearly fell off. He immediately sought help from a magic healer. The magic healer wrapped his thumb with herbs and chanted magic words several times. The chant was repeated for several days. A week later, his thumb was completely healed; not even a scar could be seen.[16]

Ua khawv koob is believed to be the world of men, as women are not considered clever enough to learn the secret healing power.[17] However, as a magic healer told me, it is mainly because magic healing techniques need extensive training, and women do not have the opportunity to do this because of their domestic and other responsibilities. Most training sessions take place at night because of their secret nature, and this is the time when women have to put children to sleep and attend to other family chores before retiring. Thus, it is not that women are not clever enough but because their responsibilities—which are greater than those of Hmong men—prevent them from being magic healers.

In learning to magically heal a certain condition, a person must first personally experience the affliction; otherwise he may not be able to obtain and keep the knowledge. Some health problems are more difficult to learn about than others, and there are certain situations in which a magic healer cannot experience the problem at all. This is particularly so with childbirth problems, such as a difficult birth. In these cases, a higher fee must be given to the healer's teacher. In the learning process, a magic healer learns one verse at a time. He must remember the verse by heart, as there are no written or recorded words for him to refer to.

Like a medicine woman, a magic healer needs to learn from his teacher. To obtain knowledge from a teacher, one must pay a fee. The more difficult the magic healing technique, the higher the fee. When another person wishes to learn magic healing from the teacher, the fee will be the same amount as the fee the teacher paid to his master, as a magic healer explained:

> If they want to learn all of the *khawv koob* like I have learnt from my teacher, then the fee will be the same as what I have paid him to learn from him. I have paid the fee to learn my knowledge from my teacher; they will have to pay the same fee as I have paid to learn these magic things.

A magic healer also keeps an altar at his home. In seeking help from a magic healer, people must come to ask for help at his house. They also need to bring a bunch of incense sticks tied with a narrow piece of red cloth and some silver coins to be put on his altar. For minor healing such as headache and stomach pain, it is not necessary to pay a magic healer a fee. However, for a difficult situation such as childbirth, being struck by evil spirits, broken bones or deep cuts, the fee is required.

Of all the traditional healers in Australia, the magic healer seems to be the most affected by the Western medical system, mainly because of the nature of the magic healing process. For instance, in the healing of a burn, a blow of magic water on the burned area is needed. However, this is opposite to the Western approach, which prohibits contact of the burned area with water during the healing process. A magic healer commented that when there is an emergency, most people will immediately seek help from a hospital, partly because they have access to health services. He compared this to women in childbirth:

> Hmong has a lot of ways to help women in childbirth. But comparing Laos to this country there is a minimum use of our traditions here. When our country had not fallen we lived far away from the city and so we were able to help them many more times. . . . In Laos there were no hospitals because we lived far away from the hospital so we had to rely on our own methods when it comes to having children. When we came into Thailand, there were doctors so we used it [Western medicine] to help with the difficult cases. When we come to this country, as soon as the woman goes into labor we start to call the ambulance to take her to the hospital. So this is why we don't have a chance to use it.

This is more obvious with children who require treatment, since if treatment is delayed, parents may be charged with child neglect or child abuse by authorities in Australia. But when parents become unsatisfied with Western treatments, they will seek help from a magic healer. This can be illustrated by the case of a Hmong child who was burned by hot water and taken to the Royal Children's Hospital for treatment. To his parents' mind, the hospital did not do enough to relieve the pain. The child was taken home and assistance from a magic healer was sought. Only a few days after, he was completely healed.

CONCLUSION

As Bliatout (1991) has pointed out, most traditional Hmong healers are dedicated, since they make a personal effort and use their knowledge to help other members of the community. They are respected in Hmong communities, whether they are still in Laos or resettled elsewhere. This chapter shows that traditional healers still play a vital role in Hmong health and illness. It is clear that the loss of the Hmong traditional healing system would affect much more than the health and well-being of the people. In their discussion about the continuity with tradition among the Hmong in the United States, Conquergood et al. (1989: 50, original emphasis) pointed out that:

> If the Hmong who have resettled in America lose their traditions of shamanic healing, they will lose something much more fundamental than a set of curing techniques. Modern medicine may be able to substitute for a soul-calling ritual as an effective remedy for a headache. But, western medicine can never satisfy the deep spiritual yearnings of the Hmong to participate in sacred dramas that make life meaningful. . . . A shamanic performance entails something much deeper than curing a specific illness. What is really being refurbished and recreated every time a Hmong shaman performs is the system of meanings and web of symbols that grant coherence and comprehension. Whether the sickness abates or lingers, the shaman's real accomplishment in every performance is that she or he *establishes the world.*

I believe Conquergood et al.'s points are also applicable to the Hmong in Australia, as we shall see in the chapters that follow.

NOTES

1. Other aspects of Hmong health and illness and the healers themselves have been published in a number of papers and books. See Chindasri, 1976, 1983; Thao, 1986; Lemoine, 1986; Bliatout, 1991; Adler, 1995; and Fadiman, 1997.

2. In Australia, there is at least one shaman in each of the main states in which the Hmong live. In Melbourne I know of at least four, and I interviewed three of the shamans.

3. See later chapters on seeking healing for women.

4. I have provided a story about the creation of illnesses and disease in Hmong folklore in Chapter 2 of this volume.

5. See Lemoine, 1986; Conquergood et al., 1989; and Cooper et al., 1995, for examples.

6. This original cave is believed to be in China, where the first shaman *Siv Yis* resided. See Quincy (1995) for further details about the origin of Hmong shamanism.

7. Since shamans do not release their *neeb* spirits at the same time, there will always be a shaman who can help people in need.

8. There are some older men who are knowledgeable about herbal medicines as well. See, for example, a life history of Paj Txos Lauj in Mattison et al. (1994: 17). Paj Txos Lauj claims that he is a medicine man and gained his knowledge from his father, who was also a "herbal doctor."

9. I also observed this among the Hmong in Thailand, when I did my preliminary fieldwork on another research project in a Hmong village in the Chiang Mai province in early 1999.

10. After being honored and paid a fee, a Hmong medicine woman in Chiang Mai also provided me with a recipe for curing prolapsed uterus that comprised dried herbs and animal parts. All ingredients are put in a cup of warm water and drunk as tea. The undissolved parts should be used to rub the woman's abdomen.

11. This is confirmed by my observations during fieldwork in a Hmong village in the Chiang Mai province in Thailand. A medicine woman who I interviewed had been passed on the knowledge of herbs by her mother, who is still practicing medicine in the same village.

12. This is similar to my experience in northern Thailand. When I asked a medicine woman if I could talk to her about herbal medicines, she initially said, "yes." However, once I started to ask for details of each herb, she told me that she could not tell me unless I honored her and paid her some fees. Without the fee she would become ill. And so I paid her.

13. See also Chapters 4, 5, 11 and 13 in this volume.

14. According to Cooper et al. (1995), magic healing is not particularly Hmong despite the fact that many Hmong are knowledgeable about magical rites; many magic healers say they learnt this craft from other hill tribes or the Thai and Laos.

15. See also Chapter 9 on beliefs about breast milk among the Hmong.
16. He showed me his thumb to verify his claim. It is true that there was no scar, as he claimed.
17. Hmong women themselves actually said that only men are able to learn the art of magic healing, because women are not smart enough to learn difficult tasks involved in *khawv koob*.

Part Two

Women and Childbearing

Chapter 4

Conception and Pregnancy

INTRODUCTION

> Because pregnancy did not signal a major change in a tribal woman's activity, there was little concern about knowing for sure if it had started. Unlike modern Western women, who rush to their doctors for a laboratory test the moment pregnancy seems evident, tribal people took the whole event quite casually. This was possible in part because they identified pregnancy in other ways. (Goldsmith, 1990: 7)

Childbirth is a universal human experience. However, the birth experience takes place in a cultural context and is shaped by the views and practices of that culture. According to Cosminsky (1982), many rituals and symbols associated with childbearing signify the transition from one stage of life to another for both mother and newborn. They, however, "reflect values and themes of the culture" (p. 205). As such, pregnancy, birth and the puerperium

> are each experienced differently in different cultures. . . . Accordingly, behavioral and dietary restrictions to prepare the woman for birth and to help her recover after it . . . the way of birthing . . . the involvement of others, the position of the parturient during labour, and the use of traditional and other medical personnel prenatally and postnatally—are all culturally determined. (Manderson and Mathews, 1981: 1)

This is also true within traditional Hmong culture. In her work on childbirth among the Hmong in Thailand, Symonds (1996) demonstrated that it exists in parallel with the Hmong cosmos and the concepts of what it means to be a man, a woman and a family in Hmong society.

Childbirth in Hmong culture is closely associated with supernatural powers. Fertility, infertility, the birth of a child and his or her survival are interconnected with nature and the supernatural. The Hmong, therefore, adhere to many cultural beliefs and practices related to the process of childbearing. These cultural beliefs and practices, as Manderson and Mathews (1981: 1) have stated, "provide the woman with a social framework within which she is able to deal with the physiological-medical and psychological-personal changes brought about by her pregnancy and delivery."

As McClain (1982) and Steinberg (1996) have pointed out, in most societies traditional childbearing beliefs and practices are changing rapidly in order to respond to larger cultural forces. What happens to Hmong women who are no longer in their cultural environment and who have been uprooted from their familiar society? Does childbirth still take place within its cultural context? This, largely, has not been documented. In this chapter, I will discuss the cultural beliefs and practices related to pregnancy. Those related to birth and the puerperium will be presented in the two chapters that follow.

BIRTH AS A RITE OF PASSAGE

Childbirth in many societies is seen as dangerous, powerful or polluting (Kitzinger, 1978). A woman is not yet a mother, yet she is clearly different from the state prior to her pregnancy. It is a time when the woman is in "a liminal state, separate from the safe categories of ordinary existence" (Homans, 1982: 254). This liminal state is referred to as "rites of passage" (Van Gennep, 1960). The theory illuminates patterns of childbearing in many traditional societies.[1]

In rites of passage, people are separated from ordinary society. This can be seen clearly in women in childbirth. In most societies, parturient women are usually separated from normal social activities. However, in most cases the separation is not physical but behavioral and dietary. This is an attempt to safeguard the woman from danger as well as to protect others around her from her liminal and polluted state of health.

In discussing birth as a rite of passage, Kitzinger (1982: 182) referred to the "transitional rites." She pointed out:

> Transitional rites define and regulate the passage from one social status to another. They guard the threshold between social categories of being. The individual on the journey between two kinds of social identity is controlled

> and protected and the behaviour of everyone involved carefully circumscribed to achieve an orderly transition.

Kitzinger (1982) contended that "transition rites consist of separation, trial and re-entry in a newly defined social state. With separation, the initiate is physically and symbolically set apart from peers and removed to a different place." Pregnancy restrictions and dietary rules can be seen as parts of rites of passage transformation. Kitzinger stated that in pregnancy, birth and the puerperium, "each culture has its own transitional ceremonies and draws its own map, as it were, of significant points and milestones to which behaviour is linked" (p. 183).

In rites of passage, Van Gennep (1960: 46) also pointed out that the social component of childbirth is more important than the physiological aspect:

> It is apparent that the physiological return from childbirth is not the primary consideration, but that instead there is a social return from childbirth, just as there is a social parenthood which is distinct from sexual union.

In this sense, as Kitzinger (1982: 182) remarked, if we see childbirth "as a rite of passage, the patterns of interaction between individuals and social groups comes clearly into focus." I contend that this may also hold true for Hmong childbearing.

In this chapter and the two that follow, the examination of Hmong childbearing will be based on the rite of passage theory as proposed by Van Gennep (1960).[2]

CONCEPTION: WHERE IS THE BABY FROM?

At one level, Hmong women believe that for conception to occur there must be *lub qe* (the egg) of a woman and *tus qab* (the seed) of a man. The egg and the seed must meet for a baby to be conceived. The meeting of these two components occurs during sexual intercourse. However, conception will occur only when the egg and the seed are of equal strength. If the egg is stronger than the seed, it will eat the seed and, hence, there will be no conception. The egg will eventually dissolve and leave the woman's body as menstruation.

At another level, however, Hmong women believe that conception cannot occur solely because of a meeting between a woman's egg and a man's seed. Conception can only take place when *Txoov Kab Yeeb*, the spirit parents, give permission to a soul awaiting rebirth to be born from a woman who has the right to be a mother, and this is indicated on a piece of paper (mandate of life) that she brings with her upon her birth.[3]

> I think that if you have no husband, you would not have any children. But I also think that it must be from heaven as well for you to be able to have children.

Conception, in Hmong women's views, thus involves more than biological components of men and women. It is connected to the spiritual world, as are other aspects of the Hmong world view.

SIGNS OF PREGNANCY

> In your heart, you know that for two months you do not bleed then you are pregnant.

A common sign of pregnancy for some women is missing their period. However, the pregnancy will not be confirmed until they start to have other symptoms, such as tiredness, morning sickness, and an aversion to certain foodstuffs.

> I don't know really, but when you miss a period and you get tired and feel like you don't want to eat some things like spring onion or chilli or any sort of sour spicy food, then you will realize that you are pregnant.

Several women mentioned that they did not know about their pregnancy until they started to feel pain in their abdomen or the movement of the baby. This was because they had breastfed their older children and had not resumed menstruation at all after the last birth.

> All of my children, when I became pregnant, I didn't know that. . . . I didn't have menses because I breastfed my children. . . . Only when I began to have stomach pain and could feel the baby move then I knew that I was pregnant. I had no sign of pregnancy like tiredness or vomit, so I didn't know.

Craving is believed to be a common sign of pregnancy.

> As a woman if you have a husband and you miss your period and after that you start to get tired and have cravings, then you must be pregnant.

Nevertheless, having certain dreams is commonly seen as a sign of pregnancy. Many women mentioned that they knew about their pregnancies prior to the missing of their period because of their dreams. Others said they would dream after their period had stopped and that this dream was a definite sign of pregnancy. In addition, most women stated that different dreams could tell them about the sex of their babies.

> Yes, I did dream of things. I don't know about other people but for me I would dream. If a boy, I mean before I conceived, I would dream of finding or stealing a gun, a knife and running into snakes and they bit me. This would be a couple of days before my period stopped. Then after that period I would not have any more period and I was pregnant. This would be a boy. If it was a girl, then I dreamt of finding embroidery needles and picking cucumbers. . . . Different sexes have different dreams.

Another woman told me:

> When I have not conceived I do not dream of anything but after I conceive I do dream. When I was pregnant, . . . if it was a girl then I would get cucumbers or pumpkin, that sort of things; if it was a boy then knives, bows and arrows and any sort of thing that symbolizes the male sex. But I don't dream of these things before I get pregnant. . . . Yes, I dream like these; for all my sons I would see knives.

It is interesting that one woman who had difficulty conceiving after giving birth to her first child mentioned that she had dreams like other Hmong women but she dreamt something else:

> For women who are very good at conceiving they dream of seeing knives, guns, snake bites and melons or pumpkins. For me, the reason why I could not get pregnant easily is because if I see a melon than I eat it and if I see snake and it is going to bite me then I kill it. So that is why I haven't got any more children. The old people say that this is because I don't have any baby spirits and that is why when I dream of it I eat it or kill it.

And this is why, in her belief, she had not been able to conceive another child.

DIETARY PRECAUTIONS

The Hmong do not practice dietary restrictions during pregnancy. Women said that they continued to eat normal food throughout their pregnancy, although some women who experienced morning sickness might not have liked eating certain foods.

> When you are pregnant and you like to eat it then you can eat anything you like. If you hate that food and cannot eat it, like if you eat it or smell it then you will vomit then this is the only time you will not eat certain food.

However, women are prohibited from taking Western medicines during pregnancy since this can cause miscarriage.

> If you are pregnant you can eat anything. Only you should not take any medicine that can harm the baby . . . those medicines, western medicines . . . for fever and for infected spleen. . . . If you take these medicines early in the pregnancy, the baby will miscarry.

Although the Hmong do not have dietary precautions, they do take cravings seriously. It is believed that when a mother craves certain foodstuffs, it is the baby who wishes to eat, not the mother. Hence, her craving must be fulfilled lest some physical abnormalities appear on the baby upon birth.[4]

> The old people say that it is the baby's craving. If you don't eat then it will make the baby abnormal. When you give birth, there will be something physically wrong to tell you that you have craved for that thing and you didn't eat it. . . . Like, if she has a baby and about three to four months she is very tired and she craves for ginger and if she doesn't eat it then when the baby is born then he will have an extra digit on hands and a growth on the ear.

More importantly, craving needs to be fulfilled so that the baby may grow well.

> If you are pregnant then whatever you crave you should eat so that the baby will grow well. . . . If you crave meat or chicken or pork then you need to eat them. If you crave sour fruits then you should eat them. . . . If not it might contribute to the growth of the baby; the baby will not grow well if you don't eat them.

On the other hand, hating food during pregnancy is also seen as the wish of the baby inside the womb.

> If I do crave then I must be able to eat it so that the baby does not have any growth on his hands or feet or anything like that. For anything that I don't want to eat then it means that the baby doesn't want to eat. If the baby wants to eat it then you need to eat it.

ACTIVITIES AND PRECAUTIONS

Traditionally, Hmong women continue their daily routine and work on the farm throughout pregnancy. However, women do take some precautions to prevent complications. These precautions function largely to prevent miscarriages and stillbirths.[5] For example, women believe they should not work too hard or carry heavy loads, since these activities may disconnect the placenta and, hence, cause miscarriage. Similarly, women are warned not to reach up high or take a big jump lest miscarriage occur.

> In Laos even if you stay at home you cannot take it easy that much. Even if you have older children [to help] you would still do the chores and work on farm except that you should not lift anything that is heavy or reach too high so that it does not cause the baby to fall down [miscarry].

Another woman explained similarly.

> Hmong people, when they are pregnant they do not stop doing anything. . . . But you should not carry heavy things. If you do heavy things then it will distress the baby and then it becomes very difficult. . . . If the baby is distressed then you will get pain, pain in the stomach and sore back, and it may mean that you can't feel the baby move anymore.

More importantly, women are warned not to cross a river, a low valley or wander into uninhabited areas since they may be struck by evil spirits which in turn will make them miscarry.

> When you are pregnant you have to be careful, like if you are pregnant then you better avoid going to the lowland areas, where there is a landslide, and rock caves on mountains. . . . If you go you will be hit [by spirits].

And another woman explained:

> For Hmong people, for our tradition, when you are pregnant, the old people say that you should not go across a low valley where it is muddy and a swamp. If you do that the baby will miscarry . . . because you will be hit by spirits . . . so you do not do that.

Although carrying on their daily routines, women mentioned that they were particularly careful about their activities. The most common concern was making sure not to fall over. Falling over can distress the baby and may lead to miscarriage.

> With work, the Hmong go to work on the farm. As soon as you have breakfast then you carry the back-basket and to the farm. Nothing is wrong with that. But then you have to avoid falling over. If you fall over then the baby will be disconnected with the food supply and the baby will not grow and so the baby will miscarry. . . . You have to watch your step and not to step on anything that is slippery. You have to step somewhere that is not slippery so you will not fall.

The fall also causes the baby to turn into a wrong position. The Hmong believe that a baby stays in an upright position from early pregnancy until late pregnancy, when it will turn upside down. If a mother falls in early pregnancy, the baby will turn upside down. This is referred to as "the turned liver and kidney," which means that the baby's internal organs, such as the liver and kidneys, will collapse. This will make the baby lose its appetite and, hence, it will not grow properly.

Pregnant women are prohibited from entering the home of a new mother during her confinement period (the first 30 days after birth).[6] It is commonly believed that a pregnant woman will cause the cessation of breast milk of the new mother. This is seen as a serious matter, since the newborn infant may not receive enough breast milk for his or her growth. Since the Hmong traditionally do not have access to infant formula, this can greatly jeopardize the infant's health. This prohibition extends to the husband of the pregnant woman as well. Therefore, pregnant women and their husbands are extremely cautious about entering a new mother's home in the first 30 days after birth.

The Hmong do not practice sexual abstinence during pregnancy. It is believed that sex during pregnancy has no impact on the baby, and women continue to have sex throughout their terms. However, sexual intercourse is strongly prohibited during the confinement period.[7]

> When you are pregnant and you sleep with a man [husband], there is no problem with that. We can have it throughout pregnancy.

In their new home, there is no river to cross, as in Laos. However, women continue doing their daily chores throughout their pregnancies and take special care not to lift heavy loads, reach up high or fall over. They still strongly believe that these acts could cause complications in pregnancy.

ACTIVITIES FOR EASY BIRTH

Hmong women are taught by their mothers-in-law and mothers not to lie down or sit down too much during pregnancy. This is believed to make the baby's head big and round, which makes birth difficult.

> You have to walk around and not sleep or sit down too much. If you do so it will make the baby's head too big and round, making birth difficult. . . . So you have to walk around so that the baby's head will be long and skinny, and this makes birth easy for you.

Another woman related:

> In our country, the old people say that you should not sit down or lie down too much. If you lie down and sit down too much then the baby is too big and the birth is going to be very difficult . . . so you keep doing the work and go to the farm every day.

In late pregnancy in particular, lying down or sitting down too much may prevent the baby from descending downward, leading to a difficult birth.

> If you lie down too much and you sit down too much then you will have a harder birth because it makes the baby stay up very high here. . . . It is like the baby come up here [chest] instead of going down there [cervix].

Because of this belief, Hmong women are told to continue working throughout pregnancy. However, women are warned not to carry a heavy load in late pregnancy, since this can make the baby turn into a wrong position and hence make birth difficult.

SUPPORT DURING PREGNANCY

Hmong women continue their daily chores and work on their farms throughout pregnancy. Because pregnancy is seen as a natural part of childbearing, women do not receive any extra help from others unless there are complications such as bleeding and illness.

> There is no one to help me. If you are tired you have to go and do it. There is no one to help you. With housework it is all yours, with the farm it is all yours, and with the livestock it is all your duty to do them all. My husband was in the army so all the work was basically all mine. On a hard day work from the farm you still have to clean the house, you have to feed the animals. That is the way it was. . . . You never stop, you keep on working on the farm and only come home when the pain starts and you will be giving birth later on that day. There is nothing wrong with that. You don't need to stop. There isn't day that you can stop.

In addition, as all women and men have their tasks to perform, it is difficult to lend a hand to those who may need help during pregnancy. Therefore, during pregnancy women do not have an opportunity to rest as during confinement.

> When you are pregnant you do it [chores] all like you have always been doing right up to when you labor starts. . . . For every Hmong woman this is the same . . . if you don't do it, there isn't anyone to do it for you. So you have to do it, but you just don't do heavy things. You do this right

> until you start your labor pain and then give birth. After that you can rest for one month, and when that is over then you start it again.

However, life in Australia is not as hard as life in Laos or in Thailand. Most women do have their extended family near by to help during pregnancy if needed. However, most women mentioned that there was not much to do in Australia and, therefore, help during pregnancy was not that necessary.

> There is not much to do here so if there isn't any one to help it is okay. Living in this country is easier than living in Laos, so you don't really need anyone.

SEEKING HEALING AND PREGNANCY: THE HEALERS

> When you are pregnant and if you have pain then a shaman will *ua neeb* to see what the problem is, and you also go to see a medicine woman who will help by using their hands to *theev* [manipulate] to help the baby inside and they will also make herbal medicines for you to take so that you will get better.

When complications occur during pregnancy, particularly when a woman feels tired or ill, when the baby does not grow properly, when the baby ceases movement or when bleeding occurs, Hmong women and their families seek help from several traditional healers. These are discussed in this section.

Hmong Herbal Medicines and a Medicine Woman

Hmong herbs are used only when there is a problem in pregnancy.

> Hmong herbal medicine can only be used when you have a particular type of sickness which is suited to that particular type of medicine. So even if you are pregnant but if you are not sick then you do not use the medicine. . . . I didn't use any since my pregnancies were good. . . . But there are medicines for the pregnant women such as medicines for the baby to be strong so that the mother will not become too tired.

Herbal medicines are used particularly when the mother feels very tired.

> If you are pregnant and you get tired then you can use Hmong medicines to steam with egg to eat. . . . The old people say you have to take it for three times and if you do not feel tired after that then you do not need it anymore. . . . The purpose of the medicine is to bring the baby to life [give the baby strength] so you have to eat it when the baby is still very small

> and when you feel tired. . . . It is for the baby to have life and so that you will not feel very tired.

Hmong herbs are also used when the baby does not grow properly or does not move much.

> When you have a baby in your stomach and if you have no problems then the baby will move at about two months. If the baby is three or four months and does not move then the baby is not very strong . . . so you have to use Hmong medicines to cook with egg and you make it like soup or you can make it dry [steam]. . . . Sometimes you have to take it three or four times and if the baby moves, then you stop, but if it doesn't, then you take some more till the baby moves.

Since most people do not have a good knowledge of herbs, they need to obtain them from a medicine woman.

> In Laos, I was a medicine woman and if women were pregnant, at about three months or so, they would become very tired and they would come to me and ask me to help give some medicines. If I had them then I would give them some. They would ask me like to help give some medicines so that the baby would grow and when it was time [to give birth] then they just gave birth.

The medicine woman will prepare herbs and instruct the woman in how to take them. Usually each herb, with its own healing property, will be boiled or steamed with eggs. In addition, herbs can be boiled and drunk as tea. The herb needs to be taken for at least three mornings. However, some women who are often ill may have to take them until they give birth.

> I have used them in early pregnancy. There are some herbal medicines used with eggs to make the baby grow well and the mother not too tired or become sick. . . . If you are healthy then you take the herb only three times. If you often get sick, then you take it many times even till you give birth.

Some medicine women can also manipulate (*theev*) the woman's abdomen if she falls and the baby turns into a wrong position and/or bleeding follows. The Hmong believe that in early pregnancy the baby lies in an upright position so as to grow properly. If any accident occurs, it will make the baby turn upside down. In such a case, the baby will be unable to grow properly, because the baby's internal organs (liver and kidneys) collapse (see earlier section also). A manipulation by slightly twisting the abdomen is needed in order to turn the baby back to its normal position. *Theev* can also be performed by an old lady who is knowledgeable about birthing techniques.[8]

Shamanism

The Hmong seek help from a shaman during pregnancy to prevent any complications that may occur. A shaman will perform at least three *ua neeb*. The first *ua neeb* is performed at one month to receive the soul of the baby. The second *ua neeb* is done at six months to see if the soul of the child has come to the parent's house. The last *ua neeb* is done near the due date to separate the "life aura" (a metaphysical explanation of the essence of life) of the mother from the baby as well as to make their life auras equal in strength.[9] The Hmong believe that if the life aura of the mother is stronger than that of the baby, the baby will die at birth and vice versa. Hence, it is most important to separate the life auras prior to birth.

> A shaman plays a big role in pregnancy . . . to receive the soul from heaven, to see if it has come to reside in the house of the parents, and to see if the life auras of the mother and the child are equal, if not then to divide them equally.

Ua neeb is also performed if the mother has abdominal pain or bleeds during pregnancy, since it is believed that in such cases the mother has been struck by evil spirits and miscarriage may ensue. *Ua neeb* will help to separate the spirits from the woman's body. A shaman explained about one woman that she had helped:

> She has pain in her stomach she need to come to have *ua neeb*. You *ua neeb* to help her to get better. You will *ua neeb* to remove the spirit from the pregnant woman.

During pregnancy, a woman may become tired or ill because her soul has escaped from her body. When this happens, a shaman must perform *ua neeb* to call her soul back, so that she will be healthy and able to carry the baby to term.

> When the mother is pregnant and she is unhealthy then she will ask me to do *ua neeb*, so I will do it to bring the soul home. . . . This is for a woman who has lost her appetite, she won't want to eat anything so she is very skinny, and so the baby inside the womb is not growing well.

CONCLUSION

Pregnancy in Hmong culture is perceived as a natural process in which minimum precautions are taken, and one requiring few changes in a woman's daily life. This contrasts greatly with the puerperium period. Women continue to perform their daily routines until labor begins. This pattern is similar to that of women in most traditional societies, as Goldsmith (1990: 5) has pointed out: "Pregnancy does not signal an abrupt change for women in tribal societies. They take it in their stride, going on with their everyday activities even to the last moments before birth." This, as Vincent Priya (1992) and Laderman (1983) have stated, is to ensure that women will have an easy labor and birth. As discussed, Hmong women provide similar evidence. They continue normal work and fully expect to have a trouble-free pregnancy and an easy birth.

Despite the fact that pregnancy is a normal condition, it is also a "period of special vulnerability for the both the mother and her unborn child" (Vincent Priya, 1992: 22). Hmong women take special care with their pregnancy as soon as it is confirmed. For example, they avoid heavy lifting and performing rigorous activities, they do not go into uninhabited areas for fear of evil spirits, and they fulfill their cravings and undergo shamanic rituals to prevent any complication that may occur. Women are concerned with how they may protect their unborn child from harmful influences. To do this successfully, women, according to Vincent Priya (1992: 23), need to "pay attention to emotional, social and spiritual as well as physical needs." Manderson and Mathews's work with Vietnamese women in Australia more than a decade ago (1981: 6) has shown that women strictly observed dietary and behavioral precautions in order to "guarantee a successful pregnancy." Hmong women are no exceptions.

Why do Hmong women take special care with their pregnancies? This needs to be examined within the context of Hmong society. Becoming pregnant is important for Hmong women. First, pregnancy signifies the ability to procreate; in other words, that a woman is fertile and able to bring new lives to extend the Hmong society. Being able to carry the baby to term and give birth to a healthy child is even more important. It means that a woman can ensure that there will be another member added to the family and the society. Children are important to the Hmong, because children will continue their traditions and look after them in old age. As Raphael-Leff (1991: 5) has pointed out, procreation, for society, means survival. In any society, "if women cease to become pregnant that society would die out." In the Hmong society, children are also needed so that society will continue its existence. However, children are significantly more important for women than for men. As Vincent Priya (1992: 15) has pointed out, in many cultures "pregnancy and birth are the primary arenas in which women have status and prestige which is denied to them in the society as a whole." Hmong women are no exceptions. Their status increases markedly when they become pregnant and give birth to their first child.

It is interesting to note that a pregnant woman is not only in a vulnerable state, but that she is also a source of danger to others, particularly to a new mother and her newborn infant. Cosminsky (1982) has speculated that this may be due to her "heated state," which might inflict ill health upon a newborn infant. However, the prohibition against visiting a new mother and child may be interpreted as a restriction placed on the pregnant woman to compell her to restrict her mobility in order to prevent any complications that might compromise her ability to carry to term. This is another means by which the Hmong ensure that there will be another baby added to the society.

Although pregnancy is seen as a natural process and, in general, women do not receive much assistance from their family members, they do get help when needs arise. For example, when complications such as bleeding occur, medicine women and shamans will be summoned to help the woman, so that the family can ensure that the pregnancy will not be threatened and the woman will be able to carry her pregnancy to term. This, again, is a means of ensuring that there will be another person added to the family and the society can be replenished. This is important for Hmong society, in which many lives have been lost due to Hmong involvement in the wars in China, Laos and the ensuing displacements. It is crucially important for the Hmong today, who are trying to establish themselves in new countries.

It is interesting that Hmong women do not see morning sickness as a symptom of pregnancy, and yet cravings are taken quite seriously. As Goldsmith (1990: 11) has pointed out, in many traditional societies a pregnant woman's wishes for certain foods are "treated sympathetically and carefully indulged." The Hmong are no exceptions. Women who crave certain foods are given what they wish, as cravings are seen as the wish of the unborn infant. Although these foods provide important nutrients for the growing baby, women receive a good share of them too. The Hmong live in high, mountainous areas where food is not always readily available. Hmong women have to share food with the whole family. When food is in short supply, pregnant women may not receive enough essential nutrients. The satisfying of cravings ensures that pregnant women receive good nutrition during pregnancy (McGilvray, 1982). Vincent Priya (1992: 38) has provided a succinct explanation for this:

> [Cravings] have the social effect of setting the woman apart from other non-pregnant women and emphasizing her condition. As she is encouraged to ask for what she wants, the pregnant woman has the opportunity

> to get more of what she likes and wants than she probably does normally. In many places women are the least well-nourished members of the society; they are responsible for feeding everyone else and must go short themselves if there is too little food to go around. Often pregnancy is the only time when a woman may have the chance to indulge herself and whatever the other restrictions, pregnancy can be a time of comfort and privilege with extra care and attention from relatives as well as whatever extra food she feels she wants.

Up to now, the discussions provided in this chapter point to the need to see pregnancy as a rite of passage, as proposed in the earlier section. Pregnancy is seen as a transitional state, during which a pregnant woman is not yet a mother but is clearly different from other women. Her behavior and diet are set apart from those in everyday life and from other members of the society. These behavioral and dietary distinctions function to protect her from danger, giving her the best possible chance to carry her pregnancy to term.

Hmong women, like many other women in traditional societies, see pregnancy as a normal condition and healthy state of life. Hmong women take responsibility for the health of their unborn child as well as their own health during pregnancy. However, they are not alone. They receive assistance when needs arise. This will, however, change to some extent when they move to a new society in which pregnancy is seen as a pathology requiring medical care (Rothman, 1991), and pregnant women are encouraged to rely on medically qualified professionals during pregnancy (Vincent Priya, 1992). As I will illustrate in Chapter 7, many Hmong women observe the rules of their new home, but some women resist, because their system of pregnancy and birth places an emphasis on a woman's own instinct and autonomy over her pregnancy rather than reliance on experts.

Nevertheless, beliefs and practices related to the pregnancy of Hmong women are in contrast with those promoted in the midwifery training programs that are based on the biomedical model of birth (Cosminsky, 1982). It is, therefore, important to view many practices discussed in this chapter within the context of Hmong lives and traditions. This will prevent misunderstandings and avoid a "victim-blaming" approach, and consequently, more sensitive pregnancy care for immigrant women can be achieved.

NOTES

1. See Holm and Bowker (1994) for rituals associated with rites of passage in different religious including Buddhism, Christianity, Hinduism, Islam, Judaism, Sikhism, Chinese and Japanese religions.

2. See also Romalis (1981) for rites of passage of birth in the United States for comparison.

3. See also Chapters 1 and 11 in this volume about the influence of *Txoov Kab Yeeb* in women's fertility. Similar accounts among Hmong women in northern Thailand have also been discussed by Symonds (1991, 1996).

4. Laderman (1983) has pointed out that women in many Southeast Asian cultures tend to have cravings during pregnancy. In the Philippines, for example, unsatisfied cravings are believed to cause miscarriage or deformity of the baby. In Thai culture, a craving mother will drool uncontrollably. In Trengganu, it is believed that it is the baby who craves the food, not the mother. See also Hart et al. (1965) for food cravings during pregnancy in Southeast Asia.

5. See also Chapters 11 and 12 for more details on miscarriage and infant death in Hmong culture.

6. See also Chapter 6 on Hmong confinement and Chapter 9 on beliefs about breast milk in Hmong culture.

7. See Chapter 6 on Hmong confinement in this volume.

8. Her tasks are discussed in greater detail in Chapter 5, on Hmong birth.

9. See also Chapter 11 on the life aura and miscarriage.

Chapter 5

Birth

INTRODUCTION

> And when the baby had arrived on earth, then the midwife shouted; she gave war cries, which meant that the little woman had fought a good battle, had become a brave warrior, had taken a captive, had captured a baby. (Sahagun: cited in McClain, 1991: 1)

> Birth, like death, is universal, but the way that it is experienced, interpreted and explained is not. The physical process is similar for everyone, but an individual's experience, how a woman interprets the meaning of the events for herself and explains what is happening within her, varies widely. (Vincent Priya, 1990: 5)

In this chapter, I will first discuss traditional beliefs and practices related to birth. I will also look at patterns in the Hmong community which have changed in response to the new living situation in Australia.

WHEN THE LABOR BEGINS

Hmong women continue to perform their daily chores until their labor begins. The most common signs of labor are stomach sickness or pains (referred to as *mob plab* in Hmong).

> Oh! With a baby when it is the time you will have stomach pain. If you start to have stomach pain then you know that it is the time for the baby to be born.

A similar explanation was given by another woman:

> You always out there doing farming so when you start to feel sick in the stomach or when you start to have stomach pain then you know it is a time for the baby then you just come home to give birth.

In contrast to pregnancy, when women are told not to sit down or lie down too much for fear of having a difficult birth, Hmong women are instructed not to move around too much when labor begins, since movement may make the baby turn into the wrong position.

> When you start to have the contractions, the mother-in-law and your parents will come to see you and tell you not to move around too much, just sit there [on the stool] because the baby might turn.

THE BIRTH

The Hmong see birth as women's business. Those who may be present at birth must be women. The only man allowed at a birth is the woman's husband. For their first birth, all Hmong women said they were assisted by their mothers-in-law. Some women who had had difficult births also received assistance from an elderly woman who had good experience in childbirth.

> With some women experiencing difficult labor, there have to be one or two women present as well as the husband and mother-in-law. One of the women will hold the mother and the other to deliver the baby. So there is more than one person present at birth. Sometimes the husband will deliver the baby while both of the women hold on to the mother if it is a long labor.

Hmong husbands are usually with their wives if they are around at the time of birth.[1] Men who have fathered several children may assist at a difficult birth by holding the woman's body to assist in pushing for example. They may also cut the umbilical cord. These men bear the main responsibility for burying the afterbirth and the placenta, washing the newborn infant and preparing the confinement period for their wives.[2] However, most Hmong women said that inexperienced husbands (e.g., first births and young husbands) might only observe the birth from a corner of the room. They do not know what to do. As one woman related:

> There are old people around and then when it is time then your mother, your mother-in-law and also the older relatives will help. My husband, he doesn't know anything. So when your pain starts then you call those old people and when the baby is born they will pick up the baby and cut the cord. All the husband does is watch because he doesn't know about birth. It has to be the elderly ladies who know about it.

Another stated similarly:

> My sister-in-law and my mother helped to deliver the baby. My husband was there but he did not know how to deliver the baby. Even if he was not there. If your husband is busy or he has gone somewhere but if you have a sister-in-law or an elderly there it was ok. If he was there he wouldn't know what to do anyway. If it was a mature male member of the household like my brother-in-law then he would know what to do. But if it is the young ones like my husband he would not know.

With subsequent births, most Hmong women mentioned that they gave birth by themselves, particularly if their husbands were not in the village. However, most women said they were embarrassed if their husbands were too close to them at birth. Unless the labor was difficult, they preferred to give birth alone, although their husbands might be with them in the birth room. Their husbands would do the rest after they had given birth to the newborn.

> Hmong people are very shy people. When they go into labor they sit by themselves and when the baby has already been delivered then the husband will come to take the baby. The husband does not sit there with you and help you giving birth. Only in some cases when the mother is having a difficult labor then the husband will play that supportive role, otherwise he will just sit at a distance and look at you. If he wants to help then there is nothing to stop him.

Several women in this study said that their husbands were very active at birth. These husbands were seen as caring husbands who would do everything to help their wives give birth safely. One woman elaborated:

> I don't know about those husbands that do not really worry about their wives. Some say that it is only just giving birth. They don't know how to worry so they don't come to support. But mine, he is very worried about the baby and me, and when I am nearly termed he will *ua neeb* to help me. If I have pain then he will always be there with me to see what is going on. If I am in a lot of pain then he will *fiv kab yeeb* [requesting help from the parent spirits] and house spirits and if this doesn't work he will *fiv yeem ntuj* [the sky spirit] to help.

It is important to note that only old women are allowed to check the woman's body and check the vagina when it is absolutely necessary, such as when the labor is prolonged and in breech birth. No young women or men at all are allowed to look at the mother in this way.

> If the birth has been a prolonged one and it is a breech delivery and the mother is in a lot of pain then only the older people will look but no young ones or men can have a look. Only very old women can look at them.

BIRTH POSITION

Hmong women traditionally give birth in a kneeling position.[3] Women give birth on the floor, on which soft cloths or rags are laid. A small stool is placed on the floor, and the woman sits on the stool while resting between each contraction. When she feels the urge to push she will then kneel on the cloth to give birth.

> When the baby is coming out, your body feels different. It makes you shiver and there is an urge to push. When the baby is nearly out you have to kneel . . . then the baby will fall in your arms. . . . In our country we all do this. It is very different from this country; you have to lie down.

Hmong women believe this kneeling position will make birth easier. As one woman related:

> When we start to have the contraction the old people never let us lie down. We have to sit down and kneel to give birth. Sitting to give birth is easier, the old people say. When you give birth and if you do not lie down then you are not obstructing the baby from coming out so you can give birth easier. So when the contraction becomes painful the old people will say to sit down. This is what we do. They say not to lie down; lying down makes giving birth harder.

In addition, women believe that giving birth in a sitting position is not as "dirty" as lying down, since the blood runs down onto the floor.

> If you give birth by sitting on the floor it is much easier and better because after birth you are not dirtied with the blood. But if you lie down to give birth, it is very yucky because the blood will soak on your clothes.

PLACE OF BIRTH

Traditional Hmong birth takes place in the husband's home. It is prohibited for Hmong women to give birth in their natal home, since it will weaken their natal clan's spirits (*dab qhuas*). This is considered a serious matter in the Hmong culture. To weaken the clan spirit will lead to misfortune and illness. Therefore, all Hmong births must take place outside the women's natal homes.

> Hmong women cannot give birth in your mother's home. . . . You are born as a daughter who will live outside your parents' home. So when you go out [to marry] then you will have a different *dab qhuas* from your parents so you can't give birth inside your parents' home. . . . If you do it, your parents will die and their livestock will be no good. . . . Your mum and dad will have a different *dab qhuas* to you and if you have the baby inside their house, then your wrongdoing will haunt their *dab qhuas* and these *dab qhuas* do not like you. They don't like you so they will go away from your parents' home. Then your parents are open to all sorts of health risk.

A woman who becomes pregnant out of wedlock will be given a shelter outside her parents' home when giving birth. She must remain in the shelter until confinement is finished (a month later) before she can move back into her parents' home.[4]

When Hmong women stayed in a refugee camp in northern Thailand, most of them continued to have home births. Only one woman who had a long labor gave birth in the hospital in the camp. Common reasons given were similar to the following quotes:

> I had my baby at home in the camp because there were too many people but limited hospital beds, which were not enough for everyone. Some people did not want to give birth in the hospital and they would only go if it was a difficult labor. Otherwise, giving birth at home was much preferred.

> We traditionally give birth at home. That is how we have given birth and if you have a difficult labor or the labor is prolonged then people will take you to hospital. If you can give birth on your own then you just give birth at home.

PREMATURE BIRTH

Premature birth is seen as being caused by spirits. For a normal birth, the baby must come when it is time to come. The Hmong say that a full-term baby must be in the mother's womb for 9 months. However, the Hmong recognize that some babies may come at 7 months, and this is seen as normal. The baby will survive because it knows how to suck milk from its mother. However, a child born at eight months may not survive. There is no specific explanation for this phenomenon apart from the fact the baby will not grow.

> There are children born at seven months and they do have the ability to drink milk so you don't need to help them. The ones that are born at eight months you cannot help them. . . . They won't grow so you don't know how to help them.

Babies who come before 7 months are believed to be the work of spirits.[5] As one woman explained:

> If it is not time [for the baby to be born] yet and the mother is going into labor then it would have to be caused by the spirits. In this case you have to *ua neeb* to help so that the spirits will not come close to her and this will stop the labor until it is termed.

For the Hmong, spirits are everywhere. Therefore, it is very easy for people to be "hit" by them. Sometimes, this happens because pregnant women are merely on their path.

> The spirits, you can easily get hit. When you go across their path when they wake up, you might just bump into their path or touch them by accident. . . . You can't see them, but because everyone lives amongst each other [including the spirits] you can just bump into them or touch them. . . . That is when you get hit.

DIFFICULT BIRTH: WOMEN'S PERCEPTIONS AND EXPERIENCES

Most Hmong women in this study had easy births, with the exception of two women—a mother who experienced placenta previa in late pregnancy, and another whose baby was in a transverse line (these two women had caesarean births). When asked what contributed to their easy births, Hmong women explained that it was largely due to continuing to work throughout their pregnancy, which their living conditions required.[6]

> In our country the majority of women have easy births. There is only a few that experience hard labor. . . . I feel that because we are farmers, we go to the farm, crush the rice and so on. This makes the baby not too big and the head not too big. Therefore, we have easy births.

One woman, when asked if she did anything to make her births easier, said:

> I did not do anything to prepare for easy birth. I do walk but I always walk when I do my work. We believe that if you are pregnant and you do

your work as usual it will make the baby not too big so when you give birth it is easier.

Another woman described her easy births as follows:

For me so I didn't have difficult labor. Other people, some do have difficult labor and some very easy. But for me, all of my children were fairly easy, none were difficult and demanded a lot of people to come over and help me giving birth. It would only be my husband and me. . . . We Hmong are farmers and we would go every day to our farms. At the end of the day we would rest and late at night my contractions would start and for a little while then I gave birth. . . . It wasn't long at all; one hour at the longest, but sometimes not even one hour for all my children. . . . Yes, it was painful but this would go on for a little while and then the baby would come.

Difficult and long births do occur. When this happens, the Hmong are greatly concerned for the well-being of the mother and the newborn baby, as they may not survive.

If the birth is difficult then sometimes the woman cannot be helped. Sometimes you may lose the mother when you have the baby or lose the baby and only have the mother. It is very difficult for Hmong people. . . . Some women have a long labor and they will die. . . . In the Hmong village if the labor was difficult then you would worry a lot.

The Hmong have several explanations for difficult labor. These are discussed in the following subsections.

Accident

A woman may have a fall in late pregnancy, causing the baby to turn into the wrong position. When this occurs, the baby needs to be turned by a medicine woman or an old lady. One woman related her experience:

When the baby is nearly due and the mother has a fall, this causes the baby to go into the wrong position. Then that is when you need an old lady who is very experienced in turning the baby to come to help turn it. She will need to turn the baby so the baby will be born. . . . All my children were easy except the first one that I fell over and the baby turned into the wrong position. . . . I was in pain for seven days with my first child and the baby still didn't come out so we went to ask Aunt "C" to come and turn the baby before I could give birth. . . . I nearly died. After that birth I could not walk for three days.

Women's Behavior and Difficult Birth

Another reason commonly given to explain a difficult birth is that the woman may have committed bad acts, such as saying bad words, being rude and not paying respect to her parents or to other older people. A difficult birth is therefore seen as a "curse" on the woman. A breech birth in particular is seen as the baby begging the heaven for forgiveness for the mother because of her bad actions.

> For women who have a breech birth, the old people say that these women have said bad things to their parents and any other person older than they are. It is a curse to them. . . . Some people say that if the hands and legs come out first then that means that the baby is begging heaven because the mother has done bad things. . . . The baby is begging for the mother's sins. She swears at them, yells at them and says very bad things to them . . . so when she has a baby this is what happens to her.

The Hmong believe that any bad actions the mother has done must be paid for with the baby's life. This has led Hmong women to behave respectfully toward their parents and the elderly. In the Hmong culture, respect for the elderly is extremely important.

> Yes, Hmong people, if they are the older one, if they are your parents then they are regarded as your world. If they are the older ones then you have to regard them as your parents. So you have to respect them and if you follow our rules you will have a good life. . . . In your clan, if they are older and you are the younger one then you must not say anything that is unacceptable by them. Whether they are your aunt or uncle or your parents, you must not say anything unacceptable to them.

A woman's bad behavior toward her husband can also contribute to a difficult birth. This is particularly true for women who have a "bad heart" toward their husbands or those who hide things from their husbands.

> She has a bad heart toward her husband. Like she does very bad things to him and she hides things from him. When she gives birth she is cursed and has difficulty in giving birth. Because the husband is the one who is on top [the head of the family] so you must respect his status. If the woman has a bad heart toward her husband then she will be cursed.

Spirits and Difficult Birth

Another cause of difficult birth is being "hit" by the spirit of wives of clan members (from the male side) who have died in childbirth due to difficult labor. A Hmong shaman explained:

> If a family member has a wife who has died in an attempt to give birth, her spirit will come to the new mother and cause the mother to have the same sort of difficulty as what has killed her.

In addition, the Hmong believe that a long and difficult labor may be caused by the presence of bad spirits from outside. Another shaman told me:

> If the baby is having difficulty to come out then this means that there is the presence of bad spirits. These bad spirits will have come to make it difficult for the baby to come out. So you have to *ua neeb* to remove them so that the baby will be able to come out.

SEEKING HEALING IN DIFFICULT BIRTH

The Hmong have several ways to help women who have difficult births. One common way is to hang a piece of rope from a post or ceiling of the house—the woman will grasp on the rope while pushing.[7]

> For women who are big and have difficult labor, a rope will be hung from the ceiling for the woman to hold on to. And there will be women to help support her underarms and there is another one to deliver the baby.

Another traditional way to help women with difficult labor, also borrowed from lowland Lao, is to open door(s) to symbolize the "opening of passage" for the baby. It is believed this will help the woman give birth more easily.

The Hmong also use magic healing (*khawv koob*) in combination with the symbolic action of opening the passage. This can be done by placing a digging instrument made of metal pipe called *taum txhob* at the door ledge, after which a magic healing is undertaken. *Taum txhob* is used symbolically to dig the ground (it only touches the ground) at the door ledge, from inside to outside the house, three times.

> If the birth is difficult then they get a metal instrument and they use that to open the door for her to give birth. . . . They bend like digging action without digging and they chant and soon after the baby is born.

The Hmong use herbal medicines to help women with a difficult birth. Usually, a medicinal drink made from green herbs is given to the woman. These herbs can be obtained from a medicine woman or another elderly woman who knows the healing property of the herbs and how to prepare the medicinal drink.

> There are herbal medicines to help someone with difficult labor. They do use herbal medicines so that she will deliver quickly. These herbal medicines can be given by anyone who knows about it; it does not need to be obtained from *kws tshuaj*.

Another common way to help a woman with a difficult birth is to seek help from a magic healer (*khawv koob*). This only occurs when nothing else will help.

> For some that have very difficult labor and their faces become pale to the extent that you begin to worry about the women's lives, then they will do *khawv koob*. My husband did this to one of my aunts. She gave birth okay after that.

Lastly, the Hmong seek help from a shaman for a difficult birth. The shaman will perform *ua neeb* to remove the spirits or ask *Txoov Kab Yeeb* (parents' spirits in the spiritual world) to help facilitate an easy birth.

> For some women who have difficult labor there will be a few people come to do *ua neeb* or *fiv yeeb* so that they can be helped to have quick delivery.
>
> There is no hospital that is close by. There is no hospital at all. All the Hmong can do is *ua neeb* to help.

Most women mentioned that they would have to do many things to help a woman in labor. Usually, a combination of tasks is undertaken, as one woman explained:

> For prolonged labor, the doors will be open and we also give her magic water and medicinal water to drink. This will make the labor a bit easier for her.

And according to another woman:

> If you have a long labor and cannot have the baby quickly then you drink herbal medicines to have a quicker birth and you can also do *khawv koob* to have a quicker birth as well. . . . If *khawv koob* is done on the baby then after you drink herbal medicines for a little while then you must give birth. A while like five minutes or so.

When a difficult birth occurs, the mother must admit that she has done bad things to her parents or the elderly and she must ask them to forgive her. The curse will then be removed and this will free the baby and the baby will live. In addition, in some cases, the woman must drink the water that has been used to wash the hands or feet of the person that she has offended. In this way, she admits she has done wrong and promises not to continue to commit such bad acts. When this is done, the baby will be born safely.[8]

> If the labor is difficult then maybe she has been uttering disrespectful words to the elders and so the elders need to come and rinse their hands for her to drink so that she can give birth. . . . She must come to beg for forgiveness from the elders. She must beg on her knees and beg them and they would say, "If your mouth has said too much and you have criticized us too much and it has cursed you then now we will rinse our hands for you so your baby must come out." They would do this, and after taking this she will give birth.

It is commonly believed that if a woman has done bad things to her parents, she will be likely to have one or two difficult births. When she recovers from a difficult birth, she must ask for forgiveness and show her respect for the elderly. Only then may she no longer experience difficult births. It is also believed that a difficult birth caused by not paying respect to the elderly cannot be helped by other means. A common story I was told is that people have attempted other healing processes such as applying herbal medicines, using magic healing and shamanic rituals, but these did not help. Only after the woman asked for forgiveness and drank the water was she able to give birth.

As a woman must do for her parents if she has displayed bad behavior, so must she ask forgiveness from her husband and drink water used to wash his feet and hands in order to recover from a difficult labor. The same woman contended:

> I have seen a woman who had difficult birth and she had to beg her husband and her husband had to get a bowl of water and wash his heels and his fingernails for her to drink. Only then she would give birth.

When all else fails, the last resort for the Hmong is to take the woman to the hospital. Apart from it not being the Hmong custom, the Hmong are reluctant to go to the hospital because of its distance and the costs associated with Western health care.

> For some women if they have a prolonged labor then you need to take them to hospital. If the placenta does not come out and it makes them very weak then you need to take them. After giving birth she is very weak and the baby is very weak then you need to take her too. This is what I have seen with other people but I have never experienced these things.

When the Hmong women were in a refugee camp in the north of Thailand, they had access to hospital birth. However, all but one gave birth at home, mainly because it was the Hmong tradition to give birth at home. In addition, the hospital is seen only as a place for very sick people. Since birth is seen as a natural process and a laboring woman is not a "sick person," it is not necessary to go. The hospital is only for women who have difficulty giving birth like the one woman in the study that had to go to the hospital:

> I gave birth in the hospital. For people who have quick birth they will just have it at home but for me I had a long labor. . . . It was not very painful, only that it took a long time . . . two days and two nights.

DANGER AND ILL HEALTH ASSOCIATED WITH BIRTH

When a woman has given birth, complications may ensue that may have an impact on the woman's health and well-being, and perhaps her life.

Obstructed Placenta

An obstructed placenta is seen as highly dangerous for a woman after giving birth, since the condition can be fatal. As one woman related:

> If the placenta does not come out then it will stop the [childbirth] blood from coming out and then you cannot live. This can make the woman die.

It is believed among the Hmong that a woman may experience obstructed placenta at birth because she has insulted the elderly people who have taken care of her, particularly her parents and parents-in-law.

Further, the Hmong believe that an obstructed placenta is caused by the spirits who capture the soul of the mother when she goes into labor. Because of the absence of her soul, her body does not function properly and this complication occurs. A shaman told me:

> Sometimes it can be caused by the spirits. They may have taken the mother's soul and hidden or taken to lock away and this is what causes the mother to have complications with her body. . . . Like when the mother goes into labor her soul has left her and not stay with her body when the baby is born. . . . When it [the soul] goes it will come across some spirits which are bad and they may imprison it. The soul is able to leave the body any time to look for food and water like a person.

There are several ways to assist with an obstructed placenta.

> Sometimes with some women after the baby is born the placenta does not come out. The elderly people will have to retract it by hand and also give her magic water and medicinal water to drink. In some cases women have

> to drink water used to wash the hand of an elderly who love her and has taken care of her and whom she has insulted.

Most Hmong women feel confident that the Hmong ways work. However, Hmong women also mentioned that if using Hmong procedures to get the placenta out proved unsuccessful, the last resort would be to take the woman to a hospital or seek help from medical doctors in lowland Lao towns.

> For the ones [women] that their placenta won't come out, they will get an old lady to shake the body to get it out. After doing that then you try *khawv koob* and herbal medicines and if it still doesn't work then you need to go to the doctors.

The Hmong women say that if it happens in Australia, the woman would be taken to a hospital immediately. Fortunately, there has been no incidence of obstructed placenta among Hmong women in Australia.

Excessive Bleeding

Similar to an obstructed placenta, excessive bleeding after delivery is believed to be dangerous. When this occurs, only a magic healer (*khawv koob*) can help.

> For women who have excessive bleeding, they become pale and they would have to be helped by magic string to stop the bleeding. . . . If it is hemorrhage, it is difficult to help. Only *khawv koob* can help her. They will use a piece of white and red strings mixed together and tie on her hand and perform *khawv koob*. . . . Only people who understand the magic words can do this.

Tear at Birth

In Hmong culture, it is believed that a tear occurs when "heaven" opens its door for a new life to emerge. It is, therefore, normal for a woman to have a tear. Since heaven opens the door, it will then close again, and this means that the tear will heal by itself. Human beings should not interfere with this process, as one woman explained:

> When you have a tear, it is said that heaven opens, heaven heals. So after you give birth then it will stick together like normal; there is nothing that is left unattached. . . . You don't do anything. Because it is like this; it stretches and tears and then the baby comes out, then it will come together again. It will heal up back to normal.

If a tear occurs at birth, Hmong women may use herbal medicines to heal the tear. As one woman explained:

> With Hmong people, if after birth there is a tear then there are herbal medicines used. We wash the tear with the boiled concoction and also crush the ingredient and place it on the area. In a few days it will heal and no longer swelling and we feel better. This means that we don't need a doctor [to sew the tear].

The herbs are applied three to four times until the tear is healed. However, some women mentioned they sometimes had to apply herbs for a longer time if the tear did not heal properly. These herbal medicines are usually grown in the woman's garden. If the woman does not have these herbs, she needs to ask for them from a medicine woman.

Afterbirth Pain

Some Hmong women experienced severe afterbirth pain, whereas others said they had only minor pain. Afterbirth pain only occurs with a subsequent birth, not usually with the first. It is believed that afterbirth pain occurs because of the nature of a woman's blood—in other words, whether she has "good" or "bad" blood.

> If your blood is good then you won't have it. But if your blood is not good then you will. . . . With the first one you usually don't get it. It will have to be after two or three births.

When this happens, there are several herbal medicines women can take to relieve the pain. The herb will be boiled and drunk as tea. In addition, the herb may be used in chicken soup for women to eat with hot rice during the confinement period. Each herb must be prepared separately and must be taken for three mornings.

CONCLUSION

In Hmong culture, birth, like pregnancy, is treated as part of the childbearing process which is a normal event in a woman's life. Despite this, birth can be a critical event that may "imperil her well-being" (Laderman, 1983: 172), and, in some cases, may end with the death of the woman and/or her newborn infant. The Hmong have established certain beliefs and practices to prevent this and to assist women who have difficulty giving birth, as has been discussed throughout this chapter.

In discussing childbirth in Malay women, Laderman (1983: 124) pointed out that childbirth is "not only a physiological event," but also "a stage in a rite of passage requiring spiritual prophylaxis and ritual expertise." This is similar to the Hmong view of birth. In a normal birth, a woman separates from others by retreating into her bedroom and giving birth with a minimum of assistance. However, in certain circumstances, such as a long and difficult labor, a woman may require not only physical support but also spiritual and ritual aid from traditional healers, and there are people around her who are prepared to give her assistance.

In most traditional societies, a laboring woman is usually assisted by other women or by birth attendants (Sargent, 1982; Goldsmith, 1990). The Hmong have a similar practice, but only with the first birth, when women are seen as not having enough experience to give birth by themselves. With subsequent normal deliveries, Hmong women attempt to give birth alone rather than expecting help from others. But should a woman require help in time of difficulty, other women and healers will immediately step in. In one sense, then, Hmong women do not give birth unassisted but rather are given autonomy to take responsibility over their own deliveries. This is in great contrast to giving birth in their new country, where they are placed in the hands of their Western health care givers, particularly obstetricians. Under these conditions, their autonomy seems to diminish (Laderman, 1983).

Goldsmith (1990: 25) has pointed out that in most traditional societies, women do not give birth among strangers. Women carry out their "intimate act" among those whom they "know well and trust." Women most often give birth with the assistance of their mothers-in-law and their husbands. Even the healers who are called in when complications occur are those whom the women know. Goldsmith (1990) has stated that familiarity with the people around them helps women in traditional societies have "a positive attitude toward the birth process." Such an outlook may assist women to give birth more easily. This argument may also be applicable to Hmong women who give birth among those whom they know well and trust, and it may explain why most of them have easy births.

Although birth is seen as a woman's affair, it is also related to the family, the community, the society and the supernatural world. This can clearly be seen in the case of a difficult birth entailing healing processes involving many people and supernatural beings. These "helpers" relieve the woman's difficulties in bringing another life into society.

It is interesting that the Hmong relate a difficult birth to a woman's behavior toward her parents or older people in the community. If she has exhibited poor behavior toward her parents or other elderly people, she will experience a difficult birth. This belief points to the importance of respect for the elders in Hmong society. The Hmong practice filial piety as it is practiced in the traditional Chinese culture, in which older people are respected and valued for their seniority and wisdom.

The Hmong do not have a written record of their history and culture, but rely mainly on oral traditions handed down by older generations. Old people are very knowledgeable about all kinds of ceremonies and rites essential to the well-being and the continuity of Hmong culture. This makes them highly valuable to the Hmong society. In addition it is parents who give life to and raise children. In return the children—particularly the sons and their wives—are expected to look after their parents in their old age. This reciprocity requires the acknowledgment of the children. Lastly, the Hmong are a patriarchal society and practice patrilocality, where by a daughter-in-law moves into her husband's home. It is usual that the husband's parents live with him. It is the tradition in this society that a mother-in-law has the right to dominate her daughter-in-law in all aspects of her life, including childbirth. Respect for elders exists to control the behavior of the younger woman, who is seen as having a lower status than the rest of the family.

Similarly, women's behavior toward their own husbands also determines the nature of their birthing. If the woman has "strayed from her prescribed feminine role" (Laderman, 1983: 151) by, for example, disobeying or attempting to dominate her husband, she may find it hard to give birth to her baby. This is similar to what Laderman (1983) has pointed out in her work on childbirth among Malay women: "Malays believe that since women are naturally passive and follow their husbands' lead, a woman who reverses her role may have difficulty in carrying out her normal womanly functions" (p. 151), in other words, giving birth. To symbolically ensure reproductive success, a woman who has treated her husband poorly must drink water that has been used to wash his hands and feet. After she drinks the treated water, "her husband's dominance is re-established and her submission to her wifely duties may facilitate delivery by placing her in her proper position as woman and wife" (p. 151). The Hmong are not exceptions. When a difficult birth occurs and the wife is accused of bad behavior toward her husband, she must drink water used to wash his hands and feet. It is believed that as soon as she has done this, she will be able to give birth. This belief is symbolic of the value of patriarchy in a male-dominant society like the Hmong.

It is clear that birth in Hmong culture has social meanings that are a part of the larger social system, which involves not only the woman, but also her family, the community, the society and the supernatural world. As Lefkarites (1992: 385) has pointed out:

> Childbirth is a significant human experience, its social meaning shaped by culture in which birthing women live. Cultures throughout the world express the meaning of childbirth through different beliefs, customs and practices. These diverse cultural interpretations are part of a larger integrated system of beliefs concerning men, women, family, community, nature, religion, and supernatural powers.

Although birth in Hmong culture is surrounded by cultural taboos (Camey et al., 1996), it should be noted that birth as well as pregnancy are not seen as "pathological processes" (Sargent 1982: 195), as in the West. A normal birth is not defined as a disease "in the sense of 'an undesirable deviation in the way a person functions'." With a normal birth, the assistance of a specialist is not necessary. However, when complications arise, birth becomes a "life-threatening crisis requiring a specialist's intervention" (Sargent, 1982: 195). Birth, then, is a period of danger, and giving birth carries the risk of death.

Laderman (1983: 172) has contended that "every society has priorities that shape the ideology and conduct of childbirth." In Western societies, birth is treated as "a potentially life-threatening illness," so that possible dangers to the mother and her child may be minimized. However, the mother's autonomy is also diminished when her health and well-being are placed in the hands of health professionals. In contrast, Hmong birth is seen as a natural part of a woman's life. The birth process respects a woman's autonomy, and if she requires assistance in a time of difficulty, there are caring people around her to lend their hands.

Although the Hmong have many beliefs and practices related to birth that are different from those of the West, these should not be seen as strange or nonsensical. On the contrary, Hmong birthing traditions may offer lessons for the modern obstetric caregiver in Western maternity hospitals.

NOTES

1. Most Hmong men were soldiers in Laos and they might not be in the village at the time of birth.
2. See Chapter 6 in this volume on the role of Hmong husbands during the confinement period.
3. Usually referred to as a "sitting position."
4. A similar practice has also been observed in northern Thailand by Symonds (1991). During my fieldwork in a Hmong village in Chiang Mai in early 1999, I was told of several cases of young women who had had premarital pregnancies and had to give birth in a small house behind their parents' houses. After 30 days they moved back into their parents' home.
5. The Hmong, in a study conducted by Kunstadter et al. (1987: 75) in northern

Thailand, said that babies born prematurely are "hot hearted" or they are "impatient" and "eager to be born." These babies will be weak and may have birth defects. Babies born after due date, however, are believed to be "cool hearted," and they will grow up to be strong.

6. See also Chapter 4 in this volume on Hmong pregnancy.

7. This practice is believed to be borrowed from lowland Lao tradition, as it is more common for Lao women to do so when they have a difficult birth.

8. See also Laderman (1983) for a similar belief and practice among Malay women.

Chapter 6

Nyob Nruab Hlis: Thirty Days Confinement

INTRODUCTION

> In most societies birth and the immediate postpartum period are considered a time of vulnerability for mother and child; indeed, frequently a time of ritual danger for the entire family. (Jordan, 1978: 2)

In discussing the confinement and convalescence of Chinese women after childbirth, Pillsbury (1978: 15) contended that:

> Doing the month is clearly part of China's folk medical tradition. It is something "everybody" does to get well and remain well after parturition, and its specialists generally are simply mothers, mothers-in-law, and older women who are experienced in such matters.

Similar patterns of the puerperium practices has been observed in many traditional societies.[1] But is Pillsbury's argument applicable to Hmong women? Symonds (1991, 1996) has demonstrated that it is so in her study of Hmong women in Thailand. In this chapter, however, I will examine cultural beliefs and practices among Hmong women who have migrated to Australia. This chapter covers several important points about the puerperium that were made by the women during the course of fieldwork.

NYOB NRUAB HLIS: THIRTY DAYS CONFINEMENT

> After birth, you have to confine yourself because your body is still new and you must restrict yourself with eating and limiting your jobs that you do.

In the Hmong tradition, the first 30 days after birth is seen as the most dangerous period for a new mother. During this time, a woman is seen as vulnerable to all sorts of illnesses and misfortune. Therefore, she must "confine" herself and observe several prescribed treatments and practices.

Confinement Practices

Traditionally, a woman sleeps on a sleeping area made of several layers of straw covered with a piece of soft blanket near a fireplace for three days after birth. The Hmong believe a new mother and newborn infant need warmth after birth. This may prevent some forms of ill health.

> You should sleep there [near the fire] so that it will be warm for both the mother and the baby. A mother needs warmth to prevent her from having swelling on the body. This is a Hmong traditional belief that no warmth will cause swelling and pale and yellowish if she does not keep herself warm . . . and the way to keep herself warm is to lie near the fire and burn wood for heat.

Another woman elaborated:

> The fire provides warmth for the baby so the baby will not be cold. The mother must do this for heat too. And if you cannot have this heat to warm your hands and feet during the thirty days then your feet will swell. If there is no fire to provide heat then it will make your hands and feet swell. Warmth during confinement is important; if you do not do this then when you are older you cannot bear the coldness. . . . Hmong traditionally believe in keeping warm by the fire so that your limbs will not swell up with water inside. . . . So during the first three days after birth you must sleep there so the heat will warm you.

There are two reasons for using straw as a bed. First, straw will absorb childbirth blood, which flows more heavily during the first few days. On the third morning, the straw bed will be burned and the woman can move to her own bed. This, according to the Hmong, helps them cope with the scarcity of blankets.

> The first three days you sleep on straw bed and after that you change to your mattress. This is because there is not enough bedding stuff so if they get dirty [from childbirth blood] then there is nothing to change to. The purpose of the straws is to catch the blood and after three days you change it with your blankets.

The use of straw also helps the Hmong avoid washing material containing childbirth blood in a river or stream. The Hmong live in high mountainous areas where clean running water is scarce. This practice helps to maintain their clean running water system.

Second, a straw bed is near the ground. This avoids exerting excess energy in getting on and off a bed in the first few days.

> After the birth, you just sleep next to the fire place . . . because the bed is high and if you climb on and off it might irritate your body. That is why you have to sleep in a low place for three days so that your body is tighter and then you can sleep on the bed.

Although lying near the fire is commonly practiced for three days only, women mentioned that they could lie by the fire for the full 30 days if they wished. This is particularly beneficial in winter, when women may need fire for warmth if there is any scarcity of blankets.

> You could sleep for up to thirty days . . . depending on whether if it was winter or summer. If it was in winter you could sleep there for the whole of thirty days and then go back to your bed after that.

The straw bed must be burned. The Hmong believe that leaving straw containing childbirth blood on the ground will produce a smell, attracting animals and insects. This is seen as dangerous to a new mother's health.

> We have to burn the straws after three days because if you leave them somewhere they will smell and animals might come to eat them. This will make you sick in the stomach and feel unwell. . . . It will give you stomach pain and hemorrhage and you can die from that . . . so you have to burn the straws.
>
> We have to burn the straws. At that time we didn't have any pads like in this country, there was nothing to use. There is blood on the material and that has to be burnt. If the insects lick it then you will have tummy problems. . . . If you have tummy problems then your tummy will always be sore and never get better. Sooner or later that will kill you.

In addition, leaving straw with childbirth blood around may attract the attention of evil spirits, and women may be "struck" by these spirits. These women will have poor health after giving birth.

> With these things you have to burn them. If you just take them and put them somewhere then after a while they smell and then you will be hit by spirits because the spirits will smell the blood and they see it and they follow you.

During a confinement period, Hmong women also practice abdominal binding. This is an effort to bring the woman's abdomen back to its normal shape. It also makes the woman feel more comfortable after eating because the abdomen does not become overly expanded.

> You bind the tummy to help making the body feel tight. . . . When you are pregnant the tummy gets bigger. You bind it so that the belly skin doesn't fall down low. . . . If you don't do that then with every meal that you eat and feel full your tummy will expand to the size that you were when you were pregnant. . . . When you eat and feel full your tummy will not be too big. You bind it to make you feel comfortable.

Another woman explained:

> You do it so that your tummy will not be big. If you don't do it then with each child your tummy will be bigger and bigger and then you will not look good. If you want your tummy to be slim then you will tie your tummy up so that it will not look fat. . . . If you don't do it then after one month your tummy will look big and not nice and you won't like it.

Prescribed Food in Confinement

A Hmong woman's first postbirth meal is poached egg with white pepper. A chicken's egg is quickly cooked in hot water, then mixed with white pepper and a bit of salt for taste. It is believed this will give back a woman the strength that is lost during the act of giving birth. White pepper contains a "hot" property, so it helps to induce childbirth blood and leftover placenta in the uterus and makes the womb clean. This also helps in the relief of afterbirth pain.

> The first meal is made with an egg and pepper, then after that you eat hot rice and [chicken] meat. . . . We must do that so that it will stop the stomach pain. The truth is that the pepper is the most important. The pepper will help to wash your body so that it won't give you afterbirth pain.

> For us, when we were still in Laos and gave birth at home, soon after you give birth they [family members] will take a pot and put one cup of water in it to boil and then crack an egg in it to make egg and pepper soup for you.... You grind three peppercorns and add salt.... The egg soup is to stop you from having afterbirth pains.

During the confinement period and after this first meal, Hmong women only consume hot rice and chicken soup cooked with several kinds of green herbs.[2] After ten days, however they are allowed to eat some pork and fish.

> Before ten days, you should eat only chicken meat, not the old ones but the young ones. You eat only hot rice and drink hot water. After ten days you can eat pork and fish too, but you must not eat chilli, green leafy vegetables.

The Hmong place an emphasis on consuming "hot" food after giving birth. This is to allow the body to rid itself of as much childbirth blood as possible. Retained childbirth blood in the body is seen as a contributing cause to women's ill health after birth.

> The elder says that you must eat hot food so that your blood will run properly. Later, after the thirty days you will be able to gain weight and be strong. But if you eat cold food then your blood will clog after birth. Because you haven't changed your blood then when you finish your thirty days you cannot gain weight and also you will be unhealthy and be sick all the time. This will stop you from being able to support yourself.

Another woman told me that:

> You eat this [hot food] to help remove the things from inside your body so that you will have good health.... If you drink cold water then the cold water will mix with your blood and your blood will clot.... Your body is still new and still has a lot of blood inside and if you drink cold water into your body then your blood will clot.... If the blood doesn't come out then you will be very pale and you have no energy.

Rest

Hmong women do receive good assistance and support during confinement, so they are able to rest properly. Women mentioned that their husbands and other family members take care of household chores and other work.

> You stop from doing work. If you have to do some then you only do the very light work and you only look after the baby, the one that you have just given birth to. With cooking and anything else you leave it to them [family members].

Hmong women believe that during the confinement period their husbands will take extra care of them. This makes it possible for them to rest properly.

> When you have a new baby, if you don't do that [rest] then later on it will cause you to have bad health. Hmong believe that when you have a new baby your husband has to take special care of you. He will not let you carry water or firewood and will not let you eat cold food or food that is not good for confinement. He always makes warm food for you and wash your clothes for you . . . You can't do all these things so your husband has to do that. Your body is still new.

However, this does not mean that all women have the same help during confinement. These women will try not to do too much so they can rest. Anything which is seen as "too hard" for them, they will not attempt.

> If your husband can do it then he will do it, but if there is no husband to do it then you must only do a bit of it like cooking for your children. Anything that is heavy then you asks your children to help you.

In general, the women said they were able to carry on "light" work around the house such as cooking and looking after the baby and other children. However, they added, this work should not be undertaken until at least ten days after the birth.

BEHAVIORAL AND DIETARY PRECAUTIONS

The Hmong believe after giving birth, a woman's body is "new," and hence can be damaged easily. The Hmong, therefore, have several restrictions on new mothers' behavior during the confinement period.

> The elders say that we should not do these things because the body is still new. They do not allow us to touch cold water and during confinement you should wear thick clothing and wear a scarf on your head and not let your head be hit by the wind.

Physical Activities

Hmong women avoid performing "hard" physical activities during confinement. These include carrying heavy loads and doing rigorous activity.

> When you are in confinement, you should not lift heavy things, not brushing the floor, not picking up your older children. Anything that you have to use a bit of weight, you can't do it.

It is believed that performing heavy activities can lead to a prolapsed uterus, known as *hlauv duav* in Hmong. As one woman related:

> If you lift heavy things then you will have *hlauv duav*. It is like when the womb has collapsed and come out. The womb has collapsed and if it has been like that for a long time then it would be protruding outside. It is not painful but when it is like that it is very uncomfortable.

It is interesting that the avoidance of heavy physical activity is closely related to a woman's sexuality and reproductive capacity. Women mentioned that if they overexerted themselves during the confinement period there was a danger of prolapse of the uterus, which would leave them unable to produce more children.

> If you do heavy things then your body will not be pretty anymore. After you give birth to a baby your internal body is very loose. And if you carry these heavy things, if nothing happens then it is good, but if bad things happens [prolapse] then you will not be pretty . . . as well as not being able to have more children . . . and your life will not be worth living.

Apart from heavy physical activity, there are other activities that can cause ill health in a new mother. For example, combing hair during confinement is also prohibited. The act of brushing puts an exertion on the skin and is seen as a "hard" physical activity.

> Hmong women should not comb their hair after having a baby. The reason why they do not comb the hair is that the action of the combing will pull on the hair and this will cause the skin to be very sensitive.

Dusting the floor or blowing into the fireplace while cooking is believed to cause coughing in old age.

> You must not blow the fire or lift firewood. . . . If you blow into the fire the dust from the fire will go into your lungs and when you are old you will cough and wheeze a lot and you can't walk.

During the confinement period a new mother should restrict herself to remaining within the household. Going outside the house exposes the woman to wind, which is believed to cause blindness in old age.

> If you go [out] then the wind will blow into your eyes and this will cause you to go blind when you are older.

Avoidance of Sex

The Hmong practice sexual abstinence during the confinement period.

> When you are pregnant you can, it doesn't matter. But when you are in confinement then you cannot, in confinement, definitely not. I don't have the experience but I have seen some women whom their husbands do not restrict themselves and women do not restrict themselves. Then their lives are destroyed. Then it is not good for them.

It is believed that resuming sex before the end of thirty days may cause *hlauv duav;* a prolapsed uterus.

> After having a baby, traditionally we have to stop it [sexual intercourse] for one month. If we do it before this it can cause you to have collapsed pelvic floor. . . . They say that it is a piece like intestine will come out. . . . I have not seen it but the old people say that it will make them [women] have sore lower back and it is very hard to walk up hill because a piece sticks out from that area [vagina] so you cannot walk.

Having sexual intercourse too soon after childbirth is considered a potential health problem. Women who do are thought to be beyond the help of even herbal medicines.

> If the man sleeps with you and that thing happens then there is no way to fix it, there is no medicine to fix it and if you cut it off then you will die. So you cannot fix it until you die. But if you work or eat something wrong and that happens then there are herbal medicines that are crushed on put on that area. There are some herbal medicines to drink as well and that will move that thing back into the vagina.

Warmth after Birth

The Hmong are particularly cautious about "coldness" during confinement. The Hmong see warmth as essential for a new mother to regain her strength after giving birth. Therefore, coldness must be avoided during the confinement period.

> Using cold water soon after giving birth, in your old age, it can cause you to have cold and aching bones, a chilling sensation from within your bones. This will make you unable to withstand the coldness.

Touching cold water is also prohibited in Hmong culture.

> When you are still bleeding and you touch cold water, the cold will go into your body making your blood clot. Then it causes you to have bad health and you will not bleed and this bad health makes you sick . . . very sick. When the blood clots inside your body you will be very pale and you cannot gain weight and you have no appetite. . . . And if it is like that soon after it can be fatal . . . because the blood cannot come out and it stays in your liver.

Cold showers are particularly prohibited in the Hmong culture.

> If you have a cold shower then it will cause lumps on the skin, skin tightness and stiffness. You will walk stiffly like you have no energy.

> If you have a cold shower then when you get old you will have sore bones constantly. . . . It won't happen when you are still young, but when you get old like me [a grandmother] you will get that sickness.

Most women mentioned that touching cold water or having a cold shower causes ill health.

> You cannot have cold showers. In confinement you touch and shower with warm water only. I don't mean only shower but the ones you touch as well. Not talking about when you are older but when you have a few children and you touch cold water it will itch. It is the same as when you take a cold shower. Later when you have given birth to a few children then you will have an itchy body. Also if you are in confinement and you touch water a lot then you will experience tenderness in your hands when you touch it for a long period. . . . Tender as in soft and if you touch anything that is a bit rough then it will hurt.

Warm water only is allowed during a confinement period. Women mentioned that if they wished to clean their bodies, they used warm water. Some women explain they avoided showers in Laos because of the lack of access to hot water. Fortunately, in Australia the Hmong women are able to take warm showers after giving birth because of its availability.

Dietary Precautions

The Hmong strictly observe dietary precautions.

> During confinement you can't eat anything else but warm rice, chicken with the herbs. . . . You must eat like this to help your body recover and be healthy. The old people say that other foods will lead to health risk in your old age.

All women mentioned they adhered to their traditions so that bad health and even death would be avoided. Dietary precautions are taken to protect "a new body" from illness.

> Other foodstuffs! No, you cannot eat them. If you eat them because your body is still new and if you eat them it can make you sick. That is why we should not eat anything apart from Hmong confinement food. . . . Sometimes if you eat them then it will give you heartburn so you don't eat these things. It is frightening to eat them because of the sickness you may get.

Certain food is considered potentially fatal. The Hmong refer to this as *fab* and it happens because the food is "wrong" or "poisonous" to the woman's new body.

> If she does not eat according to what the Hmong eat traditionally . . . it is *fab*. If she eats like that it can be fatal because it is wrong to the body. . . . It can be anything that you are not suppose to eat during confinement but you want it. Things that are cold and things like banana and bamboo shoots, things like that.

"Cold" food and drink in particular are seen as causing *fab* because they cause the blood to clot. Ice and cold water are believed to cause death if a new mother takes them: "If you eat ice it can kill you." The main reason for this is that cold water may congeal the blood, and a new body cannot rid itself of "old blood," which is seen as poisonous because of its polluted nature.

Green vegetables and fresh fruits are seen as "cold" and are believed to cause asthma, coughing and swelling in old age. However, women are allowed to consume some boiled vegetables, such as green beans, 20 days after birth.

> With vegetables, after birth we do not eat fresh vegetables. It must be after twenty days that we can eat some beans but not green stalk vegetables and no cabbages. . . . Green vegetables make you get asthma and that is why we can't eat fresh vegetables, but if it is boiled we can eat it.

Certain fruits, vegetables and meat, which are seen as "wrong" food, such as bananas, eggplants, and an echidna-like animal, are believed to cause *hlauv duav*; a prolapsed uterus. One woman told me of her aunt's experience in Laos:

> After birth and if you eat something wrong then you can end up with the *hlauv duav* as well. I have an aunt, she ate meat of the echidna-like animal and she had that problem. You cannot eat banana and eggplant; they can cause this. When she [aunt] ate that the first time my father gave her some medicines and she got better. The next time she ate that she could not get better. It made her unable to recover and made her not being able to pass urine. She was like that until she died.

Other vegetables are also seen as "wrong," since they produce "wind." These include, in particular, pumpkin, melons and cucumbers.

> When you have the baby you don't eat pumpkins and melons, like watermelons . . . because they make wind. The wind will enter into your body . . . it makes the body swelling up . . . and this makes it difficult to walk.

In addition, pumpkin and melons contain high levels of water, which is seen as dangerous for "a new body," since the body is in the process of adjusting back to its normal state.

> Because they have water so if your body is not yet one month old the body is like . . . is trying to get rid of blood and making a new one, and if you eat them then this will choke your system and when you get old then you will get swelling like the melon and pumpkin.

Fruits that are seen as "sweet," such as bananas, are also believed to have a harmful effect on "a new body."

> Banana is sweet and your body is very new from giving birth, if you eat before you are one month old then the sweet thing will go into your intestine and this will cause pain and infection in your internal organs. Hmong call it *kem plab* [heartburn or ulcer] in your body.

Consuming foodstuffs which are "hard" (meaning not tender and difficult to digest) will cause indigestion and heartburn during confinement or, more commonly, in later life.

> You eat only young chicken's meat not the old chicken. You eat the soft and hot rice not the hard rice. . . . If you eat old chicken because it is very hard [not tender], when you get old you will have a painful chest. So you will not be able to eat anything at all. . . . With rice, you have to make it soft so that it is good to eat. It has to be made softer than usual.

This is why Hmong women do not consume glutinous rice (known as sticky rice) at all during their confinement period.

> With sticky rice your body is still new from having the baby so your internals are very lose and if you eat the sticky rice then later on it will cause *kem plab* [heartburn/ulcer] and it will be very painful.

Food that has a burned smell or is burned when cooked is also seen as dangerous.

> Eating burnt meat will choke you and make you sick immediately. . . . Any sort of meat, if you burn it by grilling or by boiling when all the water has dried up, you must not eat it. . . . You will be coughing and unable to breathe and this can kill you.

Grilled food is therefore prohibited during the confinement period, as it can be poisonous or wrong for the body.

> If you eat grilled meat like that and because it smells, the smell will go into your body and it can cause you to *fab* or *phiv* [allergic]. Then this will make you sick. And also when you get older it can give you trouble too:

Interestingly, although Hmong women eat hot rice that has to be cooked until soft, they are not allowed to drink rice milk (water used to wash rice before cooking) or rice porridge. It is believed this will cause any remaining childbirth blood to clot.

> If eating wrong food during confinement, something which is wrong to your body then there are medicines to help. But if you drink rice milk or eat rice porridge this will make the childbirth blood inside to clot. . . . This rice water you can't even drink when it is hot. Two Hmong have died from that. As soon as they drink the rice water the blood rumbles, rumbles inside and as soon as the blood clots they die.

Restrictions for Lactating and Pregnant Women

During a confinement period, there are some restrictions with regard to visitors. Pregnant women, lactating mothers and the husbands of pregnant or lactating women are dissuaded from visiting during confinement.

> In your confinement if other people come to visit you then that is okay but only the ones that are pregnant they are not allowed to come. And if they come then it is believed that they will take away your milk so your baby will not have any milk to drink.

Those who enter the house during the confinement period should not carry bags or wear shoes. This is believed to take away the mother's breast milk. This is a serious matter in Hmong culture, since traditionally Hmong women breastfeed their newborn infants—they do not have access to infant formula.

> In your confinement, doesn't matter if it is a man or a woman, if they know that you just have a baby and is breastfeeding then when they come they must take off their shoes outside and not to wear them inside. If they carry a bag then they will leave it outside, and if they carry a basket then they must leave that outside too. They will come in with nothing like that on their body. If they carry the basket inside then they can bring the milk away and if they wear shoes they can carry the milk away too. If the person has taken your milk away you have to go to bring it back or you have to wait until they give birth themselves before your milk comes back . . . so your baby will not get milk at all.

In some situations, there is a way to counteract this violation.

> If you know the person who is pregnant and who has come to take the milk away from you, you have to go and get some of their salt, rice grain and cooking oil to cook for you to eat. This will help you to have milk again.

Another woman elaborated:

> If a woman is pregnant and comes to see you, after they leave you find that your breast has no more milk then you know that it is her. You will then ask someone from your house to go to her house and bring it back from her house. When you go you say "When you came I think that my baby's milk followed you home so I am here to bring baby's milk back." They then will get some salt and if they have eggs then they will give an egg as well and one spoon of salt. They will then say: "When I came to visit you your baby's milk has followed me home so here I give baby's milk for you to carry back to the baby." If you have rice then you give a bowl of rice too. So you will have to bring these back and prepare it for the mother to eat and if the milk comes back then your breast will swell up and have milk again.

However, many women mentioned that once their breast milk was taken, it could not be retrieved.

> If they come and after they leave they take the milk away you have to wait until their baby is born then you will have your milk back. You and your baby will have a very hard time. . . . So this is why the Hmong people restrict themselves.

THE "POLLUTED BODY": WOMEN IN CONFINEMENT

During confinement, a woman's body is seen as particularly "unclean," "dirty" and "polluted." This belief is reflected in the restrictions placed upon a woman's behavior.

Prohibited: Entering Other People's Homes

During confinement, a new mother is prohibited from entering other people's homes, particularly if they are from a different clan. It is believed that because she is still bleeding, her "polluted" body may weaken the clan spirit (*dab qhuas*) and bring bad health, illness and perhaps even death into that household.

> If you have just given birth you are not allowed going into other people's home. Similarly, other people who have just had a baby they are not allowed to enter my home either. If they do that then their *dab qhuas* will not be good anymore and they cannot earn money for living.

It is strongly believed that a new mother who has committed such acts will not die easily in old age. This is seen as a "bad" death in Hmong culture.

> If I am still in confinement I can't enter other people's home, and must stay only in my own home. . . . If you are still in confinement and enter someone else home then in the long term when you are dying it is very hard for you to completely die. You have to wait till someone burn incenses and gold paper to wash your foot steps at the door and inside their house and only then will you die. This is the Hmong way.

Because of this belief, Hmong women restrict themselves to their homes for the entire 30 days after birth. If they do enter another house, they must pay a "penalty" to counteract any misfortune. This penalty is a considerable amount by Hmong standards, as one woman elaborated:

> You should not enter into other people's home. But if you do go into their home and through their door because they have different *dab qhuas* then it will make their *txhij meej* [household spirit] weak. This will make them very unhappy toward you. If you forget and you go into their house then you have to go and have *ua neeb* [shamanic ritual] to heal the house and to clean out your uncleanness, your blood so that the spirit *txhij meej* will come back to live in their house. This *ua neeb* is a heavy duty one and when you go to ask *txiv neeb* [shaman] to heal it you have to pay him a piece of money [bar of silver] before he will come to do the *ua neeb* . . . and you have to buy a pig to heal the family and a chicken to dust off your

> uncleanness that you have brought into their home. . . . It you don't do this, they can't achieve anything. If it was still in Laos and they have livestock then these animals will not grow well and they will die; all sorts of things can happen to them. This will make them very angry at you.

Not Going Through the Front Door

Women are also warned not to go through the front door of their own house. As is believed about her effect on other's homes, it is thought that a woman's "polluted" body can weaken her own household spirit, known as *txhij meej* in Hmong. Once *txhij meej* is weakened, it cannot take good care of the family members and their animals.

> During confinement if we need to go outside the house we cannot go through the front door. . . . They say that because your body is still bleeding and it is unclean. Hmong are spirits believers and there is a spirit at the front door and if you go through the door then the spirit doesn't like it and it will go away. So there won't be anyone to look after the door, no one to look after your house. Hmong say that the spirit is called *txhij meej*, he is the one that looks after your house, your children, and if in Laos it looks after your livestock too. So that no one will get sick.

Childbirth Blood and Restrictions

Any material that comes into contact with childbirth blood during the confinement period must be washed within the house. This includes clothes used during birth and women's clothing used during the bleeding period after birth. Hmong husbands will usually dig a hole in the ground inside the house (Hmong houses in Laos and Thailand are built on a dirt ground). All clothes and materials are washed, and the "unclean" water is thrown into this hole. When the confinement period is finished and when a woman's bleeding stops, the hole is covered. These clothes and materials are not allowed to be washed in a stream or river. It is believed that doing so will attract a spirit's attention, who could then trace the woman through the smell of her childbirth blood and "strike" her. This would lead to illness and perhaps death for the woman during the confinement period. The Hmong are particularly cautious about this.

> You will have to dig a hole inside the house for you to bury or wash your clothes that you have the baby in and when you have no more birthing blood then you fill up the hole. . . . You can't bring them to wash in the river because if you do that then *dab* [spirits] will follow the smell of your blood to you . . . and it is not good for you.

As previously mentioned, during confinement women are restricted within their own household boundaries. This is related in part to the woman's body, "polluted" by childbirth blood. The Hmong believe that the woman's body after birth has a smell that will attract the spirits outside the house, and that if she goes outside, she will be struck by these spirits.

> If you are still in confinement you must not go out. . . . There are a lot of spirits and like your body is still new and you still smell bad . . . from your bleeding, your childbirth blood . . . and you might get hit by spirits.

HMONG HERBAL MEDICINES IN CONFINEMENT

The Hmong rely heavily on their green herbs during confinement. Herbs play an important role in maintaining the health of a new mother. There are several common green herbs, known as *tshuaj qaib* (chicken herbal medicine), used in confinement. They serve a number of purposes, including relieving aches and pain after birth, producing extra blood after birth, washing out childbirth blood and remaining placenta from the uterus, replacing energy and strength lost during birth, promoting a good appetite, improving weight lost during birth and enhancing breast milk.

> You eat them so that your body will settle back to normal stage quicker and if you don't use them then it will take you a long time to get back to normal. The bleeding will go for a long time and that will make you very thin. That is not good. . . . If you bleed too long the body won't get back to its regular again and this can make you pale and skinny. If you have the chicken herbs to eat then your blood will be good and you will feel stronger more quickly. . . . You eat them to give you strength and also to wash out your blood quickly too.

If a woman does not have any health problems after giving birth, she will only consume chicken soup cooked with several green herbs to help "heal" her body. As a medicine woman told me,

> If she has given birth and she is well then all we need to do is give her the herbs to help her body heal and then she will be healthy. She will eat the chicken with herbs and she will be healthy and the baby will be healthy. You don't need to help her with anything else.

However, if the woman has afterbirth pains, herbal medicine needs to be used to relieve the pain. It is believed that afterbirth pains occur because the body is not clean from the childbirth blood and placenta remaining in the body.

> If it is because of her body, because it is not clean then we give her herbs to wash her body. . . . You must use herbs to wash it out. This medicine must be made with chicken for her to eat. . . . If she has very bad pains and clots then there must be three chickens, have to make three chickens with herbs for her to eat . . . and she must not eat anything else.

In addition a woman may become ill during confinement if she does not restrict her diet. When this happens, the Hmong use green herbs to help restore the woman's health.

> When you are in confinement and you eat something wrong and it gets stuck inside your chest. You can use *lauj vag*; you cook it in chicken to eat. It is quite effective. If you are in confinement and you eat something that give you heartburn then you take the leaves to make it with chicken.

Apart from using herbal medicines to assist in healing and maintaining the health of a new mother, massage is also employed to help rid the body of any remaining blood and placenta. A medicine woman may perform this. However, an older woman whose task is similar to that of a traditional birth attendant may be asked to perform the massage.[3]

In the case of ill health arising from failure to keep the body warm enough, the Hmong will resort to herbal medicines. The herbs are used in combination with hot rocks, a method known as *tshuaj txhawb*—the steamed herbs method. Herbs are boiled and the rocks are heated up in a fire. The rocks are then put into the hot herbs, which creates hot steam. The mixture is placed near the body of the woman and a blanket is placed on her body. The heat is trapped inside the blanket and is absorbed by her body. This assists the woman to regain heat lost from her body and relieve her from any ill symptoms caused by coldness of the body.

CONCLUSIONS

> The postpartum period is the liminal stage in a woman's passage through the rite of childbirth. As in all such transitional stages, the person on the threshold is in an extremely vulnerable position and must be segregated from her community. (Laderman 1983: 174)

Laderman's statement is particularly applicable to the Hmong. For the new mother in Hmong culture, the segregation is behavioral rather than physical. Women are restricted from certain activities, foods and social contacts until the dangerous period is over, largely because both mother and baby are seen as being in a "precarious state following the birth" (Fuller and Jordan, 1981: 46). This is similar to many other cultures throughout the world, where the puerperium is seen as the most vulnerable period a new mother and her newborn endure (Jordan, 1978; Pillsbury, 1978; Sich, 1981; Laderman, 1983; MacCormack, 1982; Cosminsky, 1982; Townsend and Rice, 1996; Symonds, 1996; Cheung, 1997; Rice et al., 1999).

In writing about childbirth in rural Korea, Sich (1981) points out, "It is considered to be extremely dangerous for the health of a mother if the rules for post partum care are not observed as they should be." The Hmong see things similarly and follow many confinement practices to enhance good health. One woman put it succinctly: *"The Hmong do these things for good health."*

The Hmong place an emphasis on "prevention" during confinement. This is clearly seen in many discussions with women who speak of being particularly careful about their activities and diet.

> If your blood has clotted then you have to look for medicines to help your body get better. If you are not being careful you have to use some money to buy these medicines to help yourself. If you are not careful this is what will happen to you. . . . You have to pay a lot of money for them before you get the medicines. So that is why you have to make sure that after giving birth you have to eat hot food and you have to restrict yourself so that it won't kill you either.

In a similar vein, another woman explained:

> If you do heavy work then your body will be destroyed because you have just given birth and your body is still new and has no strength. If your body is destroyed then your life is also destroyed. . . . You must know what will happen. The old people say that you have to be careful with your body. You do not carry heavy things. If you destroy your body then your husband will not want you anymore. That is all. If I say this much you should know what I am talking about.

It also appears that Hmong women feel restricted somewhat by traditional practices, which they consider to be related to their reproduction. As one woman related:

> Because women are the ones that bear children so they have to be careful of everything.

However, on closer examination, we see that these practices have functional purposes. This can be seen in the dietary practices of the Hmong. As previously discussed, Hmong new mothers only consume chicken soup with hot rice for an entire 30 days, although after 10 days they are allowed some fish and pork. Mathews and Manderson (1981: 15) have pointed out that high protein foods are "channelled to those in need, who because of their sex and for economic reasons may at other times receive very little protein." In their everyday lives, Hmong women do not receive much meat because of its scarcity and the inferiority of their gender. However, after childbirth, which is seen as a depletion of their strength and health, the women are treated with more equality. This practice, therefore, exists to restore the health and well-being of a new mother (Pillsbury, 1978). It is not detrimental to the woman despite the arguments of many researchers that dietary restrictions during the puerperium may put new mothers at risk of inadequate nutritional intake (Wilson, 1973; Eichinger Ferro-Luzzi, 1974; Weise, 1976).

Although women are secluded during confinement primarily because they are considered polluted and in a "socially dangerous state" (Mathews & Manderson, 1981), the avoidance of many activities during the confinement period protects the women from poor health. Avoidance of physical activities, for example, gives a new mother both adequate rest before resuming her household duties and protection from infection. Similarly, the avoidance of sexual intercourse during the first 30 days helps restore her physical health to its normal level and prevents possible further illness. This may be seen as unnecessary from the Western perspective. However, a recent study (Carter, 1998) has shown that resuming sex too soon after birth can be fatal.

Fuller and Jordan (1981: 46) found that "the period of seclusion has important consequences for the mutual adjustment of mother and child." Relieved of everyday normal activities and household chores, a new mother can give her exclusive attention to her newborn. It is at this time that a mother may learn about her baby. In addition, this seclusion ensures more successful breastfeeding, as she does not have to meet the demands of other children and housework. The mother will put her baby on her breast whenever the baby makes a noise. When she emerges from her confinement, breastfeeding has been established, and she has learned about her newborn. The period of separation during the puerperium may assist women to cope with childbirth better and, hence, enable them to move into the motherhood state smoothly.

An interesting practice during the puerperium is the use of heat. According to Goldsmith (1990: 80), "at this time, as tribal people understand, the mother is cold, weak, and exhausted, her uterus is full of harmful fluids. Heat it is said, shrinks the uterus, restores her strength, and stimulates the production of milk; it is also, of course, comfort to the new mother." The Hmong hold similar theories about heat in confinement. These seems to persist in many cultures throughout the world (e.g., Kitzinger, 1982; Laderman, 1983; Goldsmith, 1990). Goldsmith (1990) has pointed out that the reason for the use of heat is practical rather than symbolic, since the heat assists women to recover quickly from childbirth. She also remarked that "evidently the treatment was quite effective, for the tribal mother rarely suffered from hemorrhage, recovered quickly after birth, generally regained her former figure, bled for only a short time, and usually had no problem with her milk supply."

Pillsbury (1978: 17) identifies three main reasons why Chinese women carry out postpartum rituals. These are "curing the pregnancy-induced imbalance, preventing future illness, and preventing future misfortune to themselves and those with whom they interact." Similarly, Cheung (1997) states that the practices of sitting the month among Chinese women in Scotland is a "social sanction" for the new mother that is used to ensure that she is able to rest and recover. It is also a means by which to prevent her future illness. Cheung contends that "this practice has a direct bearing upon the psychological well-being of the woman" (p. 64). As Niehof (1988: 243) points out about childbirth in Madura, Indonesia, many of the behavioral and dietary restrictions are based on two principles: "in the first place the mother and baby are thought to be in a state of transition which makes them very vulnerable to evil forces. Secondly, they are not only contaminated, but also contaminating." A new mother should therefore confine herself to the house and should not participate in normal activities so she can protect her own health as well as the health of those around her. The Hmong, indeed, hold similar perceptions. These are reflected in their beliefs and practices during the confinement period, as have been described in this chapter.

It has been suggested that the reintegration of the new mother into society is breaking down in many other ethnic groups in Western societies.[4] However, this has not happened with the Hmong, who continue to practice confinement for 30 days and keep to their customs as closely as possible. In Cheung's work (1997) with Chinese women in Scotland, she found that the extent to which women followed and observed postpartum practices depended to some extent on their needs, environment, family condition, financial state and educational status. In my study, however, all Hmong observed and followed their traditions strictly. Only a few customs had been modified, such as lying near the fire. This practice is not feasible in the Australian environment. In addition, the women had to leave the place of birth during the first 30 days, since they gave birth in the hospital and had to go home. This suggests that Western health professionals "must remain aware and respect the indigenous beliefs and practices linking the events of reproduction and the health status of women" (Pillsbury, 1978: 11).

FINAL THOUGHTS ON CHILDBEARING

In discussing childbearing in Madura, Indonesia, Niehof (1988: 239), pointed out:

> For the mother pregnancy and childbirth imply gradual social isolation before birth, and social re-integration thereafter. Especially for women who are pregnant for the first time the accompanying ritual takes on the character of a rite of passage. Interwoven in rite-of-passage symbolisms are symbols which are thought to avert danger and which point to well-being and fertility.

These three chapters have shown similar patterns of pregnancy, birth and the puerperium in Hmong culture. As discussed, all rituals surrounding pregnancy, birth and confinement exist to protect the woman, enhancing fertility and the well-being of the woman and her newborn baby. In rites of passage, segregation is clearly marked. However, segregation in Hmong culture is behavioral rather than physical. A woman is never left alone. During pregnancy, a woman begins her rites of passage pursuing certain activities that set her apart from other women, thereby ensuring that her pregnancy will go smoothly and a difficult and long labor will be avoided. When giving birth, she is separated from others but receives assistance from other women as well as her husband. After the birth, the rite of passage is markedly clear. The woman must observe many restrictions in order to avoid ill health and misfortune. During this period, dietary and other behavioral changes clearly set her apart from normal community life. After 30 days of confinement, she emerges with a "clean," healthy body. She then is able to reintegrate into society and resume her social duties and chores.

The new pair has survived the dangers of childbirth and a new member has joined the society (Laderman, 1983). At this stage, the process of transition to motherhood is considered complete, and the woman returns to society as a new mother, with a higher status. As Kitzinger (1982: 182) has suggested, if we perceive childbearing as a rite of passage, we may clearly see "the patterns of interaction between individuals and social groups." Her argument is applicable to Hmong society as well.

These three chapters have also shown that childbearing in Hmong culture is "integrated into culturally determined behavioral patterns between pregnant women and their families." In this sense, the Hmong's beliefs and practices are in conflict with "the cosmopolitan medicine which aims at the individual and knows only how to deal effectively with individual women" (Sich, 1981: 69). The childbearing process is clearly in sharp contrast with the midwifery training programs that are based on the biomedical model of birth (Cosminsky, 1982; Laderman, 1983). Many Hmong beliefs and practices relating to childbearing procedures discussed in these chapters should not be seen as "very strange indeed" (Pillsbury, 1978), "nonsense," or "problems" to be ignored or eliminated (Cosminsky, 1982). The Hmong have observed that these are ways that successfully cope with the crisis of childbirth, and they are interrelated with other aspects of their society. As Pillsbury (1978), Laderman (1983) and Cheung (1997) have demonstrated, many of the beliefs and practices during the puerperium are "efficacious" rather than "dysfunctional."

Because of modernization and Westernization, some traditional childbearing practices are being displaced by Western procedures.[5] This, however, has not happened within the Hmong society, despite living in a Western country such as Australia. This is important, since it means that health care providers will continue to come across the many traditional beliefs and practices of the Hmong when working with their community.[6]

And, since birth is "rich with meanings which have penetrated the whole of social life" (Kitzinger 1982: 194), continuing to "search for meaning in practices" of childbearing among Hmong women may provide us with insights into many facets of birth that many of us "in the West do not understand" (MacCormack 1982: 19).

NOTES

1. See, for example, Jordan, 1978; Manderson, 1981; Cosminsky, 1982; Kitzinger, 1982; MacCormack, 1982; Laderman, 1983; Chu, 1996; Townsend and Rice, 1996; Symonds, 1996; Cheung, 1997; and Rice et al., 1999.
2. See Chapter 3 on Hmong herbal medicines.
3. See also Chapters 4 and 5 for more extensive details of their tasks.
4. See, for example, Homans, 1982; Cheung, 1997; Rice et al., 1999; and Small et al., 1999.
5. See, for example, McClain, 1975; Muecke, 1976; Mathews and Manderson 1981; Rice and Naksook, 1998; and Cheung, 1997.
6. I believe an appreciation of Hmong cultural beliefs and knowledge of their expectations and social circumstances are essential for sensitive and culturally appropriate birthing care. This, however, does not mean that health care professionals need extensive training in cultural awareness or require a "manual" when working with Hmong women. One simple method is to ask individual women about their wishes and needs concerning their traditional practices. Most often, if caregivers show the women genuine concern, the women will inform them of their cultural needs during the childbearing process.

There may be some variations from one woman to another in terms of expectations and individual needs. As Cheung (1997: 64) points out, "Each individual is different. To provide a woman-centred maternity service, mutual understanding is a prerequisite for meeting the needs of an individual woman." It is essential that health care professionals ask women about their individual needs during the childbearing processes. This also helps to avoid making stereotyped assumptions about Hmong women.

I believe that only by taking these issues into account can culturally sensitive care be achieved in a birthing service. As Lazarus (1990) has insisted, good care significantly affects a woman's well-being. If women are to be motivated to return the next time they are pregnant, changes must be made in maternity hospitals. This may also make childbearing a more pleasurable experience for Hmong women in their new homeland.

Chapter 7

Birth in a New Homeland

INTRODUCTION

> A woman about to become a mother, or with her newborn infant upon her bosom, should be the object of trembling care and sympathy. Wherever she bears her tender burden or stretches her aching limbs. God forbid that any member of the profession to which she trusts her life, doubly precious at this emotional period, should handle it negligently, inadvisedly or selfishly. (Oliver Wendell Holmes, cited in Raphael-Leff, 1991: 134)

In the past decade, there has been considerable interest in childbirth experiences among women from non-Western backgrounds who are now living in Western countries. What researchers are interested in is finding out what happens to women who have to move to another social environment different from their own. Most studies point to many changes in childbirth patterns of women who migrate to another country.[1] However, what happens to Hmong women who have been uprooted from their familiar society is largely unknown.[2] We still lack knowledge about how Hmong women deal with childbirth in their new social environment, whether they have any concern about their own well-being or that of their babies, and how they see birthing services in the new home. Most importantly, we do not know the extent of communication between Hmong women and their caregivers. This chapter attempts to fill the gap.

I will first discuss women's perceptions and experience of pregnancy, birth and the hospital stay. I will then discuss the issue of communication between Hmong women and their caregivers during their childbirth process.

WOMEN'S PERCEPTIONS AND EXPERIENCE OF ANTENATAL CARE

Antenatal Check-Ups

All Hmong women in the study who had their babies in Australia attended a public hospital for their antenatal care. All women except one attended antenatal check-ups organized for them by the hospital. When they were asked if they had missed any appointments, most women said they had not. The main explanation they gave for their consistent attendance was that the hospital would arrange another appointment for them if they missed one. Women believed that antenatal check-ups were a good thing to have and an important part of their pregnancies.

> I think it [antenatal check up] is a good thing. Check up is good but because in Laos and in Thailand we didn't know so we didn't do anything about it. So if you were well then you were all right, but if you had problems then there wasn't anyone, e.g. a doctor, to look after you, and that was a big problem. Therefore, it is a good thing.

In traditional Hmong culture there is no antenatal care during pregnancy. Most pregnant women do not do anything about their pregnancy unless there are complications. Because of this tradition, many women believed that an antenatal check-up was not essential. They, however, would still attend antenatal check-ups.

Although Hmong women see that an antenatal check-up is important, they may not utilize antenatal care early in their pregnancy. Four women did not have their first antenatal check-up until they were seven months pregnant because of other commitments. As one young Hmong woman told me:

> I went for check up when I was seven months pregnant because if you went early you got tired of going and so you would wait until it was near its term. Also because at that time I still went to school, I was still studying [English for migrants] so that if I went early then I would have to miss school a lot and that was why I didn't go.

Five women arrived in Australia already pregnant. By the time they got settled and dealt with other urgent needs such as accommodations and schooling for their older children, they presented quite late in their pregnancy. One woman related that she had planned to attend an antenatal check-up but was too late, because of the early arrival of her newborn infant. Women stated that they did not know that they were pregnant, since there were no symptoms or signs until they started to feel the baby's movement. Additionally, the women breastfed their babies until they became pregnant again. By the time they knew that they were pregnant they were about four to five months into term. For these reasons, they did not attend antenatal check-ups until late in pregnancy.

Women said they had good experiences with their caregivers during their antenatal care. However, there was one woman who felt very dissatisfied with her doctor, who had insisted she take contraceptive pills or undergo tubal ligation because he believed that she had had "too many children." The experience this woman had with her doctor frightened her to the point that she did not return for further antenatal check-ups.

Vaginal Examination

All women, except three, had a vaginal examination in an Australian hospital. Women related that because they were told to have the examination for their well-being and that of their babies, they agreed to have it performed.

> With my daughter at [. . .] hospital I had the examination. They checked me and there was no problem. They told me that I needed the examination to see if there were any problems with the baby and me, so I had that done, and the result was okay.

Women agreed to have a vaginal examination because they believed that it was a common practice in their new home. If they refused it, they might be seen as resisting integration into this society. One woman explained that:

> I felt that this was the way of this country, that was why I didn't say anything and just let them do it. . . . In this country they said that the doctors would examine you internally . . . but this is not something we do in Hmong culture. But since we have arrived here they said that everyone needed to do this and because I couldn't speak the language so it was more or less like I couldn't say anything about it.

However, there were three women who insisted on not having the vaginal examination. These women mentioned that they told their caregivers they did not want to have their vagina examined. Most caregivers did listen to the women and did not insist on the examination. As one Hmong woman elaborated.

> I said to them that I didn't like the examination, whether to put the hand inside to feel the baby or to look at my vagina or to be checked by a male doctor. I only liked to have a female doctor and when I had the check up, only look at by abdomen. I said that to them but they didn't say anything bad to me. All they said was that if I didn't like that and if I was very embarrassed about it then they would not do anything like that to me.

However, one woman said her caregiver was not pleased with her decision not to to have a vaginal examination:

> They did insist that they would do the examination on me, but I refused to have that done so they didn't. They said that they wanted to examine it but I said that I didn't want it. . . . They didn't do anything to me but they looked like they were very upset. Their faces look frowning and did not talk to me after that.

One important aspect of vaginal examination is the sex of the caregiver. All women in the study mentioned that they did not wish to have a male doctor performing a vaginal examination. Fortunately, most women who agreed to have the vaginal examination had female doctors to look after them.

> I don't like male doctors for this [vaginal] examination. When I went to [. . .] hospital, I had two females to examine me.

Antenatal Classes

Nearly all the women in the study did not attend the antenatal classes organized by the hospital. Women mentioned that they were not informed by the hospital. Some related that even if they were told to go, they would not attend, since it is not their traditional practice to have a formal antenatal class during pregnancy. One woman stated:

> Hmong people do not do these things. Even if they were asked, Hmong people don't usually like to do these things. It is not our tradition.

Fifteen women mentioned that childbirth was based on real-life experience, not something that women needed to learn from classes.

> These things I didn't need it, I didn't think I liked to learn about these . . . because having a baby and learning about it well, experience was much better than being taught like that.

WOMEN'S EXPERIENCES OF LABOR AND BIRTH

The Labor

Nearly all multipara Hmong women had an easy birth and a short labor. It was usual for many Hmong women to arrive at the hospital and give birth as soon as they got into a labor ward. Women said that their labor was so quick that their caregivers were surprised about it. Two women, in fact, gave birth at their flats before they could get to the hospital or the arrival of the ambulance, because their labor was extremely quick.

However, among first-time mothers, there were two who had difficult births. One woman related:

> The birth was so difficult. They kept telling me to push hard but I didn't have the energy to push. The labor was long. It started at four A.M. and it was after 11 o'clock that I gave birth. It was so painful and so long. . . . They gave me one injection and after that I felt that my eyes were getting stiff and hard. I felt really sleepy but I still could feel all the pain. . . . I felt scared of not knowing what to expect and it was too painful.

Women felt somewhat indifferent about their birthing experiences in Australian hospitals. Because of their quick labor and inability to speak in English to communicate with their caregivers, women felt that they did not have any great concerns about it. However, one woman said she did not like one aspect of giving birth here, namely, stitching the tear. She related:

> Having children in the hospital I did not like one thing. . . . It was that I only gave birth and I only had a tear but why they had to stitch it up. . . . But we Hmong people, giving birth to a big one or a small one, we do not need to be stitched. . . . It would heal up by itself, it would be just the same, and no one had died from that. . . . They did not ask me if I wanted to have it done, they just told me that they would do it and they just performed it.

In Hmong culture, it is believed that a tear occurs when "heaven" opens its door for a new life to emerge. It is, therefore, normal for a woman to have a tear. Since heaven opens the door, it will then close again, and this means that the tear will heal by itself. Human beings should not interfere with this process.

The Presence of a Husband and Family Members

It is a common practice in Australian hospitals to have a father present at the birth. Nearly all Hmong women had their husbands with them during labor in Australia. Women explained that it is a common practice in Hmong culture for husbands to help in the labor process. Traditionally, a Hmong man assists his woman by supporting her under her arms so that she can better push the baby, particularly if she is having a difficult birth.[3] One woman explained:

> With some people experiencing difficult labor, there has to be one or two women present as well as the husband. One of the women holds the mother and the other delivers the baby so there are more than one person present at birth. Sometimes the husband will deliver the baby while both women hold on to the mother if it is a long labor.

Therefore, in the Australian hospital Hmong women did not have any objection to having their husbands at the birth. Three women, however, did not have their husbands with them. In one case, the husband had to stay at home to look after the older children; hence, the woman went into the hospital alone. In another case, the husband was asked to go home and come back in the morning, because the doctor believed that his wife would not give birth until late in the next day. He returned home, and she gave birth at four o'clock in the morning.

One woman, however, said that her caregivers did not allow her husband to be in the birthing room. Her husband and her mother came to the hospital with her but they were told to wait outside. She related:

> When I had the baby, there were two nurses and one doctor, a man doctor. My husband came but they didn't let him in. . . . They just said that they did not allow him to come inside. My mother came too but they told my mother to go outside. So they all waited outside.

When asked if she had asked hospital staff to let her have her family members at the birth with her, she said: "It was so painful at that time that I didn't want to say anything, I didn't want to speak at all."

WOMEN'S EXPERIENCES OF HOSPITAL STAY

Length of Stay

Eleven women stayed in the hospital for two or three days. Two women stayed for seven days because of caesarean birth and another stayed for four days because her newborn had to be in an incubator because of jaundice. One woman experienced placental abruption and had a premature delivery. She therefore had to stay in the hospital for one month. In addition, one woman gave birth in a family birth center and went home within 24 hours.

When women were asked about their decision to go home early, they mentioned the need to look after other children at home as a main reason. Women said that because their husbands worked or studied English, there was no one to take care of their other children. Women also mentioned that young children missed their mother and hence were miserable at home. Because of these concerns, they decided to go home as soon as possible.

The woman who gave birth in a family birth center stated that it was the policy of the center that women had to go home within 24 hours. If there were any complications, she would have had to move to a public maternity ward. She did not like staying in a ward and she did not have any health problem, so she went home within the day. However, she also gave another reason:

> I didn't want to stay there so I came home. They also said that if I was strong enough then I could go home. Because on the first floor [family birth center] you could only stay for 24 hours there, if you had a problem and you needed to stay longer then they would send you to sleep where there were a lot of people. So if you wanted to go home early it was okay. There was no one to look after my two older children at home too, so it was very hard for my husband to send food for me to eat. So that was why I went home.

Satisfaction with Care from the Hospital Staff During the Hospital Stay

Most women mentioned that most members of the hospital staff were nice and kind to them. As one women explained:

> I gave birth at [. . .] hospital they were very good to me. . . . They didn't say bad things to me. . . . When I gave birth there were two young women who looked after me. . . . After I gave birth the two left and another two came to look after me, they didn't do anything bad or say anything bad to me.

None of the Hmong women ate food provided by the hospital, because of cultural postpartum dietary restrictions. Traditionally, in the first month after birth a new mother can only consume hot rice and chicken soup cooked with several green herbs. She is prohibited from consuming food that is "cold" in terms of both temperature and humoral quality as well as other foodstuffs that can cause illness and death (such as fruits, fresh vegetables, red meat and cold drinks).

Women related that their caregivers did not pay much attention to this. Only one woman was asked why she did not want to eat hospital food, but she could not explain to her caregiver about Hmong confinement practice regarding food. However, one woman mentioned that the catering staff tried to provide her with appropriate food during her hospital stay. A member of the catering staff happened to see her eating food brought in by her husband when she returned to take the tray away. Later on, the staff member came back with food, that similar to her traditional postpartum food, although it was not the same.

> They brought in a lot of things and drinks too but I didn't eat and didn't drink. My husband brought everything from home. . . . I didn't eat any and they would have to take it back. The one that sent the food to me, she brought me the food and found that I didn't eat their food and ate my own when she came to take their food away. On the day I was coming home she didn't make the same one, but brought me a piece of chicken and some rice for me to eat.

Women also believed that they received as much attention and care from their caregivers as women from other groups did. However, three women mentioned that although they did receive assistance during their stay in the hospital, it was not enough. They wished that their caregivers had helped them more than they had. As one woman pointed out,

> I think that they were helpful, but I think it was not enough for me. . . . Like when they had just moved me to sleep in another room, I still had pain in my stomach and other areas of my body. They did not come to take the baby for a bath and they didn't give milk for the baby and the baby was crying too. . . . I wanted them to take the baby for a bath. At that time if I weren't very tired than I would be able to do it myself. But I was very tired and that was why I didn't, but they didn't take the baby for a bath either. The baby was still covered in blood and those things from birth. It was almost night-time that they brought a small amount of water and gave the baby a bath at the bed. I pressed the thing and they came so I asked them to do so. They didn't wash him properly either.

Another woman made similar remarks. She did not have a difficult birth but lost a lot of blood after the delivery; she therefore felt quite weak and as if she were about to faint. However, her caregivers insisted that she give the baby a bath. The woman could understand what the nurse said but could not speak English well enough to explain to her that she needed help because she felt weak and faint. However, she did give the baby a bath.

Three women came across nurses who were rude and treated them badly during their stay. One woman had a caesarean birth and experienced great pain after the operation. She could not walk to the toilet because she was in pain and weak and could not see properly, and hence needed help from the hospital staff to physically support her. However, she was told that she could do it herself. When the woman tried to drag a chair to support her body to get to the bathroom, she was again told to stop making noise. Her worst experience with this nurse was when she could no longer tolerate the pain and called the nurse and asked for some pain relief. The nurse dissolved three tablets in a cup of water for her to take. After that, she experienced noise in her ears and she could not hear properly. She also felt dizzy and her head spinned. Fortunately, the shift was changed after three nights and the woman said that she had nicer staff looking after her for the rest of her hospital stay.

One Hmong woman mentioned that the nursing staff did look after her well. However, there was one aspect of care that she disliked: the nursing staff changed her sanitary pads for her. Her dislike was due mainly to the embarrassment over exposing her vagina to other people, as Hmong women are taught not to do in their culture. She related:

> I didn't like them to come and change these things [sanitary pads] for me or looked at my inside. I didn't like that because being a Hmong you are very embarrassed so if you have enough strength you did not want them to come to do it for you. I could do it myself . . . I felt that after we have given birth there should be nothing else and that if I was strong enough then I would like to do it myself. I didn't like them to come and looked on me too much and if they did come to see me I didn't like them to look at my vagina.

In the Hmong culture, a newborn infant must be kept near the mother. This is particularly true for the first three days before rituals for a newborn baby are performed. Traditionally, the newborn sleeps next to the mother so that she can observe and protect the baby from dangers both physical and supernatural. In the hospital, women placed their newborns on the bed with them. The nursing staff, however, did not allow this. One woman explained her experience:

> At the hospital when I slept I put the baby next to me on the bed. When the doctors came, the nurses came to have a look at the baby, they put the baby back in the cot. They said not to do that in case I fell asleep and the baby might fall out off the bed. . . . I didn't know what to say so I just let them lift the baby and later when they left and the baby cried I took the baby back again.

COMMUNICATION WITH CAREGIVERS

Cultural Issue: Caregivers' Lack of Cultural Knowledge

In the interviews, women were asked if they thought that their caregivers understood Hmong people and the Hmong way of life. All the women responded in the negative to this question. They believed that their caregivers did not have any knowledge about their cultural beliefs and practices, since the hospital staff never asked them about their cultural needs in childbirth. More importantly, some health professionals imposed their ethnocentric views on Hmong women. As mentioned earlier, one woman was told to have her tubes tied, because her caregiver believed that she had already had "too many children." This opinion stemmed from a Western cultural perspective on the number of children one should have.

When I suggested to women who made these comments that perhaps they could try to tell their caregivers about their cultural needs, most responses from the women were similar to the following:

> I think that the doctors and nurses do not understand our customs yet. I think that if they don't understand and if we try to explain to them they would not listen to us.

One woman who had had a caesarean birth related that her husband had asked her caregivers to let him be present in the operating room with her so that he could perform a Hmong ritual to prevent ill health after an operation. His request was refused. He felt that he could not explain the need for his presence to hospital staff, because they would not understand the Hmong way, and he also feared being seen as "too different."

Language Issue: The Women's Lack of English

Nearly all Hmong women had difficulty communicating with their caregivers. Only four young mothers who had been in Australia long enough to be competent in English could communicate with their caregivers effectively. Women found their lack of English frustrating, since they could not understand their caregivers and could not ask any questions or assert themselves. They felt anxious when they gave birth, because they could not understand what went on at the hospital. One woman elaborated:

> It was very difficult because at that time we had just arrived from Thailand and I could not understand what they were saying to me. I didn't know the language so if I was in pain I could not tell them that I was in pain. . . . At that time I worried about not speaking the language; what should I do. . . . I was very worried but then I gave birth to my baby at twelve [she had a quick labor].

Another woman found it rather difficult to communicate. She also believed that her caregivers did not communicate with her because of her lack of English.

> Very difficult, difficult in that sometimes there were some things that I didn't understand but because they knew that I didn't understand them they didn't say too many things to me either.

Similarly, another woman told me that:

> It was very difficult but I couldn't speak to them and they knew that I couldn't speak so they just didn't speak to me . . . because I didn't understand English . . . I couldn't speak so I didn't think much about it. When they tried to speak to me I just shook my head to let them know that I didn't understand them.

Women mentioned that an interpreter was provided during antenatal check-ups only. For some women, an interpreter was not available to them for all antenatal appointments either. However, all women mentioned that there were no interpreters provided during their labor and hospital stay and that this made it difficult for them to communicate with hospital staff.

> They [interpreters] only came when I had check-ups for the baby . . . but when I gave birth they didn't come anymore. They [staff] didn't call any and so no one came. I didn't know one word to say and couldn't read. . . . They knew that I didn't understand English so they didn't say anything to me . . . I couldn't speak to them. I felt sad that I couldn't speak to them, but I just didn't do anything about it.

Women had to rely on their husbands who could speak some English, but most relied on their young children. One woman said that she could not really communicate with hospital staff so she had to wait for her friends or husband to visit and they would help her if she needed to speak to the staff. When asked if they wished to have an interpreter to assist during labor and the hospital stay, most women said that they would like to have someone to help them at all stages of their childbearing process.

> I would like the help of an interpreter, but when I went in there [labor ward], there wasn't any one for me.

The Lack of Respect and Choice for Women

There is another important issue emerging from the women's narratives. Women mentioned that they were treated without respect and they did not have any choice in decision making. One example is the case of a woman who was confronted with eight medical students soon after she gave birth. She elaborated:

> In the [. . .] hospital where I had my youngest son, after thirty minutes of arriving I gave birth. After I gave birth a lot of them came in and gave me internal check up, using their hands scraping internally. All of them; there were eight of them. After that they told me to go to sleep in another room. I felt a lot of pain and the area [vagina] was swollen. . . . It was after the birth that they played around with me and I felt strongly that it was that tampering that caused all the pain.

The woman said that the staff did not explain to her what they intended to do, nor did they ask for her consent and permission. Since there were eight of them, she believed that they were all medical students who used her body for practice. Because of this experience, the woman resented having given birth in the hospital. She also insisted in the interview that I, as a researcher, should write to the hospital and inform the hospital staff not to do it again if she returned for her next birth.

Another example is the case of a woman who had an episiotomy performed during labor without her knowledge. The woman said that her caregivers did not tell her about the cut until it was performed and because she was under the gas mask she did not feel anything and, hence, did not know what happened. She had a fear of being cut during birth and felt that her caregivers did not think about her but only wanted their own way.

> I didn't want them to cut me but because I wasn't aware of it they did it. They gave an instrument that had air and it was noisy. They told me to breath hard and so I did it. The noise went on for a while and then I felt like I was unconscious. And I think that was when they did it and I wasn't aware of it. They cut it and the doctor told me that they had cut my flesh. . . . I was afraid of being cut. . . . The cut was quite big and swollen and was very painful. I could not sit down at all after the cut. . . . I was like that for about one month.

Another woman was persuaded to undergo caesarean section, and she believed strongly that the doctors wanted to use her body for medical instruction. Her main reason for thinking this was that she had previously given birth vaginally to her five children without any complications at all. Why was she suddenly told that she needed an operation with this child? She related:

> I wondered why because I had so many children already, why did they say this to me. . . . They said that even if I had many in the past with no problems and with this one there was no problems but just that it was in the wrong place and they did not let me have it normally. If I tried to have it by myself I could not. I think that the doctors wanted to perform a caesarean on me and use me for an experiment for students to learn from it.

The last case is that of a woman who experienced placental abruption and needed a caesarean section. She had to stay in the hospital a month. Although she believed that her caregivers tried to help Hmong people, she felt that she was coerced into following their ways. If she refused to follow their instructions she thought they might refuse to treat her later on. As she elaborated:

> It was good too they did help me a lot but they kept frightening me by saying that if I didn't undergo the operation then I would die. . . . They said that I should sleep there, and I must do what they said. They did not let me go home because if I came home and started to bleed then they couldn't help me. They insisted that I did what they felt and that was why I didn't like it there. . . . They said to stay in the hospital so that they could help me because if I came home then if the bleeding started then they could not help me and then I would die and the baby might die. If I came home then they would not help me and if the bleeding started then they would not help me because I didn't listen to them. So if I got sick and went to see them they would not help me as if I ran away from them because I didn't listen to them. This was what they said.

CONCLUSIONS

Although Hmong women feel satisfied in general with their childbirth experiences in Australian hospitals, they also report some difficulties with their caregivers and hospital routines. What contributes to these difficulties in the hospital? There are at least three important factors.

Firstly and largely, the difficulties arise from differences in cultural beliefs and expectations. From a social science perspective, it has been acknowledged that childbearing is not only a biological event but is also determined by the social and cultural environments within which it occurs.[4] In different societies, we therefore find different patterns of childbearing.

The childbearing patterns and expectations of Hmong women seem to differ from Western norms. The case of the Hmong woman who was told to have her tubes tied, for example, clearly shows that the Western doctor did not appreciate the value Hmong people place on having many children. Similarly, Hmong women customarily put their newborn infants on the bed with them but were not allowed to do so in the hospital. Although the women wish to protect their newborns by keeping the babies near them, this practice is seen by their caregivers as dangerous. Because of the different systems of cultural beliefs and practices, Hmong women have expectations about childbirth that conflict with those of their caregivers. This contributes to their difficulties when they have their babies in a new home.

The second difficulty faced by Hmong women is the lack of thorough and effective communication between health care professionals and these women. This is partly due to the women's lack of proficiency in English.[5] As previously mentioned, most Hmong women do not have enough English to communicate with their caregivers. Some have to rely on their husbands, who also cannot communicate effectively because of their limited English. However, the health caregivers' lack of information and clarification also contributes to misunderstanding and miscommunication. The case of the woman who believed that if she did not follow her caregivers' instructions she would not receive any help later on is an example of miscommunication. Is this actually what her caregivers said to her? Or was it because of some misunderstanding caused by an unfamiliar English expression? Or was it the lack of a clear explanation of the birthing process from health professionals? The woman received assistance from an interpreter at the time of consultation. What part did this three-way communication contribute to the woman's misunderstanding? In the study conducted by Small et al. (1999), it was found that communication is essential to providing good care to women of non-English-speaking backgrounds. Women not fluent in English had problems communicating with their caregivers and, hence, had less positive experiences of care than those who could speak better English. In addition, women in the study expressed their strong desire to be able to speak English so that they could themselves communicate with their caregivers. Hmong women in this study were no exceptions.

There is also the issue of the hospital staff's lack of information about Hmong customs and consequent offering of choices that contribute to Hmong women's difficulties when having their babies in Australia. This may be because childbirth has been medicalized in Western societies. Because of this, health professionals, particularly doctors, have become experts on childbirth, and their decisions are far more important than those of the women.[6] As has been shown, women feel that when a decision about their childbirth is made, they do not have a say or any choice. They are either not informed about birth procedures or are coerced into following their caregivers' instructions. Women feel that they have no control over their own bodies and resent hospital policy and practices. The woman who was persuaded to undergo a caesarean operation strongly believed that she was coerced.

What is important here is that it is too easy for health professionals to conclude that Hmong women do not wish to adapt to living situations in their new country and that that is why most of them maintain their traditions. Because of this misconception, conflicts arise between women and their caregivers. However, the results of this study indicate that very often, Hmong women have made it quite clear that they have tried to change their lifestyles in order to integrate into this society. In Thailand many women have home births and even though they wish to do so here, they still seek help from the hospital because they realize that this is the Australian norm. They, therefore, follow the norm.

Antenatal care is a good example. Women attend antenatal check-ups unless they have other commitments because they believe that this is what Australian women do. Similarly, although they have great concerns about the future of their own health because they have to abandon or modify many traditional customs in Australia, they do so because in this way they can adapt to living situations here. Although it may be true that some women feel strongly that they must maintain their traditions, this is primarily due to their desire to maintain their good health and the well-being of their newborn, not because they do not wish to adapt.[7]

What then are the implications of these findings? As most Hmong women and their families in this study still strictly adhere to their cultural beliefs and practices related to childbearing, I believe that knowledge and appreciation of Hmong cultural beliefs, expectations and social circumstances are essential for sensitive and culturally appropriate birthing care. This, however, does not mean that health care professionals need to have extensive training in cultural awareness or a "manual" to help them work with Hmong women more effectively. A simple approach is to ask individual women about their wishes and needs regarding traditional practices. Most often, if caregivers show the women genuine concern, women will inform them of their cultural needs during the childbearing process.

Secondly, contrary to the medical and psychological approaches that consider women in "universal terms, emphasizing common aspects of their experiences" (Woollett and Nicholson, 1998: 97), I argue from the feminist perspective (Oakley, 1979; Croghan, 1991; Raphael-Leff, 1991; Lazarus, 1994; Woollett and Nicholson, 1998) that women are diverse; hence, their experiences and circumstances vary. It is perhaps essential that health professionals ask a woman about her individual needs during the childbearing processes. This may also help to avoid a stereotyped assumption about Hmong women.

Lastly, by adopting a feminist perspective, I argue that women should be offered a choice about their childbirth (Rothman, 1984, 1991; Lazarus, 1994; Yelland et al., 1998; Rice et al., 1999; Small et al., 1999). Women should not be coerced into the health professional's decision about their care, but make their own choices. Their voices need to be heard and met if sensitive care is to be provided. This will lead to greater satisfaction with care among Hmong women. It may also make childbearing a more pleasurable and less frightening experience for Hmong women in their new homeland.

Only by taking these issues into account can culturally sensitive care be achieved in birthing service. As Lefkarites (1992: 410) has said, "It is respectful of cultural diversity and supportive of policies that are truly concerned with a healthier outcome for mother, baby, and other significant family members." And as Lazarus (1990) has insisted, good care significantly affects women's well-being. If Hmong women are to be motivated to return the next time they are pregnant, the need for change must be addressed by maternity hospitals.

NOTES

1. Woollett et al. (1995), for example, compared the ideas and experiences of pregnancy and birth among Asian and non-Asian women in East London. They found that Asian women's attitudes and experiences of pregnancy and childbirth were still influenced by cultural beliefs and practices. However, they also found that Asian women had a strong commitment to Western maternity care. Thus, their traditional beliefs and practices were modified to some extent in order to adapt to new living situations. In Australia, Rice et al. (1999) found that Thai women now living in Australia were generally satisfied with the postpartum care provided for them. There were, however, problems that resulted from their inability to follow Thai traditional confinement practices in hospitals. Because of this restriction, several women decided to go home early. Traditionally, there are several customs a new mother must observe to maintain good health and avoid future ill health. Most women were aware of these cultural beliefs and practices. However, not all of them could follow these customs because of changes in their social situations. Small et al.'s study (1999) examined childbearing experiences of Filipino, Turkish and Vietnamese women, and found that many women still adhered to their traditional practices. Women were less concerned that caregivers had little knowledge about their cultural practices than they were about the care they did receive, particularly if caregivers were unkind, rushed or unsupportive. In addition, women not fluent in English experienced problems in communicating with their caregivers. These led to less positive experiences of care among these groups of women.

2. In the past decade, since the resettlement of Hmong in the United States and other Western countries, including Australia, a number of papers have been written about their childbirth experiences. In the United States, Potter and Whiren (1982) examined Hmong birth from a historical perspective. Their data was collected from one Hmong couple and a medicine woman in a mid-western U.S.

city. Faller (1985) described perinatal needs of Hmong women in the Denver and Boulder areas. Scheinberg (1983) examined interactions around childbirth of Hmong women with their health care providers in California. Nyce and Hollinshead (1984) discussed reproductive beliefs and practices of the Hmong using existing literature as their source. These four studies were, however, conducted more than a decade ago. In her paper, Faller (1992) attempted to examine the characteristics and birth outcomes of Hmong women in a small town in the southeastern United States. A limitation of this study was that it was based mainly on the opinion of health care professionals. Only one Hmong woman, who had been in the United States since she was five, was interviewed. None of these studies examined women's experiences with childbirth in great depth. Edwards et al. (1987) and Helsel et al. (1992) examined characteristics of pregnancy and birth outcomes of Hmong mothers and babies in St. Paul, Merced, and San Joaquin. Their study utilized perinatal statistics and, hence, did not represent Hmong women's opinions and feelings about their childbirth experiences. More recently, however, Jambunathan and Stewart (1995) employed a qualitative method and looked at issues surrounding pregnancy and childbirth among Hmong women in Wisconsin. Their study focused on breastfeeding, contraception, touch, communication with health caregivers and procedures performed during birth. Only a few papers have examined traditional and changed patterns of childbirth among Hmong women in Australia (Rice, 1994, 1997), and a case study discussed the experience of a Hmong woman who underwent caesarean section (Rice et al., 1994).

3. I have discussed the role of Hmong husbands in birthing in Chapter 5 of this volume.

4. See, for example, Jordan, 1978; Romalis, 1981; Lefkarites, 1992; Raphael-Leff, 1991; and Rice and Manderson, 1996.

5. Similar problems have been documented by several social researchers with other groups of immigrant women. See for example, Homans, 1982; Woollett and Dosanjh-Matwala, 1990; Rice, 1993, 1994; Yelland et al., 1998; and Small et al., 1999.

6. These issues have been found to exist even among women from Western backgrounds. See Oakley, 1986; Martin, 1987; Romalis, 1981; Rothman, 1984, 1991; and Lazarus, 1994, for example.

7. This is also clearly indicated in Jambunathan and Stewart's study among Hmong women in Wisconsin (1995), and in the studies of Dobson (1988) and Woollett et al. (1995) among Indian women in England.

Part Three

Women and Child Rearing

Chapter 8

Child Rearing and Infant Care

Come to your new mother, father, brother, sister, and relatives.
Come to live to a rightful old age.
If following a hard path then may there be a metal shield to protect you.
And if going on a hard way then may there be a metal shield to protect you.

A blessing to a newborn infant given by a Hmong grandmother

INTRODUCTION

It has been evident from social science research that child rearing practices in any society occur in accordance with the social environment and cultural norms of the society. In most societies, however, child rearing practices share a common value: the preservation of life and maintenance of the health and well-being of a newborn infant.[1] Child rearing in Hmong culture is no exception.

However, what may happen when people have to resettle in another society? An important question that needs to be looked at is whether they are able to continue their traditional practices or whether they have to abandon or to modify them. The latter two practices are largely unknown among Australian immigrants. A study by Rice and Naksook (1998) of Thai mothers in Australia showed that most Thai mothers continued to follow Thai cultural beliefs and practices. The most common reason given among Thai mothers for such cultural continuity was their fear of the death of their newborn infants, in particular death from Sudden Infant Death Syndrome (SIDS). Will the need to save the lives of children be applicable to Hmong mothers who need children to continue Hmong society? This chapter examines this issue in great detail.

In this chapter, I discuss child rearing beliefs and practices and their relation to child health in Hmong culture. I focus in particular on both traditional and changed patterns of beliefs and practices related to the care of a newborn infant among the Hmong now living in Australia.

BIRTH DATE AND TIME

The Hmong seriously take into account the date and time of birth of their newborn infants. It is believed that a child must be born on a "right" day if he or she is to have good health and a good future. A girl should be born on an even day and a boy on an odd day.[2] One Hmong woman explained:

> If the baby is born on the sixth or eight day then it must be a girl, and if ninth or eleventh day then it must be a boy.

In Hmong culture, days occur according to a lunar cycle. The Hmong count their calendar by starting with an odd day (Day 1) followed by an even day (Day 2) and continue with Day 3, Day 4, and so on, until Day 29 or Day 30. The cycle then starts again, on Day 1 of the next month.[3] The Hmong believe that children born on a "wrong" day will be sickly and will not grow properly.

> If the baby girl comes on the even day, she will always be healthy, and if the baby girl comes on the odd day, she will always be sick. But if the boy comes on the even day then he will always be sick. . . . So the dates are important [for the health of infants].

The Hmong also refer the birth date of a child to animal days. Twelve animals represent certain dates in the lunar month. Similar to odd and even days, each animal day has its own meaning. Some animal days are good days on which to be born, but not others. One woman elaborated:

> We take notice of the day to see if it is an odd day or an even day and to see what kind of animal day it is . . . so if the baby is born on the day of a good animal then the baby will grow up with good health and not become sick so often. But if the baby is born on the animal day that is not good then the baby will always be sick and unhealthy. The old people say that if the baby is born on a cow day or an elephant day the baby will be good in education. And if the baby is born on a dragon or a rainbow day then

> when he grows up he will have good fortune making profits from a business. . . . Also the baby will grow well and be healthy. . . . But if the baby is born on a chicken or a pig day, he will be sick often and not grow well.

Time of birth is also important. The Hmong believe that is either early in the morning or from late in the afternoon through the evening are good times. Children who are born during these periods will have good health and a good future. One Hmong woman explained:

> For children, the time of birth is important. When the baby is born, for example, in the morning, at about 7 to 9, it is a good time to be born; if 11 or 12 to 2 o'clock, it is not good. But, between 4 to 9 in the evening, it is also good. Between 11 to 2 is not good because that child is said to be born late. This means that other babies would have taken all the good papers [mandate of life] for prosperity on earth and other good things [from heaven] . . . so if the child is born between 11 to 2, he will be left with only the bad papers. When the child comes to live on earth he will not be able to achieve much, and his life will not be good. But if the child is born between 4 in the evening to 9 at night, it is good . . . because in the evening and at night new documents [from heaven] have already been set for the next day.

There is no way in which the parents can choose the date of birth, since this is determined by the spirit parents who send children to be born in this world. However, there is a ritual that can help to counteract the wrong birth date. In this case, a shaman will perform *ua neeb*, which will involve the spirit parents, and ask them to bless the newborn child with a good future. This will prevent ill health and misfortune for the newborn.

> The old people say that if the baby is born on the wrong day then they must *ua neeb* or name the baby to suit the date of birth and this will be able to protect the baby.

These beliefs and practices continue to be practiced even with children who were born in Australian hospitals. At least one family member, most often the father, will take note of the birth date and time of the newborn. If the baby has been born on a wrong day, a ritual will be performed by a shaman upon returning home, usually on the second day or early on the third morning.

NECKLACE, HEALTH AND LIFE

After birth, before the umbilical cord is cut, the Hmong will put a silver necklace around the newborn infant's neck (Photo 8.1).

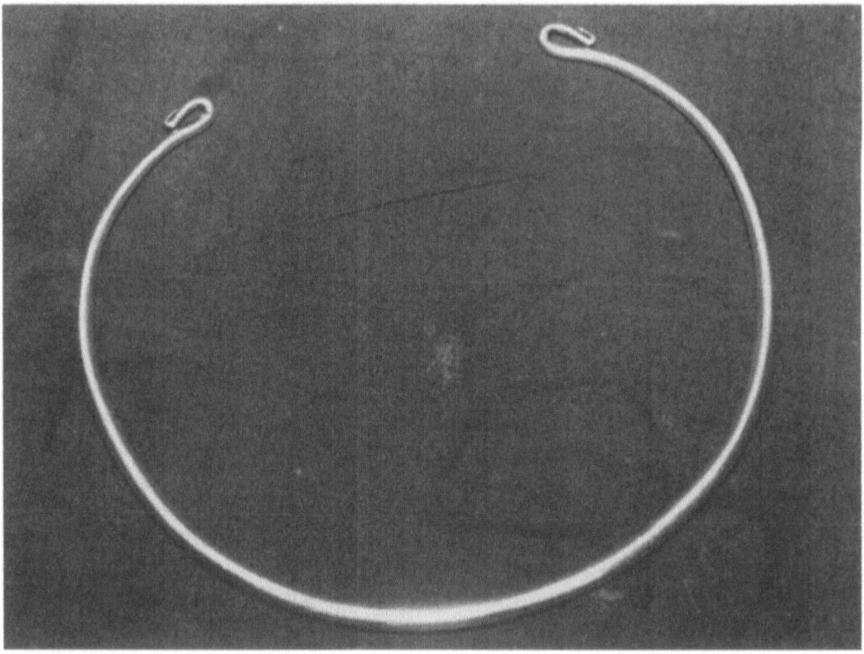

Photo 8.1 A silver necklace placed on a newborn infant and young child for protection.

> In Laos you have to make a tiny spiritual necklace and when the baby is born you put the necklace on before you cut off the umbilical cord.

According to the Hmong way, this ritual has two main functions. First, it is meant to protect the newborn infant from spirits who may wish to take the infant with them, meaning that the infant may die soon after birth. Babies still inside the womb will usually be protected by their mothers via the umbilical cord. The infant may be struck by spirits at this stage, but only if the mother acts in a way that may provoke them to strike, such as crossing rivers or wandering into a dense forest during late pregnancy. To prevent the baby from being struck and taken away by the spirits, a Hmong mother will use a necklace as a symbol of the connection between the baby and her body (womb), and as a claim that the newborn belongs to her.

> As soon as the baby is born you put it on straight away. If you were poor then you would still get a piece of string and tie it around the baby and saying, "this baby is mine." So if there are spirits around then they can't take it. . . . If you don't put that around the baby then they won't know that the baby belongs to someone else. And if they are around they will be able to take the baby. This is why the Hmong have to do this.

Secondly, the necklace is used as a symbolic mechanism for tying the infant's soul to his or her body. It was commonly mentioned by the study's informants that a person has three souls. The first soul enters their bodies at conception. The second soul comes when babies take their first breath. To secure this soul, a necklace must be put on the infant's neck, as one Hmong woman explained:

> When you give birth you have to put this one [necklace] around the baby's neck. . . . You put it on first, before you cut the cord. . . . The elders say that it is something to do with his life . . . it is to tie for his life. . . . As soon as the child is born you have to tie the child with the necklace before the cord is cut. . . . The necklace is worn so the baby's soul will be secured. It is to lock the soul with the child.

The third soul, however, will not enter the baby's body until it is called on the third morning after birth. This ritual will be discussed later in this chapter.

Although Hmong mothers still practice the necklace ritual in Australia, most women felt that they were unable to put the necklace on the newborn soon after birth. Since all of them gave birth in hospitals, a midwife or, occasionally, a doctor delivered their babies, and they felt that they could not ask the midwife or the doctor to put the necklace on the infant for them. The main reason they gave for their reluctance was that they believed it would not be permitted, since such a practice is different from the way people do things in Australia, and they might be seen as being different or odd. However, most mothers brought the necklace with them and they would put it on the infant as soon as they had the opportunity, most often when they had settled into a maternity ward and none of the hospital staff members were in sight.

> After birth, they took us to sleep in a room, but I can't remember what time when I put it [a necklace] on . . . not long after he was born. . . . They cut it [the umbilical cord] before I put it on him. I didn't ask them and also the bag that I brought with me was outside with my husband. So when the baby was born they have already cut it [the umbilical cord].

THE "JACKET": PLACENTA AND THE CHILD

In Hmong culture the placenta is perceived as an important part of a person's life and well-being. It is referred to as the child's "jacket," which he or she must spiritually wear upon his or her death in order to enter the ancestral pool, a place where dead family members stay together awaiting rebirth. The placenta is buried inside the house where the child was born.[4] One woman gave the following account:

> We have to bury the placenta so the baby knows where to look for his jacket and so when he goes back to heaven he can bring it with him so that he can be reincarnated to be another person again.

If it is a boy, his placenta is buried near *ncej cuab*, the middle post of the house, which is perceived as the most important part of the Hmong house. It is where the *dab qhaus* resides and where all important Hmong rituals must be performed. The girl's placenta, however, is buried under the birth bed.

> A Hmong house has three poles for support. They are all parallel to each other. The two on the sides are just supportive but the one in the center is the *ncej cuab*. So if a boy then your bury it at the middle one. The boy's placenta is buried at the *ncej cuab* so that the *dab qhuas* will recognise that there is an addition to the clan. If it is a girl, she is not important in the same sense, so her one can be buried under the bed.

This tradition seems to present a problem for the Hmong in Australia. Because they give birth in hospitals, they cannot bury the placenta within the place of birth as was their original tradition. Many Hmong women are anxious about what will happen in their child's future. One said:

> I am worried about it. Throughout our lives we bury the placenta at the middle post or under the bed so that after when the children are old and die they can come back and find it. But when we come to this country what they do with it we don't know. That is why I am worried.

The Hmong realize that it is no longer feasible for them to bury the placenta inside the house, because they live in a high-rise flat or in a house with a concrete floor. They therefore prefer to have it buried inside the hospital where they give birth. When they are told that they can ask to take the placenta home, one woman said:

> Bringing it home I would not be able to do anything with it. Because I live in a flat, I really cannot do that [to bury], but if I live in a ground house then I would like to take the placenta home and bury it there.

PRAISING THE NEWBORN AND SPIRITS

In the first month of life, the newborn infant is seen as vulnerable to spirits. Because they are malicious, evil spirits are particularly feared by those who have a new baby. Ancestral spirits, however, are generally protective, and usually look after family members. However, they too can be dangerous to a newborn infant, particularly when they hear that the baby is beautiful and good. The Hmong say that living people want a nice and good baby, and that spirits want the same thing. Hence, if they hear people praise the baby, the spirits will pay more attention to it. And if they believe that the newborn is beautiful and good, they may wish to have the baby, which means that the newborn will die. Evil spirits may also wish to have the baby if they hear that it is beautiful. This belief has led the Hmong not to praise a newborn infant, particularly in the first month of life. One woman explained:

> Never say thing like "Oh your baby is beautiful." The spirit will like the child because the human likes the child. If the baby is beautiful then you have to say, "Oh why is your baby so ugly." That will make you happy but if they say, "Oh why is your baby so beautiful or handsome," then you start to worry . . . get upset and feel frightened about this.

And another one remarked:

> It depends on the parents. There are some that don't like to say good things like lovable that sort of thing. Not to say this because then the living will like and spirit will like the baby, so they don't say things like that. . . . If the spirit like the child then the child will get sick. If that happens and if you don't know then the spirit might be able to get to the child and the child will die. That is why we don't say words like those.

On the contrary, they may try to say the opposite thing, such as "The baby is ugly." This is to persuade the spirits not to take the baby with them. The same woman continued by saying:

> So the way is to say the opposite things, like the baby smells like *quav* [excrement], the baby is ugly. . . . For some when the baby is lovable, they say the baby smells like *quav* so that the spirit will also say well it smells like *quav*, and it will not like the baby. So the baby will not have bad health.

The Hmong continue this practice in Australia. However, they often come across health professionals who tend to praise the newborn infant. Many women mentioned that they felt somewhat anxious about this because of their traditional beliefs. Others felt indifferent, they believe that this is a common custom in Australia, which they should also accept. A few women believed that there are no spirits in Australia who can harm a newborn. Hence, the praising did not really bother them. On the contrary, these women felt that the praise was a good thing because it showed that some health professionals admired their newborn infants.

HMONG PROHIBITION: TAKING THE NEWBORN OUT DURING THE FIRST 30 DAYS

Because the Hmong in their original homeland are extremely anxious about evil spirits outside the home who may harm their newborn infant, it is common practice not to take an infant outside during the first month of life. It is believed that the newborn still has a "milky" smell from his or her body, and that this will attract the spirits, who may want to take the baby with them. New Hmong mothers also stay inside for the whole month after giving birth. Although they may step outside the house for a short period to do what is necessary, they are not permitted to take the baby out with them.

> You have to stay indoors for one month before you take the baby outside. . . . The old people do not let them go outside. If you take the baby outside then the spirit may catch the baby, and when you come home the baby will cry a lot. That is why they don't let the baby go outside.

In Australia, it is impractical not to take the newborn out within this first month. All Hmong women gave birth in hospitals and therefore had to travel from hospital to home, which meant that they had to take the baby outside. However, most mothers mentioned that they wrapped up the newborn carefully, quickly got into the car and, again, quickly entered their homes. They felt that this might prevent the baby being seen by evil spirits outside.

> You have to go outside [coming home] so you go out and go straight into the car, out from the hospital. Your husband would drive the car to the front [of the building], and then you come out and get into the car. And when you get home, you get out of the car and straight into the house. Because it is very quick so it might be ok.

Another important aspect of Australian health care is the requirement that a mother bring her newborn to a Maternal and Child Health Center for examination. Upon returning home, usually after the first week, a maternal and child health (MCH) nurse may visit the new mother and infant and then an appointment is made for the mother to bring her infant to the center. This presents some problems for Hmong mothers because of their belief that the newborn should not be taken outside. However, nearly all Hmong women in this study were fortunate enough to have a MCH nurse visit them at home. Most Hmong live in a close-knit group, concentrated in one suburb in the inner city. It therefore was not too much trouble for the nurse to pay Hmong mothers a visit. In addition, the nurse was knowledgeable about Hmong practices, and she believed it would help Hmong mothers a great deal if she visited them at home rather than getting them to travel to the center.

SLEEPING ARRANGEMENTS

In the Hmong culture, a newborn infant must be kept near the mother from birth until the first month passes. Infants continue to sleep with their parents until another child is born. Most continue to sleep on the same bed until they are old enough to move and sleep with other siblings. This may mean that the child might be about 4 to 6 years of age or even older in some families before he or she moves from the parents' bed.

> With Hmong people, because the baby is breastfed, so the baby sleeps with you . . . sleep until you have a younger one then you move the older one away and put the baby where the older one has been sleeping.

A newborn infant sleeps with his or her mother throughout the night. The Hmong say that keeping a newborn infant with the mother is a Hmong tradition that people have followed for centuries. One woman explained:

> We, for generations, we have the baby sleeping with us, on the same bed. . . . The Hmong do not do the same as what people do in this country when they leave the baby to sleep by him or herself. We have always practiced this so that is why we let the baby sleep with us.

Hmong mothers also believe that a newborn infant needs warmth from the mother's body during this period. Mothers will wrap the infant tightly to keep the infant warm and to prevent crying.

> When the baby is very young like one or two days, because the baby just came out from your womb, you need to wrap him up. If you don't wrap the baby then the baby will be cold and cry a lot and he cannot sleep.

Hmong mothers tend to breastfeed their infants, and co-sleeping makes it easier for them to do so.

> Because the baby is breastfed, if you put the baby to sleep by himself when the baby cries you have to get up and sit to feed him. You should put the baby to sleep next to you so that the baby is warm and make feeding easier too.

However, most mothers mention that the main reason they put their babies next to them is because they are worried about the baby's safety.

Keeping their babies near them enables them to observe and protect their babies from dangers. One woman related:

> I feel that the baby is still very small and I don't feel like leaving the baby to sleep on his own. I want him to sleep with me. . . . Maybe if the baby cries, I cannot hear him. And if the baby is sick then I know. If the baby wants a drink [breast milk] or cries or wants me for some comfort then he cannot find me if he is in another room.

Another explained:

> The baby sleeps with me all night. . . . The baby has to sleep with you because the baby is still too young and so that you can hear the baby when the baby cries or if the baby vomits or gets sick.

This practice continues in Australia and has presented no problems for Hmong women at home. However, a few women mentioned that they had some trouble with this practice during their hospital stay. When these women placed their newborns on the bed with them, the nursing staff did not allow them to keep them there. One woman explained her experience.

> At the hospital when I slept I put the baby next to me on the bed. When the doctors and the nurses came to have a look at the baby, they put the baby back in the cot. They said not to do that in case I felt asleep and the baby might fall out off the bed. . . . I didn't know what to say so I just let them lift the baby and later when they left and the baby cried I took the baby back again.

RITUAL FOR A NEWBORN: *HU PLIG* AND NAMING CEREMONIES

In Hmong culture, it is essential to perform an important ritual for a newborn infant known as a soul-calling ceremony. The Hmong believe that each living person has three souls, and newborn infant is no exception. As previously mentioned, the first soul enters his or her body when the child is conceived in the mother's womb. The second soul enters when the baby has just emerged from the mother's body and taken its first breath. The third soul, however, will have to be called on the third morning after birth. If all three souls are secured in the infant's body, he or she will be healthy and will thrive. By contrast, the infant may become ill and eventually die if all souls do not reside in his or her body.

> You do this [*hu plig*] so that the baby's soul will come to stay with him and so that the baby is happy and thus the soul is happy too. The soul

will come to stay with the baby and the baby will be healthy. This is traditional Hmong belief.

Hu Plig: A Soul-Calling Ceremony and Life

> With the Hmong, when they give birth to a child they *hu plig* to give a name and to perform a custom to inform the *dab qhuas* for the baby so that the baby will grow well. . . . Every child must have this. . . . If we don't *hu plig* for the baby then the baby will not grow at all and is very tiny. Sometimes it is not that the baby will be sick all the time, but the baby will not grow and stays very tiny.

The *Hu plig* ceremony is traditionally performed on the third morning after birth.[5] The ceremony starts at dawn, before sunrise, and continues until noon when a blessing is given to the new baby and his or her parents and the feast is offered to guests and relatives. The soul-calling ceremony is usually performed by an old person who is knowledgeable about the ritual. Very often, a grandfather is the one who undertakes this task. However, a shaman is often called to perform the ceremony, because most shamans are skillful in healing rituals and other ceremonies, including the calling of a soul.[6]

At dawn, a shaman begins the ritual at the front door of the family home. The shaman will first perform a naming ceremony for the newborn infant. The Hmong believe that the name of the baby represents his or her soul. If a wrong name is given to the child, it means that the soul of the child is not called. The right name has to be chosen. This may require that a naming ceremony take place several times before the right name is selected for the soul of the child. The correct name to give to the child is determined by tossing a pair of buffalo horns on the floor. The position of the horns when they land will indicate the name chosen for the baby.[7] One Hmong woman related:

> On the third morning we make a shirt for the baby and use four chickens in the ceremony. Two chickens to *hu plig* and one for the baby's guardian spirits from heaven and another one for the spirit of the household so that it is informed that there is an addition to the family. Then you choose any name that you like for the child and if the child likes that name then the *kuam* [instrument used in the ritual] will land in the right position. If the *kuam* does not land in the right position then you must find another name for the child.

Naming is essential for the well-being and growth of Hmong infants. If a wrong name is given to the child, he or she may or will become ill often and will not grow properly. The child will also cry very often. As one Hmong woman related:

> We the parents have to choose the name. You have to give that name to the baby and if the baby does not like that name then it will be tiny and will not grow well and also will get sick often.

Another Hmong woman explained:

> After you have chosen that name for the baby and the baby has good health and grows well then you know that the baby likes the name. . . . If the baby is ill often then you choose a different name for the baby and you have to *hu plig* again. So it is a long process.

When the right name has been chosen for the baby, a soul-calling ceremony is performed later on that morning. Again, the shaman will stand at the door of the house and commence a soul-calling chant. With this ritual, the name of the baby is called to represent the soul of the baby. This ritual is performed so that the third soul of the infant will come to reside and be secured in his or her body. In the chant, there are words that will instruct the soul about his or her home, family and siblings. The chant also tells the soul of the child that his or her family wishes to welcome him or her and promises that he or she will be looked after well by the family. The Hmong believe that without this promise, the soul of the child may not be satisfied and, hence, will not come to reside in the baby's body. As a Hmong shaman said:

> When the baby is born, on the third day, you have to give it a name, whether it is Li or Mo. And then you say to the soul, "Come, you have to come and stay, your name is this and so you must come to live in your new home. . . . Yes, come to live with your parents and do not feel sorry. You have parents and family to take care of you now so you must come to live with your parents, brothers and sisters."

Thanking the Spirit Parents: Harmony with the Supernatural Beings

The Hmong believe that children are sent from heaven with the permission of *Txoov Kab Yeeb* (the spirit parents), who are responsible for the birth of all Hmong people. Without the permission of *Txoov Kab Yeeb*, a child cannot be born. Therefore, when a child is born and survives to the third day, a ritual to pay gratitude to the spirit parents must be performed. It is believed that if this is not done, the child may cry excessively, will not feed and hence will not grow. One Hmong woman explained:

> Because this couple has sent the baby to you so you must do that [conduct a thanking ceremony for the spirit parents]. If not then the baby will cry a lot and will not feed and will not grow well either.

After the naming and soul-calling ceremony has been performed, the shaman will commence a chanting on behalf of the family to pay respect and offer gratitude for bringing the child into the family to the spirit parents.

> When you have a new baby, on the third morning, you have to *hu plig* to call the baby's soul and you have to *fiv* [citing of words to thank] *Kab Yeeb*, it is to thank *Txoov Kab Yeeb* that they have brought the baby to you. There are two parents; that is why you *fiv* them with two chickens. When you *fiv*, you call out *Txoov Kab Yeeb*. The couple is responsible for bringing the baby to you and you are very thankful to them.

After citing words of thanks, the shaman will then offer some food to the spirits. In addition, some incense sticks and gold paper monies are offered to the spirit parents. This is, again, a symbol of gratitude for sending children into the Hmong society.

> When the old people do it, they cite some words called *khawv koob*. . . . You prepare some chickens for them and you give the incenses and gold paper for them by burning them so that they will be happy. It is like making them a thank you lunch.

The Blessing and the Feast: Social Support and Cohesion

At noon, after the soul-calling and naming ceremonies are performed, a big feast begins. Those who have helped with the ceremony, relatives and friends are called to join in the feast. While the soul-calling and naming ceremonies are being performed, men gather together to prepare the meat. After this is completed, the women cook dishes for the feast.

The blessing is performed prior to the feast. When all the dishes have been set on the table, senior members of the community will sit at the table while those who are junior will stand on one side of the room. One senior member, often the shaman who performs the soul-calling ritual, will start making a blessing for the couple and their newborn. Next, the shaman performs a thread-tying ritual (*khi hlaus*) by tying the wrist of the baby with white cotton threads and blesses it for good health and a good future (Photo 8.2).[8] The shaman then ties the cotton threads on the wrists of the parents. If the newborn has siblings, all of them will also be tied with the cotton threads. Tying of the cotton threads is seen as connecting a newborn infant to his or her family. As one Hmong woman explained:

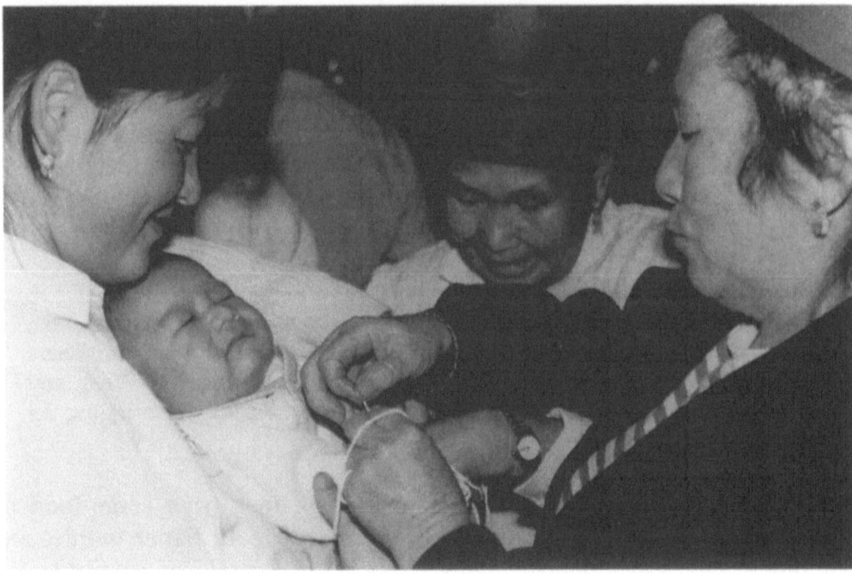

Photo 8.2 *Hu plig* ceremony for a newborn infant.

> Tying the string is like tying the baby with the parents. It the baby has siblings then it is done too. Tying with the parents signifies that he has a family to come to live with now.

The white cotton threads are then distributed to family members and others attending the ceremony. As the shaman does, they also tie threads on the baby's wrist as well as the parents' wrists and they receive the blessing from all guests. In addition, all family members and guests place some bank notes on a tray carried by the father, or in his palm, after tying the threads. Once these rituals are completed, the feast begins.

The feast represents the strong social cohesion and support within Hmong society. It is not only family members and relatives who are called to join the ceremony and the feast—friends, neighbors and other acquaintances are also invited. In fact, almost everyone in the neighborhood may be invited. As mentioned, during the blessing process, when white cotton threads are being tied on the baby's and parents' wrists, some bank notes will also be given to the parents. This is to help out with the expenses of the ceremony and the feast. The feast also acts as a public announcement, informing the community that there is a new member coming to live in the family and, hence, the community's continued existence is also supported.

This soul-calling tradition has been continued in Australia. All Hmong women mentioned that they had a soul-calling ceremony performed for their babies, even those who were born here. When I asked if all Hmong would do this, the following answer was commonly given:

> You have to *hu plig* so that you have to give the baby a name . . . and to call the baby's soul to come and live with you. . . . We have always done this. I have never seen anyone not doing this; they have always done it.

However, because of changes in their living situations in Australia, some Hmong families cannot have a soul-calling ceremony performed on the third morning after birth. Most select a convenient time to suit as many family members and relatives as possible. This may mean that some soul-calling rituals are performed in the first week and others may be done at one month, when the mother has finished her confinement practices. However, many of the families want to have the ceremony performed as early as possible. I have recently participated in the soul-calling ceremony of an infant who was four days old.

CONCLUSIONS

Hmong mothers and their families have tried to continue to adhere to their cultural beliefs and practices despite living in a new environment. Most Hmong women have managed to follow their traditions, but they have had to change some aspects of the traditions or adapt them to new living situations (such as putting a necklace on after an umbilical cord is cut, burying the placenta away from the birthplace and changes in feeding practices).

Why have the Hmong sought to continue their cultural beliefs and practices despite the change in their living environment produced by moving to Australia? The answer is clear from the study interviews: Hmong mothers and their families wish to preserve the lives of their newborn infants and maintain their good health and well-being for the rest of their lives so that Hmong society can continue to exist. Although children are important and essential in any society because they are its future, they are even more important in Hmong culture, since they are the ones who will look after their parents in old age when they are no longer able to fend for themselves. This has been an essential aspect of Hmong society, in which there are no government benefits to take care of old, aged persons. It is perceived as even more important for the Hmong in Australia now, since most of them are unemployed because of their lack of education and language proficiency. Many parents expressed their concerns that future old age pensions in Australia would not be sufficient for them to survive. They believed that they might suffer without the support of their children when they are old.

Most important, however, as I will also discuss in later chapters, children are the ones who will continue the family, lineage and clan, and this means the continuity of the Hmong society. This is very important to the Hmong, who have lost so many lives through wars and harsh living conditions in Laos and who have to re-establish their society in a new country like Australia.

Some of the traditional beliefs and practices of the Hmong are practical, but many of practices may appear somewhat bizarre to most Western health professionals. Hmong beliefs and practices may be easily seen as "superstitions." For the Hmong, however, these beliefs and practices fall within their religion and, hence, are logical and real to believers. Additionally, because they have followed these traditions for centuries, Hmong people do not see them as superstitions but as traditions that provide them with meaning and a sense of coherence. This is essential for immigrants such as the Hmong, who have to establish themselves in a new society that is quite foreign to many of them.

More important, however, some Hmong cultural beliefs and practices may be seen as "undesirable" from the point of view of Western health professionals. Sleeping arrangements, for example, are interesting. For health professionals who work in the Sudden Infant Death Syndrome (SIDS) area, bed sharing and overheating are seen as risk factors (Watson et al., 1998). Hence, wrapping up the babies tightly with blankets and placing them near the mother for the whole night, common practices among the Hmong, may be construed as harmful for the infant. For the Hmong, however, these practices are seen as protective factors. Since newborn infants need warmth and security, wrapping them up and putting them to sleep near their mothers are regarded as essential for their health and well-being.

If Western health professionals examine these issues from the Hmong perspective, Hmong cultural beliefs and practices may in fact not be harmful at all. As McKenna (1998) has pointed out, one can believe that cultural practices may have some protective mechanisms that help to prevent the death of a newborn infant. His hypothesis is also supported by several social science studies that have shown that cultural beliefs and practices and environmental factors may act as preventive mechanisms against the incidence of child death, particularly from SIDS, in different societies.[9]

NOTES

1. See, for example, Rice and Naksook, 1988; Scheper-Hughes, 1991, 1992; Castle, 1994; Green et al., 1994; and Gethin and Macgregor, 1998.
2. See Chapter 1 and Chindasri (1976) for more details of the Hmong calendar.

3. See also Kunstadter et al. (1987) about similar beliefs concerning odd and even birth dates among Hmong in the north of Thailand.

4. In Hmong villages in Laos and Thailand, a house is built on the dirt floor. See also Chapter 1 for details of a Hmong house.

5. Only the Yang clan may have it performed on the second morning. Most elder Hmong say that after the birth three days must pass before it is the right time to call a soul. The explanation given is that this is a traditional Hmong practice that has been performed from the beginnings of Hmong society and followed for centuries.

6. See also Symonds (1991, 1996) for thorough detailing of a soul-calling ceremony for a newborn infant in a Hmong village in Thailand.

7. See Cooper et al. (1996) for details of *kaum* and messages from these divination horns. This is a common method a shaman will use to perform all sorts of divinations, not only soul-calling and naming ceremonies for a newborn infant.

8. Cooper et al. (1995) have commented that the ritual of *khi hlaus* is frequently performed on other occasions as well. When a person is setting off for a long journey, and when a family has to be parted, *khi hlaus* must be performed to bless for a safe journey. In addition, when the souls of a particular family have wandered in different directions, a shaman will perform *khi hlaus* to "bind the soul more firmly to the household and prevent future 'discord' between them" (p. 61).

9. See Davies, 1985; Oden, 1986; Lee et al., 1989; Gantley et al., 1993; Nelson, 1997; and Watson et al., 1998, for example.

Chapter 9

Beliefs about Breast Milk and Infant Feeding Practices

Breastmilk holds a singular place in the human imagination.
(Mull, 1992: 1277)

For as long as there are children, breastfeeding will occupy a central, irreplaceable position in their survival, development, and well-being, in the rights of mothers, in the stability of families, and even in the economy of nations and in the defense of a clean and safe environment.
Dr. Richard Jolly, Acting Executive Director, UNICEF,
(in Baumslag and Michels, 1995: xv)

INTRODUCTION

In most societies breast milk is taken seriously "as a means of nurturance crucial to infant well-being." However, ideas about breast milk may vary from culture to culture. Beliefs about colostrum are particularly varied. According to the medical view colostrum is beneficial, because it contains antiinfective and immunological properties (Morse et al., 1990; Baumslag and Michels, 1995). However, in many cultures throughout the world, colostrum is believed to be of no value or harmful to a newborn infant.[1]

Closely associated with colostrum is the initiation of feeding, which differs among different societies. In Western societies, most health educators encourage mothers to breastfeed their newborn infants as soon as possible. However, in many cultures breastfeeding is delayed until the "real" milk appears. This usually happens on the third day or as late as the fourth day following birth.[2] Despite this delay, women in traditional societies can breastfeed successfully and often breastfeed for a long period of time (Van Esterik, 1985).

Perceptions of the quality of breast milk can also vary from culture to culture. Mothers in some cultures may question if their milk is "good" enough for their infants despite their having an abundance of it (Morse et al., 1990; Baumslag and Michels, 1995). In addition, mothers may believe that their breast milk can be affected by other physical and supernatural beings.[3]

Cultural beliefs and practices relating to breast milk and breastfeeding need to be examined within the social and cultural context of the society so that a mother's attitudes and behaviors can be fully understood. As Riordan (1993: 27) has pointed out, "Culture exerts a major influence on a mother's attitude towards breastfeeding and how she decides to feed her baby. Attitudes and patterns of infant feeding cannot be understood without placing them in their specific cultural context."[4]

An understanding of cultural beliefs and practices regarding breast milk has important implications for health promotion and breastfeeding campaigns, in terms of developing more effective promotional messages that may help women understand many aspects of breast milk and to fully breastfeed. In addition, such an understanding will assist health educators to fully comprehend why there are differences in attitudes and behaviors between cultures and why breastfeeding in many societies has not been totally successful, despite decades of breastfeeding campaigns.[5]

This chapter discusses cultural beliefs and practices related to breast milk and the relation of these beliefs to infant feeding practices among Hmong women in Australia. In particular, it focuses on the women's perceptions of breast milk, traditional beliefs and practices regarding breast milk, the approach to milk production, and behavioral restrictions related to breast milk. The implications of these cultural beliefs and practices for breastfeeding campaigns are also discussed.

BELIEFS AND PRACTICES RELATED TO BREAST MILK

What Milk Is Best?

Hmong women believe that breast milk is best for a newborn infant, since it is believed to make the baby healthy.

> Breast milk. I think if the baby is fed on it the baby will grow quite healthily. If they are breastfed then they do not have any allergies to the milk and it is healthy.

Women also mentioned that breast milk is the safest food for a newborn infant, because the food is filtered through the mother's body before the infant takes it. In this way, any "bad" thing in the food will not get into the baby's body. This makes breast milk the cleanest and best food for a newborn infant.

> Breast milk is the best thing for the baby . . . because when you eat anything your body has already filtered it. . . . So it means that the baby will get the best thing from you. . . . That is why it is much better.

Breastfeeding is seen as an easy thing to do when caring for a newborn baby.

> If you feed your own then it is easier because whenever they want to drink then you just need to pull it out for them to eat. This is for one. And secondly, whatever food you eat is made into the milk for the baby too. So it is easy.

Some women were told by their mothers-in-law and mothers that breastfeeding is good for the baby not only in terms of their health but of their well-being, since breastfed babies may need extra comfort when they are ill.

> My mother told me to breastfeed so that when the baby gets a fever or something the baby needs to be comforted so that you must breastfeed the baby. So I breastfeed.

Colostrum: Beliefs and Practices

Hmong women believe that colostrum or "first milk" is dangerous to the infant's health.

> That milk [colostrum] you squeeze it out. You squeeze it out so that the baby will not be unhealthy. They get stomach aches, indigestion and diarrhea if they drink it.

Some women believed that colostrum does not have as nice a taste as their real milk. Real milk is sweet; colostrum is not. Because of this, the baby does not want to take it. Therefore, they must squeeze it out.

> That milk, it is not sweet so the baby does not want to eat it. I have tasted a bit and it is not tasty at all. So I squeeze it out.

Women also mentioned that colostrum has a "sour" taste because it is yellowish. It is believed that "sour" milk may cause stomach problems in a newborn infant. Hence, it must be discarded.

> I squeezed it [colostrum] away. Hmong people say that the milk is sour and that is why it is yellow and so we must express it out. They say that if the baby is fed on it then the baby will get sick. . . . They say it will give him stomach ache. . . . And so I didn't give it to the baby.

Women also believed that "real" or "right" milk is white in color. Because colostrum is yellowish, it is not real milk to them. This makes many mothers squeeze it out before offering their breast to the baby.

> The yellow milk you must squeeze it out. . . . The yellow bit, I just throw it away. I think that it is not new and is yellow so I squeeze it away. . . . I didn't want to feed the baby on the milk that looks like that.

The color of colostrum is associated with "dirty" stuff, because it is similar to color in infection. Women believe that it is not clean and, hence, that it will cause ill health in the newborn baby.

> You have to squeeze all that away and feed the baby with the pure white milk only. I think it is not clean; it might be pus or something because it looks like pus and I think it is not good for the baby. I think that if you feed the baby the baby might have health problems and it makes the baby sick.

Women also mentioned that colostrum has a thick texture and is sticky. This was another reason women did not give it to their babies.

> I did not give that [colostrum] to the baby to eat because it was very thick and and sticky. . . . It looked sticky and yucky. . . . I didn't know whether it was good or not so I didn't give it to the baby.

However, all women who continued breastfeeding until the next child was born mentioned that colostrum only appeared with their "first birth." Since women continued to breastfeed, they had milk in their breast at all times. Therefore, they did not have to squeeze colostrum out with subsequent births.

> The older one will be fed right up until you give birth to the next one. Because you keep feeding the older baby like this, when you have one more month [of pregnancy] to go then your breast will have milk again. The milk will look normal because the child still drinks it. When you give

> birth to the baby you just put the baby straight onto your breast. . . . It is only the first one that you have to squeeze it. The baby won't have it.

Women who stopped feeding several months before the next birth would, however, have colostrum again and must squeeze it out before offering their breast to their newborn babies.

> For the ones who wean the older one for the last two or three months then they will have that colored milk again. You have to squeeze a bit at the front of the nipples away.

It was noted that there were a few first-time mothers who said that they offered their breast to their baby soon after birth without thinking about the colostrum. They believed that this would help to stimulate breast milk.

> The yellow one; I don't know. When the baby first came out I just put the baby straight on my breast. Yes I did that because if I didn't do that then the baby had no milk to eat so I just gave it. Your breast will not have milk but you give it to the baby because if you don't give it to the baby then this will not help stimulate milk production. So you must give it to the baby for that milk production.

Feeding in the First Few Days

Hmong women believe that with their first birth, their "real" or "right" breast milk will not appear until three days later. Only the "yellow" milk may appear on the second day after birth.

> About two or three days, but after one day there is the yellow one. But for you to have the right milk it will have to be two or three days before you have it.

Women believe that breast milk will not be produced until the baby arrives and certainly not until they begin eating their confinement food, which they do immediately following the birth.

> Soon after birth the breast milk had not come then. It was a couple of days after when I got it. Because there was no baby feeding on it so the baby must be born first and one or two days later when you eat food then you would have milk.

This raises the question of what women do about feeding before the commencement of their "real" milk. Traditionally, women asked other lactating women to feed their baby in the first few days until their own milk came.

> When you have not got your milk then you have to ask other people with young children to come and help to feed the baby one or two times.... They can be family or they can be just neighbors. Whoever has young children that are close to you then you will ask them. Then your milk will come and you feed your milk.

Another woman explained:

> Soon after birth of the first one there was no milk yet so you ask your sisters who have young children to come and help you feed and when you have it then you feed yours. You ask them to come to feed for three mornings and after the third morning you have milk or after the second morning you have breast milk then you feed yours.

Where Does Breast Milk Come From?

All women mentioned that breast milk comes from their blood. However, it must also be produced by the food they eat.

> When you have a baby and you have plenty of food to eat all the time then you will have a lot of milk. If you don't have enough to eat or you don't have an appetite then you will not have enough milk. So I think that it will have to be the food that make you have the milk.

However, only food that contains a large amount of liquid may produce an abundance of breast milk.

> I think that if you eat food then you will have the milk. If you eat food without the juice then you do not have enough milk for the baby to eat. If you make food with soup and you eat that and drink the soup too then you can feel that you have more milk.... I think maybe it is like that because like sometimes when you have your meals which have no soup with it or when you eat dry food only then you do not have a lot of milk ... but when you add a lot of water in your cooking then it seems that you have more milk.

Although Hmong women believed that breast milk comes from food they eat, they strongly believe that it is the particular food they eat during confinement (a period of 30 days following birth) that in fact helps to produce their milk.[6] It is also interesting that this confinement food, particularly chicken soup, contains a large amount of water.

> I think that if you eat rice and meat and drink its soup then you will have breast milk. If you only eat sweet things and only drink water, then you will not have milk. It must be eating meat and drinking the meat soup for you to have milk.

The Hmong believe that each of a mother's breasts represents different food. One breast represents rice and the other represents meat and vegetables. Because of this belief, Hmong women offer both breasts to their baby during every feed so that the infant may receive a balanced diet.

> The old people say that one of the breasts is rice and another one is vegetable or meat . . . so that is why you have to give both sides to the baby.

Because breast milk is believed to come from food, women were cautious about their food intake. During a confinement period, Hmong women only consume confinement food, which is also believed to prevent ill health in the newborn infant. However, during the lactation period, women were also careful about their food. Anything which has a bad odor, such as spring onion or garlic, will not be eaten, as it will also get into the milk and, in turn, make the baby ill. In addition, food that has a burned smell, such as fried or grilled chicken, will cause a similar problem.

> Traditionally if you have a young baby you must eat a lot of boiled vegetables, not to eat too much meat and no garlic or spring onion or grilled meat because that can cause coughs, diarrhea and bad temperament. Basically, you do not eat these things often, only sometimes during feeding.

When the baby is ill during the lactation period, a mother will avoid consuming fried food and certain food stuffs which have a strong odor such as garlic, onion and shallots. The mother must consume only plain food to avoid further illness in their infants.

> When you have a baby and if the baby is ill you cannot eat many things or must stop eating many things. When the baby is breastfed and gets sick then whatever you feel it makes the baby sicker you should not eat either. When the baby is sick, things like meat you should not grill or fry. You should not eat onion, shallot or garlic; none of these strong smelling foods. You only boil the meat with a bit of salt; just make it plain like that.

The Quality of Breast Milk

The Hmong believe that only certain mothers can produce good quality and delicious milk. The babies of mothers who have "good" milk will be strong and grow well. In contrast, some women may have plenty of breast milk, but because it is not "good" enough, their children may not grow well.

> My milk was delicious and my children grew very quick and were also very strong. Some women's breast milk is not delicious and it doesn't mat-

> ter how much milk she has that milk will not make the baby grow. For some that have delicious milk, their babies will drink a lot and when they are about four months they are able to roll over and you have to not let them lie near the edge of the bed because they will be strong and may roll off the bed.

It is believed that the ability to produce good milk is an inner quality that only some women have, and it does not depend on the food eaten during the lactating period.

> It is a born thing that the milk is delicious. With some women they may have a lot of milk but the milk is not delicious then the baby will not grow. . . . It doesn't matter what or how much you eat if your milk is not tasty then it is not tasty. . . . Mrs. A has very bland milk and her children didn't grow well. They were very skinny and hairy. They only started to grow when they started to eat solid. . . . They say that she has a lot of milk but the milk is very clear.

In addition, women believed that the capability to produce "good" quality milk is not an inherited trait. Even those who were born from the same family may have breast milk of differing quality.

> It doesn't matter even if they are from the same mother it will depend on themselves. For my family, my sister X and sister Y have delicious milk but sister Z has untasty milk and her children didn't grow very well at all. . . . Yes, it depends on the person.

Sour Milk

Hmong women believe that during lactation if they do not breastfeed the baby for a period of time they must squeeze the milk out before putting the baby on their breast. The milk, which has accumulated in the breasts for some time, is seen as "sour." This "sour milk" is believed to be unsuitable for the baby, since it may cause stomach problems.

> If you have a young baby and you have been out for a long time like one or two hours then when you come back and your breast is very tight then you must squeeze the milk away before you give it to the baby.

And,

> If you are breastfeeding your baby and you have to go out for about one or two hours then you have to squeeze a bit out before you feed the baby so that the baby won't get sick; won't get diarrhea. If you go out all day and your breasts feel very tight then you have to express some at the nipples just in case it is sour.

APPROACHES TO MILK PRODUCTION

Hmong women have traditionally relied on consuming "good" food as well as Hmong herbal medicines immediately after giving birth to produce breast milk. As mentioned in Chapter 6, the first meal after birth in Hmong culture is a chicken egg cooked quickly in boiling water with hot pepper and a pinch of salt to enhance the taste. It is believed that a chicken egg helps to nourish a woman who has lost her energy through birth, and hot water and pepper help to stimulate breast milk production.

During the confinement period (30 days following birth), Hmong women only consume hot rice and chicken soup cooked with several kinds of green herbs, known as *tshuaj qaib* (chicken herbal medicine). These herbs serve several purposes, including enhancing breast milk. As one woman explained:

> When the woman has just given birth we have special herbs with the chicken for the mother to eat. According to our tradition, we slaughter chicken for her to eat. You cook the chicken with chicken herbs and give her only hot water to drink for one month. You must use the herbs, put them in the chicken soup so that her body will put on weight and make her look beautiful after one month.

Herbs to Enhance Breast Milk

Hmong women mentioned that there are herbs that help to stimulate breast milk. These herbs are known as "milk stimulant herbs."

> When you give birth to a baby there are herbal medicines for the production of mothers' milk. You use these medicines in the chicken soup and to drink as a tea. These herbs help to stimulate the production of milk.

Some herbs appear as roots. The roots are cooked with chicken and consumed during lactation.

> There are medicines for milk production. They say if you have no milk then you have to purchase these medicines to eat so you will have milk. My sister-in-law has that sort of medicines too. They are roots and you have to boil them in chicken soup to eat for the milk production.

Another herb mentioned is referred to as *Xwm leej tsav* in Hmong. It is a small, cactus-like plant that has a white sap when broken. Symbolically, the herb produces an abundance of "white milk" (sap) and, hence, it is believed to help stimulate breast milk in a new mother.

> Some herbs when you pick their leaves or stems the milk sap will come out and this will make you have more milk.

These herbs are only needed when there is not enough breast milk to feed the baby. The Hmong traditionally live in areas where there are no substitutes for breast milk. Thus, mothers believed that they needed to take herbal medicines in order to stimulate their breast milk or to produce more to feed their babies. Women usually mentioned that if they took the medicines for three mornings only, they would have plenty of breast milk for feeding.

There are also other "milk stimulant herbs" that are believed to help women produce breast milk even when they have not given birth. These herbs, when the stems or leaves are broken, produce milk-like sap. The herbs, which can be in a fresh or dried form, are cooked in chicken soup, which needs to be taken twice to make milk. One older woman related:

> These herbs have to be in the chicken soup too. It only takes two times if you are going to have the milk. These medicines for the breast milk, for some people like me who are no longer conceive, if I use it then I will have milk again. . . . If you have an orphan and have no milk for the baby, the herb will help. The year I was in Laos my aunt's daughter-in-law died and left her with a young baby. My aunt was old, even older than me now. She took the medicine and make it with some chicken and she was able to breastfeed the baby. . . . She only took it two or three times and she was able to produce the milk for the baby.

Interestingly, most milk stimulant herbs are wild plants. They may grow in the forest or just along the side of the road. Only those who are knowledgeable about these herbs may gather them for the women. However, most women believed that the knowledge is possessed by older people only.

Green paw paw cooked with chicken meat in a soup form is also believed to be a milk stimulant. Interestingly, green paw paw has sap when the skin is peeled off. It, therefore, functions similarly to the herbs mentioned above. This fruit is abundant in Laos and even in Australia, and most women and families know about it.

BEHAVIORAL PRECAUTIONS RELATED TO BREAST MILK

The Hmong put a high value on breast milk. This can clearly be seen from the number of restrictions imposed on the mother's and other's behaviors during lactation, particularly during the first month after birth.

The Importance of Breast Milk

Breast milk is seen as belonging only to a newborn infant. When the next child is born, the previous child will be weaned. More often, the child will stop sucking on his mother's breast by himself. The next newborn child will then have the sole right to her breast milk. Older children, particularly adults, are prohibited from drinking breast milk. It is believed that if they do so they will be struck by lightning. In addition, the mother must be very careful not to let her breast milk drip on the ground where animals can lick it, since, lightning may strike the animal. This is bad for the family because they will lose their animals, which are considered precious.

> With Hmong people we do not let adults drink it and we do not let it drip on the ground for insects to lick. It is only for the small one whom you just give birth to . . . I haven't seen it but I have heard the older people say that lightning may strike them [adults or animals].

Behavioral Restrictions and Breastfeeding

During a confinement period, there are some restrictions concerning visitors, particularly for a pregnant woman and a lactating mother. These restrictions also apply to their husbands.

> It is a traditional belief that if a pregnant woman comes to visit you in your confinement period she has the ability to take your breastmilk away. Your husband will have to go to her place and bring it back for the baby.

Visitors who enter the house during the confinement period should not carry a bag or wear shoes. It is believed that these acts will take away the mother's breast milk. This is a serious matter in Hmong culture, since Hmong women traditionally breastfeed their newborn infants and do not have access to infant formula or other forms of milk substitutes.

> In your confinement, it doesn't matter if it is a man or a woman, if they know that you just have a baby and is breastfeeding then when they come they must take off their shoes outside and not to wear them inside. If they carry a bag then they will leave it outside, and if they carry a basket then they must leave that outside too. They will come in with nothing like that on their body. If they carry the basket inside then they can bring the milk away and if they wear shoes they can carry the milk away too. If the person has taken your milk away you have to go to bring it back or you have to wait until they give birth themselves before your milk comes back . . . so your baby will not get milk at all.

In some situations, there is a way to counteract this.

> If you know the person who is pregnant and who has come to take the milk away from you, you have to go and get some of their salt, rice grain and cooking oil to cook for you to eat. This will help you to have milk again.

Another woman elaborated about trying to bring back breast milk as follows:

> If a woman is pregnant and comes to see you, after they leave you find that your breast has no more milk then you know that it is her. You will then ask someone from your house to go to her house and bring it back from her house. When you go you say, "When you came I think that my baby's milk followed you home so I am here to bring baby's milk back." They then will get some salt and if they have eggs then they will give an egg as well and one spoon of salt. They will then say, "When I came to visit you your baby's milk has followed me home so here I give baby's milk for you to carry back to the baby." . . . If you have rice then you give a bowl of rice too. So you will have to bring these back and prepare it for the mother to eat and if the milk comes back then your breast will swell up and have milk again.

However, many women mentioned that the loss of breastmilk could not be counteracted. Once a woman's breast milk is taken away, it is gone, or it will be a long time before her milk can be brought back. This is serious for the Hmong, because their newborn infants will not have milk to drink.

> If they come and after they leave they take the milk away you have to wait until their baby is born then you will have your milk back. You and your baby will have a very hard time. . . . So this is why the Hmong people restrict themselves.

And

> If they are pregnant and come then they will take away [your milk] . . . and your child will not have milk to drink. Their baby will have to be born before your breast will have milk again. . . . By the time their child is born, your child will be unhealthy because the child has no milk.

Feeding and Gender

Although the Hmong practice wet nursing, a new mother is not allowed to feed other young babies during her confinement period. In the first month of life, a newborn infant has the sole right to his or her mother's breast milk. Once the confinement is complete, she may offer her breast to other infants. However, the practice of wet nursing seems to be more cautious with a girl infant. It is believed that if the baby is a boy the mother should not allow girl infants to take her milk. Similarly, if her baby is a girl she should not let boy babies on her breasts. It is believed that girl infants are "greedy" and will take all the breast milk from their mothers, not leaving enough milk for boy infants.

> They say because if you allow that to happen then the baby girl, like they are more greedy, they tend to take more milk and thus the boy does not have enough milk to drink.

Nevertheless, most mothers in this study mentioned that they would feed other young babies, whether boys or girls. They said that only those who are very strict would follow this practice of wet nursing boys and girls.

CONCLUSIONS

Hmong traditional beliefs and practices relating to breast milk are similar to other anthropological research findings. This is particularly true for beliefs about colostrum and breast milk quality. In Morse et al.'s (1990) world survey of the timing of postpartum breastfeeding, for example, it was found that although the reasons for discarding colostrum vary from culture to culture, most societies believe that colostrum is "dirty, poisonous, contaminated, bad or contained pus" (p. 307). Some societies hold that colostrum makes the newborn ill and causes vomiting and diarrhea. Similarly, in the Republic of Guinea-Bissau in Africa, Balanta mothers believe that colostrum is "dirty, insufficient and capable of causing any disease, in some cases even the death of the infant" (Gunnlaugsson and Einarsdottir, 1993: 284). They therefore discard the colostrum and delay breastfeeding until the "real milk" comes from two to five days after birth. Mothers also believe that mature breast milk may differ in quality from one mother to another. If the child is strong and looks healthy, the milk is good. If the milk is bad, the child will not grow properly and will always be sick.

In discussing why colostrum is so widely disliked, Gunnlaugsson and Einarsdottir (1993) have stated the color and consistency of colostrum are the main factors that seem to make mothers feel that colostrum can be infectious and stale. Baumslag and Michels (1995) have pointed out that mothers in many parts of the world distrust colostrum because of its yellow color, which resembles "pus" or "poison." As illustrated in this chapter, Hmong mothers regard the color and consistency of the colostrum as indications of "bad milk." They also use taste as a way to differentiate good milk and bad milk. However, an important finding of this study, in contrast to the findings of many other studies, is that Hmong women believe that "first milk" (colostrum) only occurs with the first birth. Since they continue to breastfeed until they give birth to their next child, they do not believe that they have produced colostrum again and, hence, do not need to discard their first milk. This means that Hmong infants do in fact receive colostrum.

Although some beliefs and practices relating to breast milk among the Hmong appear "odd" to Western health professionals and educators, many of these have functional purposes within the social and cultural environment of Hmong culture. The practice of wet nursing, for example, shows strong social support within the Hmong family and society. One women contends that the way family and community help each other is a very good practice in her culture; it helps other societal members to survive. This social support means the continuation of the family, the lineage, and the society.

Another example of a belief with a functional purpose is the belief that each of a mother's breasts represents different food. One breast represents rice and the other represents meat and vegetables. Therefore, Hmong women will offer both breasts to their baby in every feed. This belief functions to encourage mothers to fully feed the baby.

In many societies, pregnancy is a reason for complete, and very often abrupt, weaning (Hull and Simpson, 1985). A common reason for the termination of breastfeeding is the belief that breast milk may turn "bad in quality" for the nursing child (Fernandez and Guthrie, 1984; Vong-Ek, 1993). However, this practice does not exist among the Hmong. Hmong mothers continue to breastfeed their young children until they give birth to their next child. Women say that although their breast milk during pregnancy may not be as good as before, it is still "good enough" to feed the child. This practice serves a purpose in terms of infant survival. In societies where food is scarce, prolonged breastfeeding is the only way to ensure the survival of young children. Additionally, Jenkins and Heywood (1985) have pointed out, prolonged breastfeeding may be beneficial for the health of a child, since it extends the interval between births and supplies significant amounts of nutrients to the child.

It is clear that ideas about breast milk and its relation to infant feeding practices in Hmong culture fall within the "infant-centered" concept proposed by Kocturk and Zetterstrom (1989: 820). As illustrated, many beliefs and practices reflect the fact that Hmong mothers try to ensure that their infants have "good" and "enough" breast milk for growth and good health so that their children will thrive and survive. This reflects the importance of children in Hmong culture, as I have illustrated in the last chapter and throughout the book.

What are the implications of cultural beliefs and practices relating to breast milk for health education and breastfeeding campaigns? First, these beliefs and practices need to be examined within the social and cultural context of Hmong society. This may prevent misunderstanding and, hence, "blaming the victim." For example, Mull (1992) has stated that the belief breastfeeding should be started immediately after birth to establish breastfeeding is a new concept largely resulting from medical curiosity. However, this new belief has failed to take into account the fact that late initiation of breastfeeding usually "coexist with prolonged lactation" in many traditional societies. This is true of Hmong women, who do not initiate breastfeeding until two or three days after birth because they believe that colostrum is dangerous to the infant's health, but who also continue to breastfeed until they give birth to their next child, which may take place two or three years later. This practice is common among Hmong women, with the exception of a few first-time mothers. This is important for health professionals to know, as they may otherwise misinterpret Hmong mothers' intentions. As Morse et al. (1990: 394) has pointed out, "Primary caregivers especially those not familiar with the mother's cultural beliefs and not realizing that the mother's refusal to breastfeed is only temporary, may misinterpret her intentions. Thinking that she does not wish to breastfeed at all, they may not provide [her with] the opportunity to begin nursing the next day."[7]

Similarly, as Reissland and Burghart (1988) have noted, the condemnation of colostrum withholding among women from traditional societies by Western health professionals occurs largely because this practice is seen out of its cultural context. According to Reissland and Burghart, (1988) when this practice is examined in context, it "loses some of its salience." Because a woman who has just given birth is seen as being in a weakened state, she needs to rest as much as possible. This rest is essential to her ability to restore her health and well-being. The mother in this stage will not be able to establish an exclusive relationship with her child, as is encouraged in the West. Hmong mothers are no exceptions. Therefore, the colostrum taboo, as Reissland and Burghart (1988: 463) have stated, "while understood on its own terms as the prohibition on feeding stale milk to the neonate, forms part of a pattern of minimal, tentative contact between mother and child during the first day postpartum." Close contact and full breastfeeding will, however, commence later on.[8]

What needs to be done to provide messages that may help Hmong women see the value of colostrum and hence make the maximum use of their breast milk? Van Esterik (1985: 159), for example, pointed out that health promotion programs might develop messages that focus on specific beliefs, such as the belief that colostrum is bad milk. She stated that a campaign slogan such as "The sooner you breastfeed, the better the milk" may help mothers learn that early breastfeeding may help get rid of the "bad milk." Women may then try to initiate breastfeeding early.

Since Hmong mothers believe that there are confinement foods that can promote breast milk, health professionals need to encourage their families to bring these foods to them during their hospital stays. As Riordan (1993) has reported, this not only helps women to enhance their breastfeeding, but also shows women that the health care system supports breastfeeding.

In conclusion, I have argued in this chapter that breastfeeding behavior cannot be examined out of the social and cultural contexts of the society in which it occurs, and these factors are essential for better health education and breastfeeding campaigns (Kocturk and Zetterstrom, 1989). There is no doubt that Hmong women see that "breast is best." Therefore, the main message for those involve in breastfeeding campaigns needs to be "make it easy for women to do it" (Van Esterik, 1985: 159). Only in this way may women feel that they have the power to decide on the best way to feed their infants.

NOTES

1. See for example, the work of Jellife and Jellife, 1978; Morse, 1984; Conton, 1985; Dettwyler, 1987; King and Ashworth, 1987; Fernandez and Popkin, 1988; Fishman et al., 1988; and Gunnlaugsson and Einarsdottir, 1993.

2. This is also illustrated in the work of Reissland and Burghart, 1988; Morse et al., 1990; and Gunnlaugsson and Einarsdottir, 1993.

3. In Pakistan, for example, Mull (1992) has shown that the quality of breast milk can be affected by a "shadow" from the spirit world and the evil eye cast on the milk by an envious onlooker. In addition, breast milk can be spoiled by a new pregnancy and hence can cause diarrhea, vomiting and weakness in the child. Once a mother suspects that her breast milk is affected by any of these circumstances, she may stop breastfeeding, often permanently, believing that her milk is "bad."

4. As Mull (1992) points out, in Pakistan, children, particularly sons, are essential for a woman's financial and social security. The mother, therefore, will not put her infant "at risk" if she is in doubt about the quality of her breast milk. She may therefore stop nursing her infant, since she knows that she will be blamed for a child's illness.

5. As Hull and Simpson (1985: 2) have pointed out, "Cross-cultural studies of breastfeeding offer a promising tool for improved understanding of breastfeeding as a socio-biological process." This chapter intends to contribute a cross-cultural study to the literature in the area of infant feeding practice.

6. See Chapter 6 in this volume for food eaten in confinement by the Hmong.

7. Morse et al. (1990) have further suggested that health professionals need to be sensitive when assessing the woman's beliefs. They also need to think carefully when providing advice about feeding.

8. Morse et al. (1990) have also pointed to the dangers of stereotyping women

from the same culture. For example, caregivers may assume that a woman does not want to breastfeed immediately because she is from the Hmong culture, which does not feed colostrum to their infants. Morse et al. contend that women should be assessed on an individual basis and each one should be asked if she wishes to breastfeed immediately after birth. If she wishes to discard colostrum and delay breastfeeding until her "real" milk appears, culturally acceptable prelacteal substitutes should be offered to the infant. Morse et al. also argue: "It is better that an infant goes without colostrum and is breastfed from the second, third or fourth day, than is never breastfed at all" (p. 309).

Chapter 10

Childhood Health and Illness

INTRODUCTION

> Children who are often sick will look pale when they are born. They will have more fever than the healthy ones. This will be because their *plig* [souls] have left their bodies; that is why they are like that.

Illness is an inevitable part of life. Making sense of and coping with illness are therefore universal issues for human beings. However, as Brown et al. (1996: 183) have pointed out, the particular illnesses that "afflict people, as well as the way in which symptoms are interpreted and acted upon, vary greatly by culture." Childhood illness is no exception.

In this chapter, the cultural construct of childhood illness among the Hmong is examined. The focus is on traditional patterns of beliefs and practices related to the health and illness of newborn infants and young children. I also discuss the roles of traditional healers, who play an important part in childhood health and illness. Finally, I provide some suggestions for child health services dealing with immigrants such as the Hmong in Australia and elsewhere.

CHILDHOOD HEALTH AND ILLNESS

Pranee: Have any of your children experienced bad health?

Mai: No, none of my children have had very bad health.

Pranee: That is good. What do you do that they are all healthy?

Mai: Well, like when you give birth to them you wrap them up well and then when they grow up and can walk you give them shoes and clothes to wear. If they are a bit ill from cold, nothing serious, we have *ua neeb* to help them and we look for delicious things for them to eat and so they have good appetites and then they will grow up very well.

The Hmong treat children with respect. Hmong mothers consider good health an important aspect of their children's lives, since good health means long life. This is reflected in the many traditional rituals performed for both pregnant women and young children to prevent illness and the death of the child. In the soul-calling ceremony performed on the third morning for a newborn infant, for example, there are rituals and blessings for good health and longevity.[1] Another example is the prolonged period of breastfeeding. Hmong mothers continue to breastfeed their infants until the next baby is born.[2] Some may even breastfeed both if the older one is still quite young. One woman gave her reason for a long period of breastfeeding:

> Because you love the baby very much and the baby does not want to go off your milk so you just let them drink. The baby will just suck on it when they are older even when there is no milk.

However, this does not mean that all Hmong children are healthy. In their homeland in Laos, there was and still is a high infant mortality rate among the Hmong. One Hmong mother in this study had a child who died through illness, and others have had children who at one time or another became ill.

In everyday life, if a child shows signs of distress such as crying too often or refusing to feed, there will always be an attempt to ascertain what is happening to the child. This may require seeking advice from the elderly, community leaders and traditional healers. Once, the condition is known, healing processes will follow. This may involve several processes, including self-healing and seeking help from traditional healers. Since departing their homeland in Laos, the Hmong have had access to modern medicines in refugee camps in Thailand and in Australia. Because of this, most Hmong seek help from both their traditional healers and from modern medicine to help the child overcome health problems. One woman had a child who suffered from chicken pox. According to her, the symptoms were serious because the rash did not erupt externally. She sought help from a shaman and a magic man as well as from Western medicine. She said:

> The girl was taken to the doctor and had an injection and at the same time we gave her *ua neeb* and had *khawv koob* for her to drink to help her infection to come to the surface. . . . We did *ua neeb* at home and at the hospital we asked to have *khawv koob* for her and we were allowed. . . . She was very sick so you had to do everything you could to beat the sickness.

WHAT MAKES A CHILD ILL?

There are several traditional beliefs and practices related to the presumed causes of childhood illness.[3] These are presented in the following sections.

Natural Causes

Several childhood illnesses are believed to be caused by nature; the most commonly mentioned is chicken pox. The Hmong regard this illness as serious enough to take the life of a child, particularly if the rash does not erupt on the skin. When this happens, the Hmong believe that the rash is in fact expressed inside the body and that this is extremely dangerous. One woman told us of her first child's illness, which had killed him in Laos:

> The Vietnamese gathered us to live in Thong Hia and he had a rash. That rash was associated with high fever, it came after a fever. He had very high fever but he could not express the rash out and died from that. . . . The rash was expressed internally and could not come out so that was why he died.

The Hmong believe that if a child has a fever and it is likely to be a rash fever (such as chicken pox), they must avoid cooking or consuming food that has a bad odor, such as onions, garlic or anything that has a strong smell. It is commonly believed that this will cause the rash to erupt internally and it can be fatal to the child. The woman mentioned above believed strongly that what she had consumed caused the death of her child:

> The rash, when he had that, it was because of me. I had very bad diarrhea and I drank a bit of opium which might be smelly to him. I had a very bad diarrhea and nearly died myself. . . . And maybe it smelled bad to the child . . . that he died.

Another woman had a child who was ill from chicken pox when she was in a refugee camp in Thailand. Like the cases described above, the rash did not express itself outwardly and it made the child very ill. The woman described how when the baby had a fever she had cooked a dish that caused a bad odor to be smelled by the child. This inhibited the outward expression of the chicken pox and made the child sick in her liver and lungs instead.

Oily food is also prohibited if a child suffers from chicken pox. Because the illness is seen as "hot," oily food, which has a "hot" property, will aggravate the illness and may cause severe illness in children.

> Sometimes when you fry your food with oil, you must not give it to the child to eat if your baby has a very high temperature. The chicken pox is like something that is very hot and steaming and it is not evaporating from inside her body.

The quality of blood of a child is also seen as a factor determining health and illness. The Hmong believe that if a child has good blood he will be healthy, since he will not be easily infected with illnesses. This quality is believed to come with the baby from birth. A Hmong woman explained:

> You hope that the baby is born normal and healthy with good blood so that he will not get sick too often. . . . It depends on the baby's blood . . . and his ability to fight the infection thus not getting infection from someone else easily. This comes with the baby when the baby is born.

Being hit by dust and rain is also believed to cause childhood illness. A newborn infant will not be taken outside the house for the whole month after birth. Young children are also kept inside the house after a heavy rain and wind. One woman explained:

> After it rains the dust is heavy outside so you cannot take the baby outside. If you take the baby outside and the baby is exposed to the dust and rain then he will come down with a high fever. This will make the baby cry a lot, but it is a very sudden cry like it is frightened. . . . That is because he is hit by the dust and rain.

Souls, Health and Illness

As previously mentioned, The Hmong believe that each living person has three souls.[4] A newborn infant is no exception. If all three souls are secured in the infant's body, he will be healthy and thrive well. On the contrary, the infant may become ill if a soul leaves the body. This is particularly true when the soul whose duty is to look after the person while living—referred to as the life soul among the Hmong—leaves the child's body. The child may eventually die if all three souls do not reside in his body.

A soul can wander away from the body from time to time. This behavior is seen as equivalent to that of a human being who may want to wander to different places and will come home when he has had enough adventure. The human soul is the same. When a soul goes outside the body, a person may feel a lack of energy and have no interest in anything. When the life soul is not in the body, a person will be vulnerable to being struck by spirits. It is said that spirits will see the person clearly without their soul in their body. In young infants and children, paleness, excessive crying, high temperature, vomiting or lack of interest in mother's milk are signs of a soul loss.

> When the baby gets scared of something, this causes soul loss. . . . If he loses his soul then he will be very tired and sleep all day without waking up to drink or eat. This is when you know that the baby has lost his soul.

There are several ways in which the child's soul may escape from the body. Fright caused by a loud noise or an accident such as a fall can cause the loss of souls of young children. It is said that a soul is frightened away, and this will cause a fever in the child.

> When they have a fever it is because the older children scream and give it a fright. This is what gives a fever to the child. . . . Sometimes when they are asleep, like you put a bed next to the fire and put the baby there, and when the older children come in they might scream loudly. The baby can get frightened from that and this makes his soul frightened away, and so he will have a fever and cry.

A child's soul can feel miserable and not wish to live with his parents if his parents' souls do not equally like the child. The infant's soul may then wish to return to his ancestral pool. This means that the child may die soon after birth. A Hmong shaman explained:

> With young children, it has to be that both parents' souls like the children, like you as the person like them, for them to be healthy. If the mother's soul likes the children but the father's soul does not then the souls of the children will not want to stay . . . so it has to be both of the parents' souls like the children equally as they do in real life. . . . If the mother's soul likes them but the husband's soul doesn't like them when they are born they will not grow healthily and always have problem like getting sick or having some illnesses that can kill them. Sometimes the soul of the father likes them but the mother's soul does not; it will happen the same way too.

There are spirits who may come to touch or capture the soul of the baby. When this happens, the child will become pale and sick and eventually die if there is no ceremony performed to call the soul back.

Spirits, Health and Illness

According to the Hmong, spirits are everywhere and they do not wish to be disturbed. If people do not keep away from the spirits they may be struck and become ill. The most common explanation for any ill health among the Hmong and its most feared cause is being *raug dab* (struck by spirits). The Hmong say that if a young child is hit by a spirit, the child will cry excessively and become ill. The spirits that cause illness most frequently are the *theeb kawv* and *txhij suam*. These spirits live in the sky and are mostly referred to as "the sky spirits," or "the spirits of the sun and the moon." These spirits are believed to cause fits in young children. A magic healer related that:

> If the baby cries and gets sick the baby is being hit by *theeb kawv*. It is the spirit that lives on the moon. When the baby is still in the womb the mother's breast will have already been dripping milk. So after the baby is born we say that the baby has already been hit. Sometimes this can cause the baby to be sick and have fits. . . . The *txhij suam* and *theeb kawv* are the spirits that live in the sky. The sky spirits will make the child have fists, clenching fits and feet and rolling of the eyes.

Another spirit commonly mentioned among the Hmong is *dab peg*. This spirit is particularly well known for causing epilepsy in young children.[5] When *dab peg* hits the child, the child will suddenly become unconscious and fall down. As one woman explained,

> *Dab*, the one that they say if the child is going to be hit by spirit, then the spirit that makes you have epilepsy is only *dab peg* that can harm you. They say that it is *dab peg*. The symptoms are like when the child gets sick, then all of a sudden the child becomes unconscious and fall over. This is what most Hmong know.

A newborn infant may be struck by the spirit called *dab tshog tshuag* if he is taken outside the house and happens to be on the spirit's path. Since the baby still has a smell like a newborn baby (milky smell), the baby will be hit by a spirit. This will make the baby cry excessively at a particular time each day. This belief has led the Hmong not to take a newborn baby outside during the first month of life.

> For the Hmong people if the baby cries then we say that it is being teased by spirits. . . . It can be that you take the baby outside and it is teased by *dab tshog tshuag*. This is a normal street spirit. . . . When you take the baby out on the day that you should not be taking the baby out or if you take the baby out at the wrong time then the baby will be hit. . . . Being a baby

> it drinks milk and it has that milky smell and if the soul is not with it then it can be hit by *dab tshog tshuag*.

There are other spirits who are generally benevolent. *Dab po*, for example, is believed to be beneficent and generally does not cause harm to newborn infants. But *dab po* can also tease the newborn infant. If this happens the baby will cry excessively. A shaman told me:

> *Dab po* will come and tease your newborn baby. The baby can see them, but we can't and if the baby is teased the baby will cry a lot. So you have to *saib tsawv* [a ritual to shield or hide the baby from the spirit] for the baby and say "you must leave now, I am a living parent now."

Dab po is sometimes referred to as *Txoov Kab Yeeb*, the parent spirits who send children down to earth to be born. These spirit parents may make the child sick and take him back if the parents do not take good care of the child. A magic healer explained:

> *Dab po* are the ones that give you the child. They have given the child to you so you must love the child and if you don't love the child then they will make the child sick and take the child back. We have to beg the spirits and give them gold paper money and incenses, and we have to promise to love the baby, then the child will get better.

A Hmong woman said:

> If you do something wrong to the child then they [spirit parents] will come to make the child cry. . . . If you say something unrespectable to them they will come to make the baby cry . . . or if you do something bad to the baby or when you do not honor them properly on the third morning after you give birth to your child . . . they can make the baby cry a lot.

As previously mentioned, a soul-calling ceremony must be performed for a newborn infant on the third morning after birth. At this ceremony, a ritual to honor the spirit parents must also be conducted. This is referred to as *fiv Kab Yeeb* or *fiv dab po* in Hmong. If this ritual is not performed properly, the spirit parents may become angry. They may make the baby cry excessively, and he will refuse to be fed:

> When you have a new baby on the third morning you have to *hu plig* to call the soul and you have to *fiv dab po*. . . . It is to thank *Txoov Kab Yeeb* since they have brought the baby to you. There are two parents that is why you *fiv* with two chickens. . . . When you *fiv* you have to call them and because the couple is responsible for bringing the baby to you, you

> are very thankful. . . . If you don't do that then the baby will cry a lot, will not feed and will not grow well.

Ntaj Dab: Black Magic

The Hmong also believe that children can be the victims of black magic. The most familiar black magic is known as *ntaj dab;* voodoo-killing by a knife. Children who suffer from this do not provoke the accuser but are rather the targets of revenge in place of their parents. One Hmong woman whose child died because of black magic in Laos elaborated about her experience:

> My child was very lovable and very healthy. . . . He was playing and running around, then suddenly he ran to me saying "Mum hurt, Mum hurt." He ran into my lap and then dirtied his pants. He then climbed up again and then vomited. He did this for five days and then died. On the third day he was unconscious. . . . When he died, he had a red mark around the neck and there was a cracking noise came from the neck and his head was only supported by his skin. . . . This is why I knew that it was done by *ntaj dab*. . . . At that time there was a war and there were a lot of people that came to the airport. They were known to do *qe zeb* [spiritual stones] and killed a lot of people.

The woman also strongly believed that her child died because of the jealousy of Lao people because her child was a very lovable and nice baby. In addition, her husband had gambled with the Lao and he did not pay them enough. Hence, they wished to punish her husband by using black magic to take the life of her child away.

> I think that they [Lao men] were very jealous of my child. My husband also was gambling with them. Whatever they wanted I would give to them. If they wanted opium then I would give it to them. But they loved my child so much that they did that to him [killed him].

An illness caused by black magic is believed to be dangerous, since it is difficult to trace its origin and, therefore, a healing process cannot be effective. Most often, if a child is the victim of black magic, death is the final outcome.

SEEKING HEALING AND CHILD HEALTH

Kws Tshuaj (A Medicine Woman)

As I have illustrated earlier, the Hmong's first choice in cases of illness is to seek help from a medicine woman in their community. This is particularly true for minor illnesses caused by natural agents. The medicine woman usually gathers different kinds of *tshuaj Hmoob* (Hmong green herbs) grown in her garden. She will instruct the parents in how to prepare the herbs. Usually, these are finely chopped and steamed with eggs. This is done in the morning for three mornings. The herbs are believed to make the child strong and able to recover from illnesses.

Some common herbs are also grown in the backyard of the family. Many grandparents are knowledgeable about Hmong medicines and they may prepare herbs for their children for common colds and cuts. However, with more serious illnesses, a medicine woman must be asked to heal the child.

Txiv Neeb (A Shaman) and *Ua Neeb* Rituals

The rituals of a shaman for young children, as for adults, are mainly concerned with protection and curing. In the case of the soul of a young child captured by spirits, the shaman will perform *ua neeb*, a trance healing ritual, to hide the soul of the child first. The shaman then performs another *ua neeb* to chase the spirits out of the house of the child. With hiding of the soul, the shaman prepares a glass of water and puts a string of the child's hair in the glass. The child must spit into the glass as well. Then the glass is turned upside down. This is to flood the child's soul so that spirits will not see it. The glass will be placed on top of a bowl in the bedroom or cupboard and covered with a piece of cloth or gold paper that has been cut into the shape of a person; usually two pairs of people holding hands (called *moj zeej*). When all water has drained from the glass, the whole process continues again. This is believed to stop the spirits from touching the baby. A shaman explained:

> The baby's soul will be hidden inside the bowl so that when the spirit comes to look, there is water surrounding the soul so the spirits cannot touch the baby's soul.

Another way of hiding a soul is to perform an *ua neeb* to secure it under the pillows. In the trance, a shaman will ask his spirit helper to find the soul and then bring it to the place where the child sleeps. The shaman will then secure it under his pillow. In this way, the spirits will not see the child when he goes outside the house, and, hence, his soul will not be captured by the spirits again.

For children who are often sick, a shaman must perform a soul-calling ceremony called *hu plig tuam choj*. This type of *hu plig* is performed at the road intersection or at the door of the house. A shaman will prepare three wooden planks, place them in a "Y" shape at the road intersection or the door and then perform a *hu plig* ritual. It is believed that this is the wish of the soul of the child. The planks on the road or door symbolize the path for his or her soul to travel home. It is also said that *hu plig tuam choj* is particularly essential for a child conceived with the assistance of *neeb* spirits through *ua neeb* rituals conducted by a shaman.

When this path is made, people who pass by know that there is a sick child in the family. They will be invited to enter the house to tie a cotton string on the wrist of the baby and to bless him or her. The planks will be left at the spot until they rot away.

The shaman also acts as a social mediator, trying to ensure that both mother and father pay attention to and love their children equally in the physical world. In the case of parents' souls that do not like their children equally, the shaman will call everyone involved together and try to mediate to see if it is possible for the parents and the children to stay together as a family. This will reassure the souls of the children that both parents love them and will take good care of them. This will stop the child's soul from returning to his or her ancestral pool (meaning death after birth).

In the case of *Txoov Kab Yeeb* causing ill health in a child, the shaman will have to perform a trance ritual to negotiate with the spirit parents to help the baby to become better. The shaman will first *ua neeb* to beg the spirit parents and then perform *ua neeb* to heal the baby's problems. Lastly, the shaman will have to perform another soul-calling ritual to honor the spirit parents properly. When all of these rituals have been carried out, the child will recover.

Khawv Koob (A Magic Healer)

For naturally caused illnesses such as broken bones, cuts and burns, magic water must be made by a magic healer for the child to drink and also to wipe on the wound. The magic healer prepares the magic water from normal drinking water. Several silver coins are put into the bowl of water. Incense sticks are burned and waved around the water bowl while the healer chants. The magic water is made in the presence of the child and given to him or her to drink immediately. This is done for three mornings.

For illness caused by being struck by spirits, it is common for a healer to chant magic words on a knife or a leaf and place it under the pillow of the child who is ill. The leaf may also be placed at the front door of the child's house.

For the ritual of calling a lost soul, a magic healer also uses magic water. *Khawv koob* is believed to be essential for cases in which a child has been frightened and his soul has been left at the place where the fright occurred. The soul then escapes for a long period of time and is reincarnated into another living form. This is referred to as *zwm*, as a magic healer explained:

> When the child has fallen over at a particular spot and giving the child a fright and the soul is left there, the child will be small and not growing. They say that the child has lost his soul and has *zwm*; that is a soul has been left at the spot for a long time and the soul has been reincarnated into something else, then you will use *khawv koob* to call the soul back.

CONCLUSIONS

The Hmong treat the health and illness of their children seriously, partly because of high infant mortality rates in their homeland and also because the Hmong hold particular views about the causes of health and illness. As I have described, the Hmong have four main explanations of childhood health and illness: natural cause, souls, supernatural beings, and black magic. This is what Scheper-Hughes (1984) has referred to as the "naturalistic, supernaturalistic and personalistic" causes of illness and misfortune. It has been seen that for a child to become ill, not only nature contributes to his or her illness; other forces—supernatural beings and human aggression—contribute as well. As Wembah-Rashid (1996: 86) has stated, these explanations point to the influence that individuals, both the living and the dead, have on the health and illness of children. Similarly, Savage (1996: 96) has pointed out that in many traditional societies, health is perceived as a "harmonious state where the social, religious or supernatural realm clearly impinges on physical and psychological well-being." Childhood health and illness are no exceptions. Therefore, if a child is ill from whatever causes, it is "an indication of disharmony with the living and/or between the living and the dead."

The supernatural world, it is believed, acts as a social control agent to regulate the human's behavior, which may have some effects on the health of children. This can clearly be seen from the prohibition against taking a newborn infant outside the house during the first thirty days after birth for fear of being struck by spirits of all sorts. The living conditions of the Hmong in Laos are not as good as they are in many Western countries. Their environment is dusty, and animals roam around people's living quarters. The newborn child may be susceptible to harmful agents caused by these living conditions. The Hmong, therefore, use the supernatural beings as a controlling force to eliminate the possibility of childhood illness. Similarly, the value of having social harmony between the living can be seen in the belief that a child may become the target of human aggression by means of black magic if the parents are in conflict with other people. In addition, social harmony between the living and the supernatural world is reflected in the belief that even benevolent spirits such as the parent spirits, if they are offended, can cause illness in children.

These issues are important if we consider them in the context of the high rates of infant mortality of the Hmong in their homeland. The belief system may guard against the blaming of individual parents if something goes wrong. This is particularly true for the mother. In most societies and most often, if a child is ill or dies, the mother will be the one who bears the blame more than any other family member. Attributing childhood illness and death to such agents, which are beyond the control of the mother, may protect her from being seen as "a bad mother" or one who has performed "bad mothering" (Scheper-Hughes, 1984: 536).[6]

It has been noted that the Hmong in Australia adopt a pluralistic view in dealing with childhood illness. When a child is ill, both traditional and modern medicine are sought. Although the Hmong tend to resort to their traditional medicines (Hmong herbs) in their first attempt to heal the child, parents may take the sick child to a health center if the symptoms are prolonged. In addition, the child may be taken to a hospital for treatment, but at the same time parents seek help from a shaman and a magic healer to perform *ua neeb* or *khawv koob* at home. What is the reason for this help-seeking pattern among the Hmong? At one level, it may be similar to what Grace (1998: 1292) has pointed out in her work on infant illnesses in Indonesia:

> The underlying logic of the decisions parents (particularly women) make about when and where to seek treatment for their infants must be sought not only in socio-economic factors, but also in local perceptions of practioners and the appropriateness of the treatment they give for particular illnesses. . . . [This] is affected by [people's] understanding, and day-to-day experience of, the appropriateness and efficacy of the treatment they receive from "traditional" and "modern" practitioners.

This is also true among the Hmong. As I have described, the Hmong attribute the causes of childhood illness not only to nature, but to supernatural beings and human aggression as well. If the illness is seen as caused by nature, herbal remedies as well as modern medicines may be used. However, if the cause of illness is believed to be due to supernatural forces, spiritual healing processes must be sought, since the belief is that herbs and modern medicines cannot cure the illness.

At another level, however, the pattern of help-seeking among the Hmong is more pragmatic and aims to ensure child survival. As de Zoysa et al. (1984: 734) have pointed out:

> Health care decisions are influenced by a multiplicity of factors which are dependent on the cultural and socio-economic setting and their interaction

with the range of therapeutic options. Where modern medical techniques and remedies penetrate traditional societies, "rustic pragmatism" may prevail and "anything that is available and culturally legitimate" will be tried.

Although the Hmong believe in their traditional practitioners' powers of cure, they also believe in the power of modern medicines. As van der Geest and Whyte (1989: 346) have remarked, "medicines are widely believed to contain the power of healing in themselves." Anyone who gains access to modern medicines acknowledges their power in the healing process. The Hmong in Australia are no exception. Because of their access to modern medicines in Australia, Hmong parents are able to apply the power of modern medicines to help their children recover from illness. They believe that the combination of traditional and modern medicines will make their sick children recover as soon as possible. This belief may help to ensure the survival of their children so that Hmong society will continue its existence.[7]

Traditional healers also play an important part in Hmong society. Not only do they assist people in healing, but help create harmony within the society as well. A shaman, for example, mediates social relationships among the living and between living and the supernatural world. This is why the Hmong see a shaman as an important part of their lives.[8]

This discussion shows us that cultural beliefs and practices related to childhood health and illness have tied the Hmong not just to their families and their society, but also to the supernatural world.

Hmong cultural beliefs and practices concerning childhood health and illness have implications for child health services in Australia. First, Hmong explanations of childhood health and illness and their help-seeking behaviors are markedly different from the Western norms. This may create cultural conflict and confusion between the Hmong and their Western caregivers. When this happens, misunderstandings and misdiagnoses may also follow, as Fadiman (1997) has pointed out in the case of a Hmong family in Merced, California. In her study, Fadiman found that Hmong parents' explanation of the causes and treatment of epilepsy differ markedly from those of Western medical professionals. The Hmong see childhood epilepsy as the resultant symptom of *qaug dab peg,* which means "the spirit catches you and you fall down" (p. 20) Epilepsy in Hmong culture is regarded with ambivalence. It is, on the one hand, seen as "a serious and potentially dangerous condition" (p. 20). However, it is also seen as "an illness of some distinction," (p. 21), since most Hmong epileptics become shamans; traditional healers who heal illnesses through trance. Because of these cultural differences, one child was mistreated and mismanaged by his Western doctors. The child was taken away from her parents and placed in a foster home because her doctor believed that her parents maltreated her by delaying to seek help and not giving her Western medications. It is, therefore, important that health professionals take Hmong cultural beliefs and practices related to child health and illness into account when providing care for Hmong children and families. A simple method by which knowledge of Hmong cultural beliefs and practices may be obtained is to ask the parents about their cultural beliefs and practices regarding the child's illness. The health professionals may work with an interpreter if the parents have limited English, so that the parents can explain their concerns in great detail. At the same time, full explanations of the child's symptoms and treatment options in terms of Western medicine can be given to the parents so that they know what to expect when seeking help from Western health care.

Secondly, the Hmong have a pluralistic view of health and illness. To restore their children's health, they seek help not only from their traditional system but also from Western health care. This should not be seen as a lack of trust in modern medicine, but as a practice consistent with their pluralistic view. Because of this, it might benefit the Hmong, if they are able, to incorporate their traditional health care system into that of the West. For example, a magic healer might be called upon when burning or broken bones are involved. In addition, if the parents suspect that the child's illness is caused by soul loss or by a soul having been captured by spirits, a shaman might be invited to perform a shamanic ritual to bring the soul of the child back. This has been recommended by the World Health Organization (WHO) at Alma Ata, which encourages the involvement of traditional healers in primary health care in order to achieve "Health for All by the Year 2000" (WHO, 1988: 199). Several studies of different societies have also pointed to the advantages of bringing traditional healing practices into modern health care.[9] Such an incorporation would not only help the Hmong make the maximum use of health services, but also assist them to feel more familiar with Western health care, which is markedly different from their own.

What I have outlined in this chapter may be used as a starting point for developing culturally appropriate health services for the Hmong community in Australia and elsewhere. For example, it can be a resource for caregivers when working with the Hmong. In addition, it can be used as an example of a different health care system when teaching future health professionals to be sensitive to people from different cultural backgrounds. A clear understanding of cultural beliefs and expectations is essential for health professionals if misunderstandings are to be avoided. It may eventually lead to culturally appropriate and sensitive health care for all immigrant children such as those of the Hmong.

NOTES

1. See Chapter 8 in this volume for greater details of the ceremony.
2. See Chapter 9 in this volume for infant feeding practices in Hmong culture.

3. See for example, Chindasri, 1976; Thao, 1984; Westermeyer, 1988; Kunstadter et al., 1987; Bliatout, 1991; Cooper et al., 1996; Moua, 1996 and Chapter 1 in this volume for more details on Hmong health and illness and the causes of sickness.

4. See also Chapter 1 in this volume for a discussion of souls and health and illness in Hmong culture.

5. See Fadiman's book, entitled *The spirit catches you and you fall down: A Hmong child, her American doctors, and the collision of two cultures* (1997) for thorough details of *dab peg*, which causes epilepsy in children.

6. This is similar to what Scheper-Hughes (1984) and Castle (1994) have reported about child bearing practices among poor urban mothers in Brazil and rural Mali.

7. As mentioned, in Hmong culture children are necessary for one's well-being, not only in this life but also in the afterlife. Children, particularly sons, are important because they care for the family altar, feed the ancestors and carry on the clan spirit into the next generation. This ensures the continuation of the family, lineage and clan. And it is a means by which the Hmong can be sure that their society will continue its existence.

8. As I have mentioned in Chapter 3, in Laos there must be at least one shaman in every village. Without the shaman, people do not feel secure and the village may not continue to exist. In Australia, as mentioned, there is at least one shaman in each state and there are at least four shamans in Melbourne.

9. See for example, McNee et al., 1995; Nichter and Nichter, 1994; Gove and Pelto, 1994; Nichter, 1993; Hogel and Prins, 1991; and Hoff and Maseko, 1986.

Part Four

Women and Reproductive Health

Chapter 11

Unsuccessful Reproduction: Infertility and Miscarriage

> The one crowning sorrow of any true woman's life is childlessness, and there is nothing in Heaven or on earth that can fill the void.
>
> (Words from a women's advice book published in 1909, quoted in Sha, 1990: 10)

> Miscarriage represents a loss or diminishing of whatever sense of control a woman had about her life, health, or fate.
>
> (Reinharz, 1988: 92)

INTRODUCTION

Infertility occurs in all societies. Although infertility is a biological problem, the experience of it is often modified by the social construction and cultural practices within that society.[1] While it is known that infertility can be attributed to either the male or the female, it is the woman who generally bears the burden. Because of the assumption that all women are fertile, failure to conceive is usually seen as a problem inherent in the woman's body. McGilvray (1982: 62) has pointed out that among Tamil people in Batticaloa, Sri Lanka, infertility is primarily seen as a woman's problem. A supernatural agent may contribute to her childlessness, but "seldom is the potency of the husband questioned." A woman without children is seen as both "personally unfulfilled and ritually inauspicious." Similarly, Neff (1994: 477) has pointed out that among the Nayars in South India, the woman is usually blamed for her childlessness. The unfortunate woman will be an "inauspicious guest at weddings and sacred rituals" and she is "cut off from networks of sustenance and support."[2]

Some women may be able to conceive but may not be able to carry the baby to term. Miscarriage is another common reproductive failure that women in many parts of the world experience.[3] In many cultures, miscarriage is also seen as closely related to the society and the supernatural world as well as to the woman's body (Cecil 1996a).

In this chapter, I first examine the social constructs and cultural interpretations of infertility among Hmong women and then discuss the constructs of fertility, infertility and infertility treatment within the Hmong society. The chapter also explores traditional Hmong explanations of miscarriage and the ethnomedical knowledge and practices that pertain to it. In particular I examine the role of cultural beliefs and practices in response to miscarriage in Hmong society in terms of Cecil's (1996a) findings on the ways in which social and cultural factors affect the experience and management of miscarriage.[4]

THE INFERTILE BODY: A CHILDLESS WOMAN

Children are regarded as the prosperity of the family; therefore, having children is highly desirable. Hmong women are expected to be able to produce many children. Ideally, to be considered a good woman, she must bear at least as many children as her mother or mother-in-law.

Why are children important and so valued? Answering from a "social structural perspective," Inhorn (1996: 247) pointed out that children are important for three reasons. First, children are necessary in order to secure the survival of their parents and families. Second, in most patriarchal societies children are the only "valuable power resource" for their mothers. Hence, having children can improve the status of many women. Third, children are needed for the continuation of the society.

In a similar vein, children in Hmong culture are necessary for one's well-being, not only in this life but also in the afterlife. If a couple does not have sons or daughters to marry out, there will be no one to look after them in old age. Sons are more important than daughters because they care for the family altar, feed the ancestors and carry on the *dab qhuas* to the next generation. This ensures the continuation of the family, lineage and clan. Without children, neither Hmong men or women are perceived as complete.

> For the Hmong having a life together they must be able to produce one or more children so that when they grow older they will have support in that the children will look after them in their old age.

Although Hmong girls as children and adolescents do not have social or familial status equal to Hmong boys and men, their status changes when they marry and are able to bear a child. The birth of the first child brings prestige to a Hmong woman. After giving birth to her first child, a Hmong woman becomes known as its mother, and is referred to by the name of her child, for example, "Blia's mother." She is no longer addressed as "my younger daughter" by her parents, nor as the woman of her husband, as in "Mrs. Lee Xiong," by others. Women gain respect and status when they produce children.

A woman who cannot bear children in the Hmong culture is known as one who has a difficult life. She is always seen as unfortunate, unlucky and unfulfilled, not only in this life but also in the next. She is also not regarded highly in the community: "Have no children? If you have no children then other people look at you as an unimportant person."

THE EXTENDED FAMILY AND WOMEN'S POSITION

As stated, Hmong women experience pressure to produce children to ensure the continuity of lineage, to produce children who will care for them in their old age and feed their spirits when they die. If a woman remains infertile, after a few years of childlessness, the husband is encouraged to take a second wife since in Hmong culture polygyny is usually practiced if a first married wife is unable to produce children. As one informant said:

> In the Hmong culture, if after two to three years of marriage and she can not bear children the husband is encouraged to marry a second wife. This is because she cannot bear children and she is not respected among the husband's family. So they will encourage him to marry someone else to have children to carry on the clan name.

The first wife has no say in this since she is unable to bear a child, and she becomes the "big sister" among her husband's wives. If the other wives are able to produce children, she becomes the "oldest mother" to her husband's children. Her status may not be affected if the junior wives and their children respect her and treat her as their "big mother." Problems arise only when she cannot get along well with the junior wives and her husband takes sides with his new wives. In some cases, the woman may be divorced and forced to move out of her husband's home.

Most Hmong women I interviewed did not wish to become a senior wife because of the insecurity of this position. Many said that their husband would eventually favor a wife who could bear him children, and they would be seen as worthless.

> If you have no children, in a long term like up to ten years, then your husband would look at her as not worth it.

A more important issue is the need to have a son in the family. The Hmong are patrilineal and the eldest son takes care of elderly parents. Upon the death of the parents, the son must honor and feed his deceased parents' spirits to ensure that the parents' souls can reach the ancestral pool in the other world and be able to reincarnate. Sons are crucial for this important function, because women are not allowed to perform ancestral worship. If a woman is unable to bear a son, she is, again, forced to let her husband bring in another wife.

However, there are couples who wish to maintain their marriage and refuse the practice of polygyny. After years of trying to conceive using herbal medicines and shamanic rituals, these people may acquire children through adoption. Traditionally, male children from relatives of the same clan will be adopted. In this way, the child will have the same clan name as the adoptive father so that the clan name and the lineage will continue. More commonly, a couple may adopt a child of one of their sisters. The adopted child will belong to the adoptive parents throughout his lifetime although his biological parents may live nearby. He will perform his duty as a son of the family in the same way a biological son does for his biological parents, including looking after them in old age, performing rituals upon their death to bring them back to their ancestral pool for reincarnation, and feeding them after their death.

WHAT MAKES WOMEN INFERTILE?

Hmong women provided several layers of explanations about the causes of infertility. Their explanations about "ethnogynecological causes," to use Inhorn's term (1994a: 163), can be best presented following the analytical framework proposed by Inhorn (1994a: 10) in her writing about infertility in Egypt.

The Cold Womb

The Hmong believe that a woman may be infertile because her womb is in a state of "coldness." The "cold" state here refers to humoral coldness: "When *kws tshuaj* felt my stomach they all said that my womb was cold, not warm." To be able to conceive, a woman's womb must be in a "hot" stage.[5] Whether a womb is hot or cold is also believed to be related to the quality of blood in the woman's body.

> Your stomach [womb] must be warm for you to conceive. If it is cold then it is like your blood is not good and so you cannot have children. If your

womb is warm that means your blood is warm and your body is warm and then you can have children.

The Body with Bad Behavior

A woman's bad behavior toward others in the society can also make her infertile. This includes saying bad words about other people, particularly children. It also includes making comments about other people's physical appearance causing anger among those who have been offended. This also invokes a deity's anger, since the deity sees everything from the sky and keeps a record of her behavior. The deity considers a woman like this not suitable to be a parent, and so will not send children to her. In addition, because of misbehavior the offended parties may become angry and hence lay a curse on her body, causing infertility.

> She has said a bad word and *Huab Tais Ntuj* is on her shoulder and he knows that she had said [such thing]. . . . She has to remove her words and beg them with new words so that *Txoov Kab Yeeb* will give children to her.

Another woman explained:

> If she sees someone with a dumb child that could not speak and she hates him or she might say bad things . . . like the Westerners say "yucky" to children who do not clean themselves and she can't stand them. The children's parents might say, "She hates my children so I doubt she can give birth to any, not even like mine." So she is cursed with that word and thus she can't get pregnant.

Infertility and the Body with Menstrual Blood

Hmong women in the study also said that infertility is caused by having poor menstruation:

> You must have good menstruation to be able to have children. When your menstruation is good you will not have sore stomach. It gives you strength and you can conceive.

Menstruating women are also subjected to some restrictions.[6] For example, women should not perform heavy work and rigorous physical activities. This is believed to cause the uterus to "turn" into a wrong position, which results in infertility.

> Women should not do heavy work during your menses. Heavy work and running fast can make the uterus turn and thus can make the mother infertile.

In addition, women should not eat "cold" food or drink icy cold water while menstruating. The cold food will congeal menstrual blood and make the womb "cold."

However, the most common explanation for and most feared cause of infertility among the Hmong is being *raug dab* (struck by spirits). In the Hmong world there are "spirits of ancestors, sky and earth, food and water, sun and moon, and wind" (Thao, 1984: 327). Spirits are everywhere and they do not wish to be disturbed. If people do not keep away from the spirits, they may be struck and become ill.

In the case of infertility, a young woman may have crossed rivers or streams while menstruating and washed the clothes worn while menstruating in these rivers or streams. These activities are believed to disturb the waters and thus cause the anger of the spirits of the rivers or streams. Hmong women are seriously warned against these activities. The spirits are able to trace a woman through the smell of her menstruation and "strike" her. This causes miscarriage whenever she conceives. Repeated miscarriages in turn cause infertility in the woman.

A woman can become infertile after having a first child if the childbirth blood is washed away in the stream. Again, the blood is believed to cause the anger of the spirits. The woman is then struck by the spirits and she becomes infertile.

> When a woman has the first child and she has all the blood from having a baby and if she takes that to wash in the river she will not have any more children. . . . The Hmong say that she will be *raug dab* and even if she has *ua neeb* as many times as she can she will not have any more children.

Women who have bad menstrual pain will be infertile too. The reason for menstrual pain is that a woman has invoked the spirit's anger by not observing a strict rule while menstruating, as mentioned above. The pain results from spirits throwing rocks at her body. Because of the repeated injury to her body, she is unable to conceive a child. The following account provided by a shaman illustrates the point:

> When she has menses and she doesn't refrain from doing certain things like after the rain she goes across the river, so the noble people [spirits] going by will notice that she is like that and she has stepped over them. This will make them very angry and they will make her have a lot of pain in her stomach when she has menses. . . . If she has menses and has pain then she can't conceive; the purpose of the menses is in order for her to have children. Why would having the menses and pain prevent her from getting pregnant? Whenever she has her menses, she always gets a lot of pain. This is because they know that she is nearly having her menses, like when she comes and does that to them [steps over them], then they will

come and throw the rocks at her and she will have those pain and not have any children.

Mandate of Life

The Hmong believe that an infertile woman did not bring "a piece of paper"[7] from heaven when she was born that indicated that she would have children. This paper is written and given out by *Txoov Kab Yeeb,* a spirit couple who are believed to assist in fertility. If the paper does not indicate that a woman can have children, she then becomes childless. "For the ones who cannot have children, old people say when they came from heaven they did not bring their paper to have children." As I have discussed earlier, the Hmong understand that to be able to conceive, a woman must have a husband or at least a man involved in the affair. However, pregnancy cannot happen solely by having a husband. It is determined by *Txoov Kab Yeeb.* A child can be born only when *Txoov Kab Yeeb* give permission, and they only direct the child to be born to a woman whom they have stated is to do so in her "piece of paper," written before her own birth.

> I think that the baby is a given thing from heaven. It must be from heaven because if it is not, then I don't think it would be possible to have children. The old people say it is by the heaven. When it is time for the baby to be born then the heaven will open the door and when it is done the heaven will seal the door again.

It is also said that a child cannot be born because *choj tub,* the path for the child to travel from heaven, has been broken. The broken path prevents the child from finding his or her parents' home and therefore he or she cannot be born.

> [*Choj tub*] . . . is there so the baby will have a path to come and she [the woman] will be able to have children. If it is not done like this then . . . it is like a jungle if there is no path and you were in it then where do you go? Like the river too if there is no bridge how do you go across? If you go then you will drown in the river and so you won't be able to go unless there is a bridge.

The Man's Body

Although women are thought to be primarily responsible for infertility, men are occasionally mentioned as contributing to infertility if they have no testicles or unevenly sized testicles.

> If the couple cannot have children then it is because of the husband. He has no testicles.

Similarly, another woman said:

> My mum says that some men have uneven sized testicles. These men cannot make their wives bear children.

Some women attempted to explain that because of the uneven-sized testicles of men, some men are not able to provide adequate seed for the woman. Because of this, these men cannot give children to their wives.

THE MEANING OF MISCARRIAGE

Miscarriage has grave consequences for the Hmong society at large. As mentioned in earlier chapters, the Hmong believe that each living body has three souls. When all three souls reside in the body, the person is healthy and well. Upon death, the three souls leave the body. One soul will stay at the grave of the person. The second soul will travel to the land of its ancestors. The third soul will travel to the spirit world and wait to return in another body. When it is time for the soul to be reincarnated, it will be given permission from *Txoov Kab Yeeb* (spirit parents) to enter the womb of a woman. Miscarriage thus means that a soul cannot be reincarnated into the family, and that there will be fewer offspring to continue the family, the clan and lineage.

A miscarriage is perceived as "the falling of the baby" or that the baby is "leaking from the mother's womb." In the Hmong ethnophysiological view, the baby is connected with the mother through the "blood line" or "food line." The mouth of the baby is connected with the feeding connection, which is referred to as the "breast inside the womb."

> The old people say that it is like the baby is sucking on the breast inside the womb and the connection is disconnected and thus the baby has no nourishment. If it has happened for a long time and you do not go to find medicine for the baby then the baby will not be good and could die in the stomach.

Hmong women also use the metaphor of a dam to represent a pregnancy: a dam full of water can support many lives living in it. Once the dam has no water, however, it cannot support life. It is thought that the baby is nourished if no bleeding occurs, which equates to having the dam full of water. The dam, however, can be damaged by certain means, including supernatural beings. As one woman elaborated:

> Miscarriage! Like . . . when you have a baby, it is like a dam that you have just made and they come to let the water out. The dam will be dry and so it can't support lives in the dam. When you are pregnant and then if they come and destroy it, the baby will not survive.

When a miscarriage occurs there is no elaborate mourning ritual, as is the case in the deaths of adults or babies, who are seen as human. A newborn baby is regarded as a full human being only after a soul-calling ceremony is performed on the third morning after birth. Thus, a "falling baby" is not human, and the body is buried in the forest without any ritual.

THE WOMAN'S BODY AND "THE FALL OF BABY"

The Hmong provided several explanations for falling babies, related mainly to their own body and behaviours. The most common reason cited for the falling or the leaking of the baby was bleeding during early pregnancy.

Vigorous Physical Activities

During pregnancy, Hmong women are cautious about vigorous or hard physical activities. It is believed that carrying a heavy load or doing heavy work can distress the baby, which causes it to cease growing. It may eventually "fall out" if there is no relief for its distress. One woman explained:

> If you do heavy things then it will distress the baby, and then it becomes very difficult. . . . If the baby is distressed then the mother will get pain in the stomach and sore back. It could also mean that you can't feel the baby move anymore, this is what distress means. . . . If you know that it has been distressed and you have the symptoms and you cannot feel the baby move then you go to the old lady to feel the baby and then fix the baby for you.

Carrying a heavy load is also believed to disconnect the "blood line" or "food line" of the baby inside the womb. As one woman related:

> If you carry water and anything heavy then you can disconnect the baby's cord. . . . To what I have learnt is that if the cord is disconnected when the baby is not due it will give a lot of stomach pain and you will bleed. . . . If the baby is very strong then it won't fall, but if the baby is weak then it will fall.

Reaching up high is also prohibited during pregnancy. Jumping from a high place can also disconnect the "blood line" or the "food line":

> Don't lift heavy things and don't reach up too high and no big leap in a high place so that you use a lot of energy by doing that . . . because if you jump then you cause a big vibration, and this can cause the baby to fall down. If it falls then it will miscarry. If the baby has a strong hold then it will make the baby very small and not develop larger. . . . If bleeding is a result of the leap then it will miscarry.

When the disconnection occurs, treatment is sought immediately to save the baby from falling. A Hmong magic healer explained:

> If the mouth line is disconnected, then you will take the woman to see old people to help turn the baby. She will turn it back into the right position and also use the herbal medicines for her to drink.

Women's Falling

The Hmong believe that falling during pregnancy either because of an accident or as a result of work may cause the baby to turn into a wrong position. This, in turn, will cause pain in the abdominal area and, hence, a miscarriage may occur. Falling also causes the baby to cease its movement because the food line has been disconnected. When this happens, the Hmong say that the baby does not grow properly inside the mother's womb. Hmong women are particularly careful about falling during pregnancy. If falling occurs and there is no one to turn the baby's position and stimulate movement, the pregnancy may end in miscarriage:

> If you are pregnant and you have a fall from working, this causes the baby to turn into the wrong position then you need someone to feel you. . . . In my country we work a lot. If it is slippery when you go to the farm and you fall over quite hard, the vibration of your fall will cause the baby to turn slightly. This will cause you to become sick [have severe pain in the abdomen].

One woman related her experience in Laos:

> When I had [one of her sons], I went to the farm and I fainted and rolled down the hill for quite a distance. I rolled over and over again while I was pregnant with him. My husband knew how to turn the baby, but he was at work at another farm. I asked people to find him and tell him that I fell over and my stomach felt very tight and uncomfortable. When he came back he turned the baby and it felt comfortable immediately.

ILLNESS AND FEVER DURING PREGNANCY

Illness and high fever during pregnancy is regarded as dangerous, as it may lead to miscarriage.

> Some people experience a fever and have a high temperature, the body is very hot and it over heats the baby so the baby can miscarry. . . . It is when she becomes sick and her body becomes hot with temperature, thus overheats the baby and the baby miscarries. But if she has a headache or other pain but not that heat to steam the baby then the baby cannot fall out.

When having a fever or an infection, Hmong women avoid taking any Western medicines (known as American medicines), because they believe that Western medicines are harmful and can cause miscarriage.

> In Laos they are medicines for fever and also in Laos we often have infected spleen, you should not eat those medicines, American medicines. I mean like when the spleen has an irregular growth on it, it is the medicine for that problem. If you take them early in the pregnancy, the baby will miscarry.

THE SUPERNATURAL WORLD AND "THE FALL OF BABY"

As mentioned, the Hmong believe in many supernatural beings: gods, spirits of places, household spirits, malicious spirits, and spirits of the dead. They believe that spirits are everywhere and that they do not wish to be disturbed. If people do not keep away from the spirits they may be struck and become ill.[8]

The most common explanation for and most feared cause of a miscarriage among the Hmong is being *raug dab* (struck by spirits). As one woman elaborated:

> A miscarriage is caused by spirits, hit by the spirits. Like for example a dam and someone comes along to put a hole in the dam and thus releasing the water and the fish in it would die and come out as well. It is the same thing with miscarriage; it is always caused by spirits.

The spirits may strike the mother or the baby. In the case of the mother, it may occur when she travels near a landslide or crosses a river or a valley. Because spirits can be anywhere, it is difficult to know if she will cross their path while they are active (awake). If she happens to cross the spirits' path at this time, she will be hit and this may cause bleeding. To be struck by nature spirits is therefore seen as a matter of chance.

> The spirits, you can easily get hit when you go cross their path when they wake up. They and you have your own house and paths and you will go your way and they will go their way. But sometimes you might just bump into or touch them by accident, and this is when you get hit.

One woman related that Hmong women have to work on the farm and this means that they have to travel from home to their farm, which makes them prone to being hit by spirits.

> [There are] spirits of the low lands, and spirits of landslides, rock caves on mountains. We lived in the village in the high lands, on the way to the farm we had to cross over red raw landslides, where the spirits live. So you are very vulnerable. If you don't be careful, like if you were pregnant then you should avoid going. If you go then you will be hit.

However, the Hmong also believe if a pregnant woman is not careful enough she will be hit by spirits. Her carelessness has offended spirits and they want to punish her. As a shaman explained:

> For a woman who has a miscarriage, it is because she is not careful when it rains. After it rains there is a temporary river and if she crosses that river, they [the spirits] who are not always bad, but sometimes good, believe that because she is pregnant, she is going over their heads. They will not be happy with her, and they will throw a rock at her. They throw a rock and hit her. . . . If she has only pain then it is only that they throwing things . . . a rock at her, but if she bleeds then it means that they are removing the baby.

Another reason for being hit by spirits is related to menstruation. A young woman may have crossed rivers or streams while menstruating and washed the clothes worn while menstruating in these rivers or streams, which is believed to disturb and anger the spirits of the rivers or streams. Hmong women are seriously warned against these activities. The spirits are able to trace a woman through the smell of her menstruation and strike her, leading to miscarriage whenever she conceives.

> There are some women that might have been *raug dab*. These people are the ones when they are still teenagers they wash their menstruating clothes in a marshy river where the spirits live and so the spirits would have eaten all their children's souls, thus their children keep falling.

The baby may also be struck by spirits, as a magic man pointed out:

> A miscarriage is caused by *raug dab*. Like her body is heavy with the baby inside and she goes out into the low valley or into the forest . . . then she

> and the baby are hit by bad spirits. They say that the woman is hit when the spirit is at play or when the spirits wake up and see her there and they come to touch the baby. They come to eat the baby. . . . The spirits eat the baby and drink the baby's blood, and that is why she miscarries.

Hmong women strongly believe that Western medicine will be unable to help them once bleeding occurs. It is only through *ua neeb* (a shamanic ritual) that the baby may be safe from falling. As one woman related:

> As soon as you start to bleed you have to *ua neeb* then it can help. If you leave it for four or five days then it can't help. . . . If *ua neeb* is not performed straight away to stop the spirit then the spirit is able to destroy the baby and you miscarry. . . . It is like a dam and they [spirits] have just start to put their hands into the water to stir it. You have to *ua neeb* to stop them at that time. If you don't ask the shaman to remove those hands, then they will keep stirring the water until the dam is damaged [leaking of the baby].

This is confirmed by a case told by a Hmong shaman who treated one Hmong woman by *ua neeb* and was able to save her pregnancy. She told us:

> Mrs [. . .], when she arrived, she was bleeding a lot and there was no *ua neeb* to help her and the baby was falling. When she came to live here, they didn't know me, and they didn't came to ask me to *ua neeb*. She was bleeding a lot and she stayed in Dr [. . .] 's clinic. Even she went to the hospital but they didn't know what to do for her. The doctor couldn't help her in any way and the bleeding didn't stop. At that time her mother was not here yet, she was still in [. . .] camp. Her mother recorded in a cassette to scold me and said that: "You are her aunt, why don't you help my child? When I get there I am not going to be happy with you." So I went to *ua neeb* for her. . . . That is why she has her daughter who is now at school already.

HU PLIG HLAWV THIAB: THE BURNING OF THE REINCARNATED SOULS AND BABY FALLING

Hu plig hlawv thiab is known as the ritual for calling the soul of a person, which has been reincarnated into another living being, back to his or her body. The ritual must be performed by a shaman or a magic healer. It involves positioning an egg in a bowl at the bedroom door and stringing out a string to the bedroom. After ritually calling the soul, the shaman will wrap the egg with the string and burn the egg until it breaks.

During pregnancy, a woman's soul can leave a body and re-enter any other body for re-birth. When this happens, *hu plig hlawv thiab* must be performed as soon as it is known in order to burn the reincarnated soul and, hence, bring the woman's soul back. If it is not performed, she will die during pregnancy or soon after birth. However, the baby will miscarry as a result of this ritual. A Hmong shaman explained:

> When you *hu plig hlawv thiab*, and if the person has gone to be reincarnated and you perform this ceremony, because the person's soul has gone and is reincarnated into a new thing, like an animal or whatever, if you burn the egg [in the ceremony] then the new fetus will miscarry. . . . Even if it is being reincarnated into the mother's womb, when you burn the egg [conduct the ritual], it will make the mother miscarry.

The Hmong regard this ritual as extremely dangerous, as another Hmong shaman related:

> This is Hmong people call *ntxeev taw rooj* (turn the table over). It is a difficult case to fix. With that if you try to heal them, maybe you can help the mother but then the baby will miscarry, and if the baby is alive then the mother will die. . . . You have to separate them when the baby is still very small. . . . If the baby is already big before you find out then it will be too late. This is because by that time the baby's life and the mother's life is at the same level so you can't help them. When the baby is born, at birth if the baby lives then the mother dies straight away, and if the mother lives, then the baby will be stillborn.

UNSUCCESSFUL REPRODUCTION: THE HEALING PROCESSES

Infertility

Infertile Hmong women seek help for infertility. Initially, a woman tries to resolve the problem alone by seeking help from *Kws Tshuaj* (a medicine woman). If she continues to fail to conceive, her husband and the extended family will become involved, and normally *Txiv Neeb* (a shaman) will be consulted.

Kws Tshuaj *(A Medicine Woman)*

Hmong women seek help for infertility from a medicine woman in their own villages in Laos as their first choice. The medicine woman examines the woman's womb by massaging her stomach in a circular motion. From this, she is able to tell the condition of the womb. The medicine woman then goes out to her garden and picks several kinds of *tshuaj Hmoob* (Hmong green herbs). She then instructs the woman on the way in which to take the herbs. Usually, these are steamed with eggs and then eaten. This is done in the morning for three mornings. The woman must then wait for one year to see if the treatment has been successful. During this period, the woman is not allowed to seek help from other medicine women. If the treatment has not been successful after the one year trial, the woman may then consult another medicine woman. If the treatment works and the woman becomes pregnant, she must honor the medicine woman. Traditionally, this is done on the third morning after the woman has given birth, when the soul-calling and naming ceremonies for the newborn infant are conducted. During the ceremonies, the new mother must acknowledge the medicine woman's power and kneel down to thank her. The family must also prepare a chicken for her to bring home and they must pay her several silver coins. Some of the coins will be placed on the medicine woman's altar to honor the spirit who assisted in the medicine woman's success in making the new mother pregnant.[9]

Txiv Neeb *(A Shaman)*

To ask a shaman to assist in fertility, a childless couple must go to the shaman's house, where his altar is located, and formally request help. Once this is done, the shaman first holds a ritual *ua neeb saib* to determine the factor that contributes to the woman's childlessness, ascertaining whether or not she has "a piece of paper," if she has been *raug dab* (struck by spirits) or has disrupted social relationships with in the society. If the woman did not bring her paper with her, the shaman will hold a ritual *ua neeb cais* to invoke *Txoov Kab Yeeb* to aid in fertility. The shaman must then offer *Txoof Kab Yeeb* a sacrificed chicken and some gold money as a reward for changing the woman's paper and for bringing children to her. In his trance, with the assistance of his helper, a shaman will put *daim nyias* (a traditional Hmong baby back carrier) on his back and travel to beg *Txoov Kab Yeeb* to send children to the couple. If the wish is granted, then the *daim nyias* symbolically carries the child down to earth.

In the case of *choj ntub* (a broken path), a shaman has to build a bridge or path for the child to travel to his parents' home. A roll of white material (mostly white cloth) is rolled from the front door to the bed of the couple. The shaman, in his trance while performing *ua neeb kho,* has the *daim nyias* wrapped on his back, travels to heaven and negotiates with *Txoov Kab Yeeb* to give the couple children. If this request is granted, the shaman will carry the child in the *daim nyias* and travel down through the white material. In the shamanic performance, this is done by pulling the material from the front door into the bedroom, so that the child will have a path to follow. It is believed that only through this ritual will a woman become pregnant if she has *choj ntub.*

In the case of being struck by spirits, the shaman also has to hold the ritual *ua neeb cais* to negotiate with the spirits and bribe them to leave the woman in peace, so that she will be able to conceive. Traditionally, the spirits will be offered a sacrificed pig and some gold money. If the spirits are malicious and do not wish to leave the woman, the shaman would have to invoke his spirit assistants to negotiate with them. Usually, the evil spirits will be defeated and eventually agree not to interfere with the woman's body (womb).

Where infertility is caused by disrupted social relationships, the offending woman must admit to having said bad things and vow to stop misbehaving, while *ua neeb kho* is performed by a shaman. The shaman assists in removing the bad words, and after this has been done *Txoov Kab Yeeb* will give children to the woman.

If the shaman succeeds in helping create fertility, the parents must come back after the child is born to honor him. Traditionally, they must offer a sum of money, a bunch of incense sticks, gold money and a live chicken. The shaman will continue to perform rituals to protect the newborn infant until he or she is three years old. If the child is ill during this period the shaman will be the first person to perform rituals to cure him or her.

Miscarriage

At the first sign of miscarriage, Hmong women themselves may try to stop it. The most common means of self-help is to sit in the corner of the house and pick up dried beans that have been spilled on the floor, one by one into a basket, until there are no more beans on the floor, which usually takes from several hours to a whole day. The woman is not allowed to move to another spot while picking up the beans. This is seen as an opportunity for rest, which will stop the falling of the baby.

> With the Hmong, while you are pregnant you cannot reach up very high. If you reach up for things then the blood line will disconnect and then you have to pick beans into a basket and you have to pick them all day long. . . . You pick them up and count how many so that the baby will be able to connect the blood connection. . . . The basket is a wide one like the small table. They will put the beans into a pile in one corner and you have to count them and separate them into the basket.

However, some Hmong women also seek help from traditional healers when severe bleeding or other symptoms which they believe may indeed lead to a miscarriage occur, such as the absence of baby movement and severe abdominal pain.

Kws Tshuaj *(A Medicine Woman)*

In Laos, women find a medicine woman from their own villages, but in Melbourne women can only seek help from a medicine woman who grows Hmong herbs. The medicine woman usually gathers four kinds of Hmong green herbs (*tshuaj Hmoob*) from her garden and instructs the woman on the way in which to take the herbs. Usually, they are finely chopped, steamed with eggs and then taken in the morning for three mornings. The herbs are believed to make the baby strong and prevent falling, so that the baby may grow properly to full term.

Sometimes the herbs are boiled with water and given to the women to drink as tea, usually two to three times a day, depending on the strength of the herbs as well as on the medicine woman, since each healer has her own remedy system.

The medicine woman may also prepare a pack of herbs for the woman to wear around her waist for as long as she can. If the bag becomes worn out or broken, it is replaced by another herbal bag. These herbal bags are prepared in particular for women who are more likely to miscarry from being struck by spirits. As one woman explained:

> You give her some Hmong medicines to wear. You have to sew a bag for her to wear around the waist. . . . You tie it there and if the bag is broken then you make another one for the woman who is often *raug dab* [being struck by spirits]. If she has two to three children and is likely that she will have no other problems then you don't have to do it anymore.

The Masseuse

The masseuse is an old woman who has delivered her own children, has helped other women deliver and can assist a woman who is having some difficulties with her pregnancy. The "old lady" is knowledgeable about and experienced with pregnancy and birth, but she is not regarded as a traditional midwife. There is no Hmong word to describe this role in Hmong culture.

If complications are perceived during pregnancy—for example, if a pregnant woman falls down, causing the baby turn into a wrong position and cease moving—the masseuse will *theev*, that is, reposition the baby by lifting up the woman's abdomen and slightly massaging and pushing in a circular motion. This is thought to help stop the bleeding and make the baby lie in a normal position so that it is able to move and grow. As a Hmong magic man explained:

> My grandmother knows the position of the baby. If the baby is in the wrong position she has the knowledge to turn it back into the right position. She is very good at it, too. When you cannot feel the baby move and that the baby is moved into a low position because you have fallen over then you will take it to grandma and she will say "Oh, the baby is in the wrong position," so she will help to turn it into the right position. If a child has fallen and we call it "the turned liver and kidney" [Hmong believe that if a child is turned upside down, that is the feet are held above the

head then their organs such as liver and kidney will have collapsed], then the child will lose his appetite and will not grow, and then may die and fall [miscarry].

Txiv Neeb *(A Shaman) and* Ua Neeb *Rituals*

The shaman first holds a ritual *ua neeb saib* to determine the factor that is contributing to the woman's problems, ascertaining whether she has been *raug dab* (struck by spirits). The shaman then holds the ritual *ua neeb cais* to negotiate with the spirits and bribe them to leave the woman in peace, so that her bleeding will stop and she will be able to carry her pregnancy through to term. Traditionally, the spirits are offered a sacrificial pig and some spirit money. If the spirits are malicious and do not wish to leave the woman, the shaman invokes his spirit assistants to negotiate with them. Usually the evil spirits will be defeated and eventually agree not to interfere with the woman's womb. During this period of several days the woman must stay at home, to avoid being struck by another spirit.

In the case of a miscarriage caused by *hu plig hlawv thiab*, there is no cure. However, *hu plig hlawv thiab* can be prevented in the next pregnancy by ensuring that the soul of the mother is secured in her body so that her soul may not be reincarnated in her own body.

Khawv Koob *(A Magic Healer)*

If a woman has bleeding and experiences extreme pain, magic water for her to drink is made by a magic healer. The water is also used to wipe her abdomen and back. Magic water is prepared from normal drinking water. Several silver coins are put into the bowl of water and incense sticks are burned and waved around the water bowl, accompanied by chanting. For three mornings, the magic water is made in the presence of the woman and given to her to drink. Some magic healers may also massage the woman's abdomen and back after the chanting and the drinking of the magic water.

A more difficult ritual—in which a magic healer performs the "cover water" ritual—is designed to help women with severe bleeding. The magic healer digs two holes in the bedroom dirt floor and places a cup of water upside down in each. The woman spits and places some hair in the holes. Magic words are recited by the healer and the woman crosses over the holes three times. The healer then covers the holes to trap the spirits so that they may no longer interfere with the woman's body. After this, her bleeding is believed to stop. This ritual is, however, not performed in Melbourne because houses do not have dirt floors as they have in Laos.

CONCLUSIONS

Infertility in Hmong society is seen as the woman's problem. Infertility not only affects the woman's identity, but also has a great impact on the identity of the "local moral worlds" (Kleinman, 1992) in which the woman lives; that is, of the Hmong society. The "infertile body" is a reflection of the "social body" in which it is located; the blame is located and expressed by social control over the woman's body.

In all societies, fertility and infertility are subject to social rules and cultural practices. These rules and practices are strictly observed and followed in traditional societies, which depend on having children to ensure the continuation of the lineage. Having children is crucial for the lives of Hmong people, since it means that the lineage and, hence, the Hmong society will live on. As I have stated earlier, it is even more crucial at the present time, since the Hmong population has been significantly reduced by successive losses of lives from battles with the Chinese in China before settlement in Laos, and then from the war in Laos in the 1970s. This has led to increased social pressure on the Hmong women. If they cannot have children, they have to allow their husband to take in another wife to bear him children. Women, therefore, have to try by whatever means available to get pregnant and give birth.

Hmong women, not men, are blamed for being infertile. It is the malfunctioning of the woman's body, whether because of her behaviors or the supernatural, that makes her childless. Hence, she is "socially subordinated" to her husband and provides legitimate grounds for him to bring in a second wife to bear children for him, even though he may have contributed to her childlessness. A childless woman has no say under these circumstances since she has shown to him and his family that she may endanger the continuity of the family line, which in turn threatens the reproduction of Hmong society.

Male infertility is rarely acknowledged in many societies, particularly in patrilineal societies. The Hmong society is no exception. Men are thought to govern the Hmong world. Only men can perform important tasks and only men can carry on the clan name. The notion that men may be infertile and therefore unable to have their own sons (in particular) to continue their duties is seen as immoral and is rarely acceptable. As Greer (1984: 34) has pointed out:

> The reason why male sterility is seldom recognised is precisely because the recognition would strike at the heart of morality: all order and coherence would be put in jeopardy.

Similarly, Inhorn (1994b) stated that infertility challenges men's procreative power. The most important product that men can create is a child, and this legitimates the right of men to rule the world. If their wives are unable to produce the men's creation, it is the women who must have done something wrong, whether through a fault of their own body, the interruptions of the social body or the interference of the body politic. Women are, therefore, the ones who nearly always bear the blame for not being able to bring a child into the "local moral worlds" of men. Therefore, male infertility is seldom recognised in Hmong culture, even though the women believe that the male can contribute to their barrenness as well.

As is true in many other cultures, there is no elaborate mourning ritual in the Hmong culture when a miscarriage occurs, as there is for the deaths of adults or babies seen as human. However, women and their families make every effort to prevent a miscarriage from occurring. Women say that they must be careful during pregnancy, and when there is a threat of miscarriage, processes are undertaken to restore the health of the baby and the mother. When babies do fall, women are encouraged to become pregnant again as soon as possible, not to replace what they have lost, but to provide a venue for another soul to be reincarnated, so that the family, clan and lineage can continue to exist. This is particularly important for the Hmong, who lost many lives to the secret war in Laos and need to re-establish their society in a new country.

Understanding the causes of miscarriage among the Hmong rests on knowledge of two main categories: the natural world, which is related to the woman's body and her behavior; and the supernatural world. As in the case of Tanzanian women (Wembah-Rashid, 1996), these explanations show the influence that individuals, both living and dead, have on pregnancies. Similarly, Savage (1996: 96) has pointed out that in many traditional societies, health is perceived as a "harmonious state where the social, religious or supernatural realm clearly impinges on physical and psychological well-being." Pregnancy is no exception. Therefore, if a woman is unable to bring forth offspring, whether through failure to conceive or through miscarriage, it is "an indication of disharmony with the living and/or between the living and the dead."

The supernatural world acts as an agent of social control over the woman's body and behaviors. Because sanitary pads are not available for Hmong women in the village, women frequently wash their bodies in a stream. Menstruating women are prohibited to cross the river or wash their clothes in running water. This prohibition is a means for social harmony in the Hmong society, reflecting the importance of preserving clean running water in high mountainous areas where running water is scarce.

It is interesting to note that none of the women interviewed had experienced a miscarriage. Some women may have had other relatives from the same clan who had experienced it, but not within their immediate households. This, however, may be a coincidence since this was a qualitative study based on a small number of informants and it was not specifically focused on women who had experienced miscarriage. In addition, Hmong women may not feel comfortable discussing their intimate experiences with strangers.

However, it may be that Hmong women do not want to risk losing their babies. They therefore take particular measures to prevent the fall of their babies, such as avoiding rigorous physical activities and illness as well as being cautious about going into uninhabited areas and provoking the spirits. Women know that they become pregnant when they have a particular dream such as receiving or seeing cucumbers, pumpkins, knives and needles. The pregnancy is soon confirmed with the cessation of their menstruation, changes in their body such as tightening breasts, and later on, the movement of their baby. Once pregnancy is confirmed, women take the particular cautions mentioned above.

Why do the Hmong take problems with "baby falling" seriously? I believe this is related to the value of children in Hmong society, as mentioned in earlier sections. As Wembah-Rashid (1996) has pointed out: "As pregnancy is expected to result in a new human being to extend the family, clan and lineage, its loss is perceived as threatening the parents' line with extinction." These explanations are indeed applicable to the Hmong as well.

Being fertile is a crucial element of life among the Hmong. Fertility ensures the continuation of the clan, lineage group, and family; the three important pillars in the Hmong world view (Yang, 1992). Infertility and miscarriage, therefore, have serious implications in Hmong society. Women are seen as bearers of children and they must have as many children as they can. Failure to do so, either through infertility or loss of pregnancy, results in suffering both in this life and the next. Like women in other patrilineal societies, Hmong women will try everything to ensure their fertility.

NOTES

1. In some Western societies, infertility may stigmatize many women, but it may not be their utmost problem. Many women in Western societies believe they have a "choice" regarding having children and, if infertility occurs, that they should have a "choice" not to have children (Klein, 1989). This, however, may not be an option for women from many societies who have the responsibility for bearing children for the continuation of the lineage and, hence, the survival of their society. Having children is, therefore, crucial for the lives of many women in many societies. Often, a woman is made to believe that she has been "born to be a mother." Women, therefore, seek help and even prepare to take risks to enable them to bear a child (Becker and Nachtigall, 1994: 507). Western repro-

ductive technology may help many women to conceive, but many others cannot afford such treatment (Whiteford and Gonzalez, 1995). However, women from many societies seek help from their traditional healers or a combination of Western and traditional medicines in order to conceive children and enable them to become mothers (Inhorn, 1994a). This is also true for women from Hmong society. In this chapter, the experience of Hmong women who are now living in Australia will be examined in the light of this argument.

2. That infertility is a "woman's problem" is clearly evident in Inhorn's study (1994a) among poor urban Egyptian women. Inhorn (1994a: 3) has pointed out that: "Not only are women typically blamed for the reproductive failing, but they must bear the burden of overcoming it through a therapeutic quest that is sometimes traumatic and often unfruitful. Furthermore, women face the tyranny of social judgment regarding infertility, for they are cast as being less than other women, as depriving their husbands and husbands' families of offspring, and as endangering other people's children through their uncontrollable envy."

3. Since the 1980s, a number of sociologists and historians have published studies on miscarriage in Europe and America. (See, for example, Lovell, 1983; Oakley et al., 1990; Reinharz, 1988; Cecil and Leslie, 1994). A number of these writers examined miscarriage from a feminist perpsective. (See, for example, Layne, 1997; Reinharz, 1988; Simonds; 1988; Hey, 1989; Letherby, 1993). However, very little research has examined miscarriage from a cultural point of view. Layne (1990, 1977) argued that this may be due in part to the sensitive and taboo nature of miscarriage. Recently however, certain papers have discussed pregnancy loss from a cultural perspective, providing the meanings of pregnancy loss in societies such as Cameroon, India, Jamaica, Papua New Guinea and Tanzania (Cecil, 1996b). Wembah-Rashid (1996), for example, examined beliefs relating to miscarriages and stillbirths among the peoples of southeast Tanzania. She showed that miscarriages and stillbirths are seen as types of disease and that their causes may be "personalistic or naturalistic." She also indicated that protective strategies for naturalistic causes are "embedded in the good conduct of the whole community, that is as long as individuals and family, lineage and clan members conduct themselves in a manner that is pleasing to God, nothing wrong will happen." Similarly, Savage (1996) showed that pregnancy loss in Cameroon is seen as caused by natural and/or supernatural factors. Women in Cameroon avoid excessive physical work loads and observe dietary restrictions during pregnancy to prevent deformations of the baby and pregnancy loss. Women and families also avoid social and religious misconduct that may be disapproved by ancestors, which in turn may cause miscarriage in women.

4. As Madden (1994) and Cecil (1996a) have argued, the issue of miscarriage among immigrant women in Western societies has been largely neglected, with the exception of Chalmers and Meyer's studies (1992a, 1992b). It is not known how immigrant women view miscarriage, what their feelings are about their pregnancy losses, what mechanisms they adopt to prevent or to cope with such loss, and the role of culture in protecting or reinforcing their emotional well-being. This chapter attempts to fill this gap.

5. See the findings of Kendal, 1987 and Cosminsky, 1982.

6. I will provide more details on these restrictions in Chapter 14 in this vol-

ume, but some accounts of the relationships between infertility and menstruation are also given here.

7. Thao (1984) refers to this as the "Mandate of Life" in his writing about Hmong world views. See also Chapter 1 in this volume for the mandate of life and deities in Hmong culture.

8. See Janet Sha's *Mothers of Thyme: Customs and Rituals of Infertility and Miscarriage* (1990) for an insightful account of the ways women seek help when miscarriage occurs in many parts of the world.

9. My conversation with one shaman indicated that if a woman does not bring the paper with her, even a shamanic healing process will not help her; it is she herself who does not want children, and that is why she does not bring her paper to earth.

Chapter 12

Death in Birth: Stillbirth, Neonatal and Maternal Death

> Lessons to be learned when birth turns into death, just as death turns into birth, as these trees here shedding the last of their spring and summer life will bloom again. Mothers who suffer those losses stand in the shade of an actuality where hurt and anguish can turn itself into love.
>
> (Donato, 1988: 32)

> The death of a babe, creates no common sorrow. Even the burial of one that has never breathed brings a keen pang to a parent's heart. . . . The scales in which a mother weighs her treasures, are not the same in which the man of the world weighs his silver and gold. A mother's grief is often most poignant for the youngest and faintest blossom.
>
> (Sigourney, 1838, cited in Sha, 1990: 72)

INTRODUCTION

Most writings on women and reproduction focus on successful reproduction such as childbirth and the period afterward.[1] Silence still surrounds issues of unsuccessful reproduction such as stillbirth, neonatal death and maternal death. Although in recent years some social science research has attempted to look at these deaths in birth,[2] very little research has examined them from a cultural point of view. Some anthropological studies in the past have neglected the issue of death in birth or only touched on the issue. This may be due in part to the sensitive and taboo nature of these kinds of death, which makes them difficult for people to talk about.[3]

In this chapter, I explore and discuss in detail traditional Hmong explanations for death in birth. It includes discussion of stillbirth, neonatal death and maternal death. It also examines the ethnomedical knowledge and practices that pertain to death in birth. The chapter finishes with discussions on the importance of life in birth and the value of children in Hmong society.

STILLBIRTH, NEONATAL DEATH AND MATERNAL DEATH

The Hmong see birth and death as a cycling process to which all Hmong are subject. In the Hmong cosmos, a person is born and his or her death will eventually come. Death is therefore seen as a natural and expected phenomenon. The Hmong also perceive that death is not an ultimate end of life, but a departure into a new beginning, a new life. After a proper burial ritual is performed, during which the soul of a dead person is guided back to his or her ancestral pool, he or she must await rebirth. When it is his or her turn, he or she will be given permission to be reborn into the Hmong society again. Hence, birth and death in Hmong culture is a natural process that no Hmong can avoid.[4]

Despite this, childbirth in Hmong culture is seen as dangerous, and critical to the life of a mother and her child. Death instead of birth may be the outcome of a pregnancy. The Hmong believe that an infant can die during the childbirth process. He or she may die in the mother's womb before the birth has taken place, or as soon as he or she emerges from the mother's body, or within the first two to three days of life. In cases of a stillborn child or a child who dies soon after birth, the Hmong believe that the mother suffered more ill health than is normal during pregnancy and that the pain of giving birth is much more severe than giving birth to a living baby.

> When the babies who die after birth are still inside the mother, they cause a lot of sickness for the mother during pregnancy. Even during labour, they cause a lot of sickness [pain] until birth and they will not live.

A mother can also die in childbirth. She may have good health during pregnancy but at birth may be too vulnerable. Given that many Hmong women and babies have died in childbirth in Laos, stillbirth, neonatal death and maternal death are taken seriously by the Hmong. This is similar to the ways the Hmong deal with the threat of a miscarriage; the death of a baby in early pregnancy.[5]

WHAT MAKES BABY AND MOTHER DIE?

When the Hmong discuss the causes of a stillbirth, neonatal death and maternal death, many layers of explanations are given.

Personal Attribution

Carrying a Heavy Load

During pregnancy, Hmong women are cautious about hard physical activities.[6] Carrying a heavy load or doing heavy work can cause distress for the baby. The distress causes the baby to cease growing, and it may eventually die if no way is found to relieve the baby's distress. In early pregnancy, this will lead to a miscarriage. In late pregnancy, however, a stillbirth or neonatal death may occur. One woman explained:

> If you do heavy things then it will distress the baby, and then it becomes very difficult. . . . If the baby is distressed then the mother will get pain in the stomach and sore back. It could also mean that you can't feel the baby move anymore, this is what distress means.

Another woman related:

> About this thing [stillbirth], if the mother goes and carries heavy things this causes the baby to die in the stomach, there will be no movement and the baby will begin to decay and then the mother will fall ill and then she delivers.

The Woman's Bad Behavior toward Parents

The Hmong also believe that a woman's behavior toward her parents while they are still living is the main cause contributing to her death in childbirth. Lack of respect, being rude and not looking after her parents when they are alive are the main bad behaviors of a woman. When her parents die they may come back to curse her and take her life away when she gives birth to another life in the family.

> When they die in childbirth and confinement, it may be that the parents of the mother have died and when she was younger she was very disobedient and did not talk nicely to her parents. Then her parents will come to take her heart and soul and that is what happens. . . . Because she did not talk nicely to her parents and if her parents asked her to cook or do chores, she didn't want to do them . . . and so her parents will curse and come to do that to her [take her life away].

The Labor

A long and difficult labor is seen as a contributing cause to stillbirth and to maternal death. Women base this explanation on the experiences of other women in their village in Laos and in a refugee camp in Thailand. The Hmong have their own traditional healing system that relies on social harmony among the living and between the living and the supernatural world, as well as on natural remedies, mainly herbal medicines. In addition, the Hmong in Laos live in a high, mountainous area where there is no modern medical health care to help with an emergency situation such as a long and difficult labor. Very often women do not receive help in time and this has led to a stillbirth in many cases. As one woman elaborated:

> To what I have seen, we were very naive in Thailand, we didn't go straight to the doctors at the beginning of the pain but stayed until it was unbearable and there was no possible chance to help her at home before she was taken [to hospital]. So when they went to the hospital if they [hospital staff] were able to help the mother then the baby would not survive and if she could not give birth and was given a CS then the mother would die.... They didn't go when the pain began and they waited too long and the baby might have died in the tummy and when they went to the hospital and took the baby out the baby was dead. Mrs [. . .] had twins, both babies wanted to come out at the same time and they waited until the mother nearly died before they took her to see the doctors. When the babies were removed both of them were dead.

Nature of Human Beings: The Life Aura

The Hmong believe that all human beings have their own life auras; a metaphysical explanation of the essence of life. The life auras of a mother and her baby must be equal for a safe birth.[7] The imbalance of the life auras of the mother and the baby may lead to either a stillbirth or maternal death.

> A safe birth can only occur when this life aura is in balance. If one has more life aura than the other does, it will lead to the death of the one that has less of it at birth.

And another woman related:

> There are a lot of different causes.... Some people would *ua neeb* [have a shamanic ritual] to separate the life aura when the baby is not born yet. If this cannot be done because the life aura of the child is greater than that

of the mother, then as soon as the baby is born, the mother will die and vice versa.

The Soul and Reincarnation

The Reincarnation of a Soul without Permission

As discussed earlier, the Hmong believe that each living body has three souls. Upon death, the three souls leave the body. One soul will stay at the grave of the person. The second soul will travel to the land of its ancestor. The third soul will travel to the spirit world and wait to return in another body. When it is time for the soul to be reincarnated, it will be given permission from *Huab Tais Ntuj* (the king deity who governs the spiritual world of the Hmong), and *Txoov Kab Yeeb* (spirit parents) will guide the soul to enter the womb of a woman. This is a cycle a human soul must enter. For a person to be born into this mundane world:

> You have to beg for the paper from heaven.... Their [deities] work is organized into separate tables and when you come down from the heaven you must come to pass each of these.... You will have to beg for the paper and they would have to make it for you to come down.... This is so that you have permission to come down and be born and if you don't have the permission and then you can't come to be born and live.

However, there are some souls who escape from heaven and are reborn without the permission of *Huab Tais Ntuj* and *Txoov Kab Yeeb*. At the time of birth, these souls must return to heaven; they are not permitted to live and thrive as are those who come down with permission. This means that the baby will die soon after birth.

> Up there [in heaven], when the baby comes down it doesn't bring the paper to come down and so it doesn't have any paper to live on earth.... It sneaks to come down and *Huab Tais Ntuj* and *Txoov Kab Yeeb* find out. They would say that this person doesn't have any permission to come down then we must take away the food path so that the person is unable to come to be a human being. This is why the baby is not growing [and die].... You can't stow away; they will find out.

The Reincarnation of the Mother's Soul

The Hmong believe that a woman's soul is capable of reincarnating in her own body. Her soul, therefore, becomes her own baby. When the baby is born and lives, the mother will die.

> The one that dies like that [dies at birth] the Hmong would say that when she gets pregnant her soul goes to make the baby and when the baby is born and lives the mother will die. This is what Hmong people say. . . . She has become the baby and therefore created another person and she must die.

If the mother's soul has been reincarnated into a baby and a ritual to separate their souls is performed in early pregnancy, the baby will miscarry. However, if the ritual is not performed, as pregnancy proceeds the baby's soul will become as develop as the mother's. When this happens, if the mother is safe at birth, the baby will be stillborn. On the other hand, if the baby survives, the mother will die at birth. As the shaman explained:

> If you separate their souls when the baby is still very small, when it is still in the womb, still very weak and small, it will be miscarry. . . . If the baby is already big before you found out then it would be too late. This is because by that time the baby's life and the mother's life is at the same level so you can't help them. . . . When the baby is born, at birth if the baby lives then the mother will die straight away and if the mother lives then the baby will be stillborn.

The Supernatural Being

Like beliefs about infertility and miscarriage,[8] the most common explanation and most feared cause of stillbirth, neonatal death and maternal death among the Hmong is being *raug dab* (struck by spirits). The spirits may strike the mother or the baby. In the case of a mother, this may happen if she travels near a landslide or crosses a river and its valley. Since spirits can be anywhere, it is difficult to know if she will cross their path while they are active (awake). If she happens to cross the spirits' path at this time, she will be hit and this may cause death. To be struck by nature spirits is therefore seen as the result of chance.

Spirits may also strike the baby as soon as he or she is delivered. As one woman related:

> Some babies are hit by the spirits. The baby would still be alive in the womb but as soon as the baby is born the baby soul will have already been delivered by the spirits [before the living mother who is supposed to deliver].

Another explained:

> If the baby has been *raug dab* but has not yet delivered. When it is ready to come out then the people want to catch the baby and the spirits also

want to catch it. And as the child delivers the spirits will catch it first. So this means the baby dies at birth.

One Hmong mother told us about the death of one of her babies in Laos:

The baby was *raug dab* and died. . . . The baby cried so much and gasped for air and the face turned blue and then just died. . . . Only children who are *raug dab* will do that. . . . He got hit by the eclipse spirit of the sun and the moon.

Not only can the baby be struck by spirits; his or her soul can also be captured by the spirits. When this happens, the baby in the mother's womb will become ill, and this in turn makes the mother ill. If this occurs in early pregnancy, it will result in miscarriage. However, if it happens in late pregnancy, the baby will be stillborn or die soon after birth.

The spirit has taken the soul of the baby away and thats what will make you sick and then the baby will come out. If the child is taken away by the spirit the pain is more severe than a normal delivery.

The Mandate of Life

The Hmong believe that women die in childbirth because their papers, which they bring from heaven when they are born, indicate that they will die in childbirth. As stated above, a person can be reborn only with the permission of *Huab Tais Ntuj* and *Txoov Kab Yeeb*. Each person, brings a piece of paper, referred to as the mandate of life, upon his or her birth.[9] This paper indicates how long he or she will live in this earthly world. If the paper specifies that he or she will live until old age, the person will do so. But if the paper specifies that the woman will live till the birth of her child, she will die at the birth of that child. One Hmong woman related a story of the death of her aunt in a refugee camp in Thailand. She had given birth by caesarean and died along with her baby soon after that:

In the year that I resided in Thailand, my aunt went to have a baby. She was very weak after the caesarean. . . . After the baby was delivered the mother died. When they took the baby home that night the mother died and soon after the baby died. . . . The mother died in the hospital. . . . When they took the baby out the mother recovered, but when the baby was taken home, the mother fainted and died. . . . As soon as the mother died and they [family members] heard about it, the baby started to get sick and as soon as the mother was buried the baby just died quietly. . . . I think that the mother came to take the baby, both were going back [to heaven] together because it was written in the paper in the beginning of their lives.

The mandate of life is believed to be powerful and cannot be avoided. Even if the woman follows the tradition strictly, she still can die in childbirth.

> Some that die during childbirth, it may be that their papers says that is when they will die. So after they give birth and . . . they will die even from eating egg and pepper soup [a traditional confinement food]. This will make them faint and then die.

There are no other ways to help or save the woman in childbirth. As one Hmong woman explained:

> Even using herbal medicines, *ua neeb* and other things, it won't help her . . . because she has brought her paper to end her like that.

The Wish of the Baby

The Hmong believe that if the baby dies at birth, it is because the baby does not wish to live in this mundane world. This explanation is particularly given when there are no other explanations for the death of the child. As one woman related:

> The one that dies in the womb! It is said that the child doesn't want to be born and so it will only live for the short time that it has existed. . . . If the baby has not been hit by spirits and it just happens like that then it means that it doesn't want to live and that is what happens. Some times, it only wants to live that long and then want to go back [to heaven].

Another explanation given about children who die one or two days after birth is that the baby only wants to come to taste the breast milk of the mother. Once this is done, they wish to return to heaven.

> The children who are born and stay around one or two mornings before they die, it is like they really want to come and drink some earthly breast milk; they only come to taste the milk . . . and then go back to heaven.

THE MANAGEMENT OF STILLBIRTH, NEONATAL DEATH AND MATERNAL DEATH

Stillbirth and neonatal death, similar to miscarriage, are treated as insignificant events in Hmong culture. The baby's body is usually passed through the wall of the house and buried in the forest.[10] There is no burial ceremony and there is no mourning as there would be for adults or children who are seen as true human beings. As one woman explained:

> The old people say that if the baby is born and stays for a little while and die, they do not make a ceremony and just put the baby through a hole in the wall . . . and then just bury it. In Thailand there are a lot of holes in the wall so they just remove the walling and wrap the baby in a cloth and someone has to be outside to receive the baby and bring it away. You do that quietly and not make any noise [performing a burial ceremony]. If the baby is bigger then they would make noises.

A proper burial ceremony is only performed if a *hu plig* (soul-calling) and naming ceremonies have been conducted for the baby. These ceremonies are performed on the third morning after birth.[11]

> If the baby is not yet having a *hu plig* ceremony done and it is very small then you don't need to make our traditional burial and no noises, not even crying [mourning]. So it is like a silent thing when you bury it.

Another woman explained:

> If the baby is over the confinement period then you will do it [burial ceremony]. You also do it if the baby is over twenty days and you have already given the baby a name.

Some Hmong women believe that the reason for not taking the body of the stillborn or neonatal-death baby through the door is that the family would have to perform a proper burial ceremony. One important aspect of this ceremony is to release the soul of the dead person so that he or she can be reborn again.

> Old people say that you must push through the wall. They do not let it go through the door. If you take the baby out through the door then maybe you have to do some traditional thing for it. Like for example, later on you have to release the soul ceremony after 14 days. . . . So if you just do it silently like that then you do not need to do anything else.

Others argue that this traditional practice is only observed by poor people who cannot afford the burial ceremony. Some families who can afford it may perform a proper burial ceremony for their stillborn or neonatal-death child.

> With that it is because you are poor and cannot afford a burial ceremony. Some people, if they have a lot of money and they love the baby a lot then they will do it. But it depends on the people. But the majority will just push the baby through the wall.

It is also believed that the spirit of a stillborn or neonatal-death child may follow people around if he or she is taken out through a door. The stillborn or neonatal-death baby, like a living baby, needs to be fed by his mother when he or she is hungry and therefore looks for the mother. When there are humans in his or her sight, the stillborn or neonatal-death baby will follow people until he or she finds his or her mother and is fed.

> This is what they [older generation] say. They say if you go out, the baby will follow you. The baby that follows you is the child which is taken out through the door. He wants to look for a feed and look for his mum.... Even you are not pregnant or even if you are a man and you go to that area where the baby is buried, the baby will follow. It will cry and you will hear the baby cries following you. This happens to men too. My father was in Laos and when they [the men] went to chase up some girls they said it [a stillborn spirit] followed them like that. When this happens you have to turn your back to it and say to come and you will carry it to find its mother to have some milk. The crying will stop but you can feel the weight on your back.... The baby is hungry and he has nothing to eat so he must look for it.

On the other hand, a maternal death is treated as a significant event. Since she is a true human being, a proper burial ceremony must be performed so that her soul can be reborn. Reincarnation as a human within the same clan is the utmost desire of all Hmong. A traditional burial ceremony in Hmong culture takes over 14 days. Each day has a particular event to be performed, and each day cannot be missed if a proper way is to be laid for the soul to enter his or her ancestral pool and later on to be reborn.[12]

CONCLUSIONS

Like the cultural construct of miscarriage, stillbirth and neonatal death are seen as nonsignificant events. There is no mourning to be done. There is no burial ceremony to be performed. The dead baby is simply passed through the wall of the house and silently buried in a forest. This is in great contrast with the celebration of a living baby on the third morning after birth, when soul-calling and naming ceremonies are performed. Noise is everywhere, and celebration continues from dawn to late afternoon.[13]

Cecil (1996b: 7) has pointed out that in many societies where infant mortality is high, infants and small children are not seen as "fully human or as true members of the society." It is likely then that the unborn child is regarded similarly. Therefore, a child who dies in birth or soon after will be treated with "little significance."[14]

If we consider this within the context of the high incidence of infant mortality in the Hmong society (in Laos), we may see that by treating stillbirth and neonatal death as an insignificant event helps the mother and her family to better cope with the loss of pregnancy. The mother, whose pregnancy ends up with death instead of birth, is encouraged to get on with her daily routines after a period of confinement rest and to become pregnant again as soon as possible. As I have stated earlier, when pregnancy is lost through miscarriage, the woman is encouraged not to replace what she has lost, but to provide another body for other souls to be reborn, so that there will be another birth and, perhaps, a living person born into the family.[15] The Hmong regard this as essential for the continuation of the Hmong society, as I have discussed in previous chapters.

According to Obeyeskere (1981), causal explanations that people use to explain unfortunate events are "culture-bound," and they usually are based on different perspectives of personal and societal meanings. Using this framework, and as I have shown in this chapter, the cultural constructs of stillbirth, neonatal death and maternal death of the Hmong fall into two main categories. First, they are related to the natural world, which is related to the personal attribution including the woman's behavior and the nature. Second, they are closely related to the supernatural world. As previously mentioned, the Hmong health care system relies heavily on social harmony among the living and between the living and the supernatural world. The Hmong also practice filial piety, which requires children to be obedient, respect their parents, and looked after them in old age. Upon their parents' death, the children must continue to pay them respect and feed them so that the lineage can continue to exist. Without the cooperation of the children in carrying on these tasks, Hmong society can be threatened. Therefore, social harmony between parents and their offspring is extremely important.

The Hmong believe in the supernatural world. Hmong society is governed and looked after by a king deity (*Huab Tais Ntuj*) and spirit parents (*Txoov Kab Yeeb*). All Hmong are their children. Harmony within the Hmong society can only exist if the living do not offend the deities. This is also necessary for harmony with the supernatural beings. Having harmonious relationships with nature and the supernatural beings ensures that the society will not be threatened. Consequently, the Hmong greatly value this harmony.

In Hmong society, we may therefore argue that for a pregnancy to end with life, not death in birth, there must be as Wembah-Rashid (1996: 80) has pointed out about pregnancy loss among the Tanzanians:

> A state of balance in the moral order where the physical state of the mother-to-be, the universe within which she is a member (i.e., the natural

environment), the gods, the ancestors and other supernatural powers are all working harmoniously and in coordination.

Similarly, as Sobo (1996: 42) has stated about pregnancy loss in Jamaica, Jamaican women combine their cultural understanding of how the body works with "social and moral understandings so that social causes can be found" for the loss of pregnancy or other sicknesses. This makes the loss "manageable, meaningful, and useful for discourse concerning social and moral affairs." The Hmong are no exception. Linking stillbirth, neonatal death and maternal death with social and moral orders provides the Hmong with a more "manageable and meaningful" understanding of death in birth and, hence, assists them to cope more easily with the loss of life.

An interesting finding of this study was that only one of the women interviewed had had a neonatal-death child who was struck by the spirit of the eclipse of the sun and the moon. Other women, however, have had other relatives from the same clan who had experienced it.[16] As Cecil (1996b: 9) has reported, women in many societies bear the "responsibility for ensuring a healthy pregnancy and for minimizing the risk of a pregnancy loss." This explains the particular care Hmong women take with their pregnancies and birth outcomes. They do not want to risk losing their babies as well as their own lives and, therefore, take particular measures to prevent the death of their babies, such as avoiding rigorous physical activities or provoking the deities or the spirits. In the case of the woman mentioned above, the situation was rather different; no one would have been able to avoid the eclipse. Therefore, she did not evoke the spirit nor was she careless.

This chapter offers another dimension of unsuccessful reproduction to the biomedical domain of reproductive health. Differing cultural understandings of birth and death among women from different cultural backgrounds need to be acknowledged if sensitive and culturally appropriate care is to be provided at the time of birth and death.

NOTES

1. See, for example, Jordan, 1978; Pillsbury, 1978; Manderson, 1981; Sich, 1981; Laderman. 1983; Morse, 1989; Chu, 1993; Rice, 1993; and Townsend and Rice, 1996.

2. For example, the work of Lovell, 1983; Layne, 1990; DeFrain, 1991; and Littlewood, 1996.

3. The issues of stillbirth, neonatal death and maternal death among immigrant women in Western societies have been even more neglected. We do not know how these women see death in birth, what their feelings are about losing their babies, what mechanisms they adopt to prevent or to deal with losing a child or the role of culture in protecting or reinforcing their emotional well-being.

We also do not know how these societies and their members deal with women who lose their lives through childbirth.

4. See Symonds (1991, 1996) for her illuminating discussion on the connection between the Land of Light (birth) and the Land of Darkness (death).

5. I have discussed this issue in greater detail in Chapter 11 in this volume.

6. See also Chapter 4 in this volume for more details on Hmong beliefs and practices during pregnancy.

7. See also Chapters 4 and 11 in this volume for the way the Hmong deal with this issue.

8. See Chapter 11 in this volume for more details about the causes of infertility and miscarriage among the Hmong.

9. See Thao's paper (1984) on the Hmong perception of illness, for his discussion of the the mandate of life belief among Hmong people.

10. A Hmong house is usually made of bamboo or planks, from which a wall can be easily removed.

11. See also Kunstadter et al. (1987) for similar practices concerning the death of a newborn infant in Hmong villages in Northern Thailand.

12. See also Lemoine (1983) and Symonds (1991) for greater details about burial ceremonies in Hmong society.

13. See Chapter 8 in this volume about the soul-calling ceremony conducted on the third day after birth and the involvement of men and others in Hmong culture.

14. A similar pattern is found in many societies, such as the Kwoma in Papua New Guinea (Williamson, 1983) in Nigeria (Maclean, 1971), in Brazil (Scheper-Hughes, 1991), in Tanzania (Wembah-Rashid, 1996), and in Cameroon (Savage, 1996).

15. C.f. Layne, 1990; Littlewood, 1996; Borg and Lasker, 1982; Scheper-Hughes, 1992; and Castle, 1994.

16. A similar pattern on miscarriage has been discussed in Chapter 11 in this volume.

Chapter 13

Fertility Regulation: Menstruation Regulation, Contraception and Abortion

INTRODUCTION

> Yes I am very worried because I am older now and I am sick and don't want anymore children. If I take the medicine it is so difficult. When you eat the pills it has to be at least one week before you know if it is good for you. So if you change the medicine you have to take the other one for at least one or two weeks before you can change to another one. If it is no good for you, you will get very sick before you can change to another one. This is very difficult because it is like you are carrying the sickness with you all the time. If you go to tie your tubes, even at the skin it looks very small but it is your tubes inside your body and if you don't have side effects then it is very good. But it you have side effects then you will say it is because of that and then you have to have another operation to undo it. This is too much problem; it is very difficult. I am still very worried about what I should do not to fall pregnant. Hmong medicines, there are some that stop you from having more children and ones that stop your menses, but you have to be age over forty or forty-five before it works. But if your age is not over forty or forty-five and if you take it, it will not work. The ones that will stop you having more children, for them to be effective, you will have to give birth first and as soon as the baby comes out you drink those medicines. This is the way of Hmong medicines and it is very difficult. If I want to take it now I can't because I am not pregnant yet. So if I take it, it won't work. It is very very difficult. (Hmong informant)

Throughout history women have had to deal not only with their ability to become pregnant and give birth, but also their desire to limit or control their own reproduction. Hmong women are no exception, as illustrated in the case above; the dilemma of a Hmong woman who wished to regulate her fertility, but had experienced too many difficulties in doing so. Although this is just one woman's story, it represents the experiences of several Hmong women in the study who wished to control their fertility. This chapter attempts to collate Hmong women's concerns about fertility regulation.

WHY FERTILITY REGULATION?

Women mentioned the need to space out their children. In the past, the need for spacing children was largely based on the fact that if children were born too close together, it was difficult for a woman to both perform household chores and work on the farm. Now women relocated in Australia cite the need to study English for migrants or seek employment as reasons for spacing children. Women also mentioned that if they continued to have children too close together their health might deteriorate too quickly. Having a sufficient number of children is another reason given for regulating fertility.

> I have enough children and I get tired of looking after them. I have a few children now and it is becoming very difficult so I don't want anymore. . . . I don't want to give birth anymore, it makes me old quickly and also that I feel that enough is enough.

Changes in living circumstances in a new country create uncertainty about whether they should have many children, as they would in Laos. Women believe that the living situation in Australia is not appropriate for bearing too many children.[1] Some, therefore, have tried to control their fertility using whatever means they believe to be effective.

How do women regulate their own fertility? Most Hmong women in this study did not use Western birth control, but had their own ways of managing their fertility. What women choose is what makes sense to them. The following three cases may illustrate this.

The first woman had never used any type of birth control but intended to have her tubes tied because of the reliability of this method. Her reason for choosing it was as follows:

> Before I have not used any birth control but maybe, I think, I will go to have my tubes tied. I have enough children. I don't want anymore children. And I also think for health reason which makes me not wishing to have more children. When we came here [Australia] I have been sick often.

> Tying my tubes would mean no more children and because I don't want anymore; that is why.

The second woman had never used birth control either but considered it after her last child was born in Australia. She, however, would use Hmong herbs as a first choice and if these did not work she would try Western birth control.

> I haven't use any birth control yet but will use it after this one. In this country I don't know any old lady [medicine woman] so I have asked some very experienced people [who are knowledgeable about herbs for fertility control] up north to send some over for me. They brought these herbs over from Laos. . . . I will try Hmong herbs first to see if it works. If it doesn't work then I would use the Western medicine.

The third woman wished to space her children. She therefore sought herbal medicines from Laos as a first choice. She also used contraceptive pills as a booster method to ensure that she would not fall pregnant.

> After the birth of my youngest son I used some herbal medicines to stop pregnancy but at Christmas time I was not sure if it was safe enough so I went to the doctor to be prescribed some pills.

The decisions of these three women clearly demonstrate that Hmong women use a variety of methods to regulate their fertility; modern and traditional. In the following sections, these will be discussed.

INDIGENEOUS FERTILITY REGULATION METHODS

Hmong women described several indigeneous fertility regulation methods that they used.[2] One natural method is the counting of dates after menstruation. A period of twenty days after a period is seen as a woman's most fertile "highest risk" time for conception. Therefore, women avoid sexual intercourse during this period.

> When it is at the high risk period of falling pregnant then you do not sleep with your husband. When you finish your period that is the time so you do not let the man sleep with you for twenty days. After the period you should wait for twenty days, then you can have the sexual intercourse.

Breastfeeding is seen and believed by all Hmong women to be a natural birth control method. This knowledge is passed on from their mothers, who practiced breastfeeding as a means of controlling their fertility in Laos. Hmong women practice prolonged periods of breastfeeding. Usually, women continue breastfeeding until the next child is born, which means that they breastfeed for at least two years.[3] Because of this practice, Hmong women manage to keep their conceptions at least two years apart.

> I haven't used anything at all. I am not just conceiving yet. I think maybe because I am breastfeeding. . . . My mum says that if you breastfeed then your children tend to be more spaced out. In my mum's generation, women only breastfeed; they just keep breastfeeding.

One older woman explained:

> I never used birth control. My children were spread out. My babies were all breastfed and because they were breastfed my period would return when the baby was about one year old and that is when I started to have another one.

As well as using breastfeeding as a method of controlling fertility, Hmong women practice sexual abstinence in the 30-day period after birth, known as the confinement period. During this period, women rest and avoid rigorous physical activity, including sexual intercourse. It is believed that having sex too soon results in the collapse of the uterus. Hmong women fear this complication more than any other, since it has no cure, and women can die from it.[4] Women also mention using the withdrawal technique as a way to avoid pregnancy.

> I have my own way to control my pregnancy. Because I don't know how to use the timing with the period so I use a withdrawal technique. That is what we do and there is nothing important [wrong] about that, is it?

Another traditional method women have used to control their fertility is to regulate or "bring down" their menstruation (see later section on "Fertility Regulation and Hmong Herbs"). Menstruation is seen as "bad" blood that must be expelled from the body. The circulation of "bad" blood enables the renewal of the blood, which in turn will make a woman healthy.[5]

The Hmong believe that women whose menstruation ceases for any reason will be unhealthy. Women may become pale, skinny and eventually die.

> When you have your menses it is good. If you don't have it then you are like a person who is very unhealthy. Because you don't have your menses you are very pale and look like a person who is always sick.

Menstrual clotting is, however, seen as highly dangerous to a woman's health.

> If you have clots and you don't have the menses anymore then you will die. . . . Like if your blood can't come out, it will clot inside your body and so you can't eat and become skinny and thus your blood inside your body will dry up and you will die.

Women also understand that when menstruation ceases its flow, there is a possibility of becoming pregnant. If pregnancy is not a desired outcome, women must bring their blood down. This, however, is seen as bringing down their delayed period, not as an abortion.[6]

MODERN METHODS OF FERTILITY REGULATION

Despite the fact that modern methods of fertility regulation have reached many parts of less developed countries, they have not reached Hmong villages in Laos.[7] Hmong women in this study only learned about birth control when they were living in refugee camps in Thailand. Camp administrators had a policy of controlling birth rates in the camp. All women who already had several children were encouraged to adopt some form of contraception.

> When I came to Thailand a lot of people were on the pills but I didn't have a husband so it wasn't something for me to do. In Thailand they called on the microphone everyday and asked people to pick up some pills. For those who didn't want to go on the pills they would do other ways so that women would not get pregnant too often.

Older women spoke of their lives in Laos, where there was no such thing as modern birth control because of basic living situations which were far away from modern technology.

> With my generation there were no such thing as birth control, not at all. My generation lived in the high mountains and there was no contraception. We were introduced to contraception when we came to Thailand. So the younger generation would use the contraception. When I came over I have finished my children in Laos already.

However, there were young mothers in this study who were still not using any modern contraceptive methods despite having better access to them in Australia. They believed that once they embarked on contraception, their future reproduction might be jeopardized, and they might have problems becoming pregnant in the future, when their young children will have grown older.

The majority of Hmong women in the study expressed a fear of using birth control to regulate their fertility. Consequently, most Hmong women have not used any form of contraception.

> I don't use the contraception because if you use that it might not be good. I am worried that it might do something bad to my body so I use my own method [counting days]. This way it is much better.

Condoms

The use of condoms is seen as an unreliable method of birth control. Condoms may protect once or twice but if used often, women still can become pregnant. Condoms are also believed to cause harm, since if not used properly, they can remain lodged inside a women's vagina after sexual intercourse.

> With condom, if you are not experienced it might fall inside and then you would have to go to have it out [at hospital].

In addition, women believe that condoms have been lubricated with certain chemicals. They believe these chemicals, if used many times, can accumulate in the vagina and cause disease in both themselves and their husbands.

> People say that using condom is unhealthy. I have never experienced it but for those who have used it say so. Some say that if you use it, particularly the prolonged use of it, the lubricant used in condom is not good. This causes the sickness, like sexually transmitted diseases. . . . So that is why not many people use it.

Because condoms are made in large quantities, they can sometimes cause "infections" if they are used often. This is what Hmong women have heard, and it is one reason they do not use them.

> They say that you should not use condom because using it is not good for you and that because they make a lot and they might be infected with something. I think I don't want to use condom; I never use it. . . . People also say that if you use condom too often then it is not good, both for you and your husband.

Contraceptive Pills

The contraceptive pill is believed to suit only certain women. Some may get side effects, others may not. However, from what some women have observed, the contraceptive pill creates more health problems than it solves.

> I have heard people say that if you take them and they suit you then they will not have side effects on you. But if they don't suit you then they will

> make you weak and when you have your menses it will be irregular. Some people say this but I don't really know if these are side effects or the drug or not. So I don't use them.

As one woman elaborated:

> If you eat them and they do not suit you then they can give you some sorts of side effects and cause you to be sick. In Thailand, the ones who had used them said that they got stomach pain, pain in the womb, and sore veins. They also lost their appetite, became skinny. They also had their menses all the time without stopping. This made them worried a lot. I have seen three people like this because they did not suit them. That is why it frightens me. See that they can cause those things to people, I don't want to use them. Once you get that sort of sickness, you can stop using them but the pain will still stay with you.

Hmong women believe that the contraceptive pill cannot only be harmful to the mother, but can also harm the baby in the uterus even after the mother ceases taking the pills. This is because the harmful effects of the pills may accumulate in the womb if it is not cleaned out.

> The old people always say that if you take something and it does not fit in with your body then it will cause sickness. Also if you eat those medicines then later on you stop that and fall pregnant it will not be good for the baby. . . . They say that if you eat the pills and do not get your womb cleaned before you get pregnant then it will make the baby have crippled arms and legs and their limbs will not have any energy to walk.

Although the womb can be cleaned, it needs to be done in the hospital. This is something which Hmong women wish to avoid.

Norplant

Most Hmong women did not have much knowledge of this method. A few women, however, told me there were several Hmong women in a refugee camp in Thailand who were coerced into using it. As one woman explained:

> In Thailand [refugee camp] they make a slit in the skin on the arm and put some sort of pill in there. I don't know what they actually do but I saw Mrs. [Y] had it. She had so many children and they put a slit in her skin and put the medicine in there. . . . Then she became very fat. When we were about to come here I asked her how come she did not have any more children, she replied "they put a cut in me and put this pill in here and the medicine is still here." She showed her arm to us to have a look at it too. . . . She was the only that I knew using this thing.

Like other Western contraceptive methods, Norplant was believed to have side effects. Women cited gaining weight as a major problem: "And after she had that in her arm, she got fatter and fatter."

Sterilization: Tying of Tubes

Sterilization is the contraceptive method feared by Hmong women (with the exception of the woman mentioned in an earlier section). The tying of tubes is believed to cause more harm than any other form of contraception. The following quote is from a woman who, during an antenatal check-up was advised by her Australian doctor to undergo sterilization. The woman refused. She lamented:

> When I went for a check up . . . there was one man, he wanted me to go on the pills or have my tubes tied. . . . I felt very disgusted at the idea of tying my tubes. I kept on refusing him and at the end . . . I said I would take care of my children myself. He said he suggested the pills or tying the tubes because in this country there are people who . . . after giving birth don't want the child so they kill or sell the child, and they are people who have a lot of children. . . . Having too many children will make you not wanting to look after them and not loving them and so you may kill or sell them. This is why he wanted me to go on the pills or tie my tubes because [he believed] I have enough children. . . . Hmong people say that if you have a lot of children then you have luck and if you have luck then you will have a house full; if no luck, then less children. . . . [He] kept saying that tying your tubes wouldn't require a large operation. I kept thinking the stomach is a large one how can he say it is a small thing. I felt sick at the stomach at the thought and frightened of it. I didn't want to be on the pills either. If I had more children then I would have them, and if I don't then I won't. I was very scared and that's why I did that way [did not return for check up].

Some women talked about what might occur after the operation, particularly in old age.

> If I don't want to have any more children I don't want to have that [tying of tubes] done. I will look for Hmong herbal medicine to drink. Maybe if you have your tubes tied then when you get older the area [of operation] might have something wrong and you might have some sorts of sickness in old age.

Many women mentioned the loss of a soul resulting from being unconscious during the operation as a main concern.[8] An operation of any type is greatly feared by the Hmong. They believe it is a way for the soul to be frightened from the body, causing ill health and, eventually, death.[9]

> It is only good if nothing happens afterwards. Side effect to the cut on your skin is all right and if you have no side effects to it then it is good. But you may get sick and if so you would think that it is because of that operation; that is why you get sick. . . . The most important thing is that they are going to make you unconscious and my soul may leave my body and this is not going to be good for me.

This belief was also expressed in an interview with a woman who talked about the experience of her own niece, who had an operation and then became ill. She believed strongly that the operation was connected with the loss of the soul of her niece.

> After my niece had the operation done she is often sick and pale. I am very scared of that. If I am not sick until I need a life saving operation then I do not want to have an operation. Having an operation has something to do with soul loss and that is why people get sick most often. People who have had operation now complaining of having some sorts of sickness.

EXPERIENCES WITH MODERN FERTILITY REGULATION METHODS

All women (except one) who used contraceptive pills experienced side effects. Loss of appetite was given as one problem arising from using Western birth control pills.

> I have used some before and they didn't make me sick but they made me lost my appetite. With food I could go for the whole day without any and I did not feel hungry. When I ate I didn't feel anything and not feeling full. I went to weight myself and I didn't gain any. That was what happened to me when I took those pills.

Other severe side effects women experienced were pains in the body.

> It was painful. Taking the pills gave me a lot of pain when I was nearly having my period and even when I had the period. It went on like that for a long time before the pain stopped; like one week or six days.

The irregularity of menstruation and the change in its color were also cited as side effects of birth control pills.

> When I came to Thailand they [camp administrators] said that I had too many children and they told me to use contraception. So I went and they gave me those medicines to eat and I had very irregular menses; like in one month I would have it two or three times with excessive bleeding. It kept on going like that so I got scared and I stopped eating them. . . . I think that taking the pills made my menses irregular because I had never had that problem before until I came over there [camp] and used the contraceptive pills.

Another woman told of her experience with menstrual irregularity after taking contraceptive pills:

> I was on some contraception before and it wasn't good for me because after taking it the blood was black and only a little bit of it came out. Also I felt a lot of pain in my stomach and lower back. When I stopped the pills I went back to normal; no more pain. At that time the blood that came out was like dead blood. It was very black and that is no good. Yes taking the pills did that to me. So I stopped and a couple of months later my body was normal again.

At the time of this study, only one woman was using birth control pills. The other three women had stopped because of their side effects. One woman explained:

> I have tried a lot. In Thailand whatever I tried wasn't good for me and in this country I have tried three to four times already and none of them seemed to suit me. So I have given it up.

Another woman related:

> After I gave birth to my youngest daughter I began to take the medicine from this country. I took them for 6 months and my menses became lighter and lighter up to the point when it nearly disappeared and I began to have the stomach pain. So I stopped that and my menses stopped too. . . . It took a long time, up to five months, before I had one. Now I don't have the pain anymore.

ABORTION: WOMEN'S PERCEPTIONS

Since Hmong women rely more on indigenous fertility regulation methods and some herbal medicines to control their fertility, some women become pregnant even when they do not want to. Most Hmong women continue with their pregnancies, even if they are premarital. Yet, there are times when a woman may not wish to continue a pregnancy. When this happens, Hmong women seek abortion as a way to control their fertility.

How Hmong women perceive abortion is largely dependent on who the women are in the context of Hmong society. To some women, abortion is seen as the right of "certain" women to control their reproduction, particularly older women who have produced many children—enough for carrying out essential tasks in their culture. Women who tend to have ill health after giving birth also have the right to abort their next pregnancy. Women in these situations will not be condemned by society, and herbal healers will be able to assist them to abort the baby.

However, if a woman is still in childbearing years and may want children in the future, abortion becomes a moral issue. In such cases, it is seen as morally wrong to kill a baby that one has conceived, and a woman may be punished by having to give birth to an "unhealthy" child the next time she conceives. The "unhealthy" child may just be sickly or may be crippled. It is believed that the baby feels sorry that its mother did not wish to give birth to a new life. The mother is judged by what she has done with her previous children. Women, in this situation, will be talked about and condemned by others in the community, both men and women.

> For the ones who abort their baby, if they do not want anymore children then it is okay. But if you are still wanting more and you keep aborting them then when you have the next one then that one will be unhealthy. ... Because you keep doing that then it is like the baby feels sorry that you don't want to give birth to them. Then when you give birth then they will be unhealthy.... So it is like a punishment for the mother too that she does this thing.

Another woman offered the following reasons for not wanting to have an abortion:

> I think that abortion is not good because for a child to be conceived it does really want to live. If you got it [become pregnant] then you must have the baby. For the ones who have abortion I think that they are punishing the baby and the baby will come to punish the mothers too. I think that the baby will do that; that is why I don't believe in abortion.... I think it will make the mothers sick and pale or become a person who cannot work, have sore arms or legs and their limbs are useless, unable to work. I think this would happen.

Abortion is also a health issue, since it is believed to cause ill health in the mother.

> Hmong people if they are pregnant and they don't want the child they still have to give birth to it. Being in this country, some [Western] women need to go to work and when they become pregnant they do go to have abortion.

> But for myself if I do not want to have it then I try not to fall pregnant. And if I do fall pregnant then I will give birth to it because if you have an abortion then I think that this can cause bad health in the mother.

If a young woman becomes pregnant prior to marriage and then seeks an abortion, she will be socially vulnerable and the target of gossip, since premarital sex, although acceptable to some extent in Hmong society, is also seen as a moral issue. Only girls who behave "badly" become involved in premarital sex;[10] worse still if they indulge themselves to the extent of becoming pregnant. However, this does not mean that they may not be married in the future. Abortion, therefore, only presents a short-term social problem for young women.

> These girls I don't know about them. People will say bad things to them and about them but the boys will still marry them if they like each other. Even if people talk about them and if they like each other then they [girls] will be married.

Although people judge women differently, they also agree that in reality women who choose to abort their baby will be thought of as having a "bad heart." If they can abort their own baby, what else are they capable of? Woman with "soft hearts," will not consider abortion as an option, but continue with their pregnancy. Because of this, people will still talk to them and treat them as members of the community.

> If taking something to abort the baby then it is a bad thing. Only if you don't want any more then that doesn't matter much. If a person does this then other people will consider her a very bad person. I think that they will still treat her the same but deep inside they will think that she has a bad heart and that is why she has the ability to kill a child or a person. This is what they will think but they will still talk to her.

Unlike birth control, which women may seek from Western medicine, abortion is strictly confined to the use of herbal medicines, the help of a medicine woman (see later section) and hard physical manipulation through a firm massage on the abdomen.[11] Abortion, however, can only be done during the first trimester. It is believed that after three months, performing an abortion will be dangerous. If the abortion is not successful, the mother may have a difficult time giving birth to the baby.

> For some people when they have become pregnant and when they are about two to three months and they don't want to have it then they use the Hmong herbs to get rid of the baby. If the baby is five to six months and you use herbal medicine to get rid of the baby then it will be very

hard; very difficult for you. The baby will die but you will have a very difficult time to give birth too.

FERTILITY REGULATION AND HMONG HERBS

> But the best method is to take herbal medicine; that is if you do not want any more children then you take herbal medicine. It is much better than taking the pills.

As mentioned, Hmong women fear using Western contraception. However, this does not mean that they do not use other medicines. Hmong herbs are usually used to regulate fertility and for abortion.[12]

For fertility regulation there are herbs that can be used to space children and those that can halt a woman s fertility. To space children, the herbs must be eaten soon after birth and continued until the confinement period ends (usually 30 days).

> Hmong medicine, yes there are medicines that you use to stop having children altogether and there are medicines for you to use so that you will have children further apart. . . . If you want to have children further apart then when you are in confinement you will put those herbs in the chicken soup and take it. . . . You take it for the whole month but you may forget so you may use it a few times only, it will still work.

However, this practice must be done for at least two births before it can be effective.

Herbs that stop reproduction must also be taken soon after birth for up to nine days.

> Hmong medicines, there are ones which you eat and have no more children but you have to take it when you have just given birth to a new baby. For it to be effective, you have to take it straight after giving birth.
> This medicine, you must drink it as soon as the baby is born. You boil it like a tea to drink. You have to take three roots, one piece you boil it and drink for three days. So three roots you need to take it for nine days and that is all you have to take.

An interesting point among Hmong women's beliefs is that herbal medicines will only work with a woman who is over forty years of age.

> Hmong medicines, there are some that stop you from having more children and ones that stop your menses, but you have to be age over forty or forty-five before it works. But if your age is not over forty or forty-five and if you take it, it will not work.

Most people obtain herbal medicines from a medicine woman, particularly for abortion, when women must seek her help. In giving out herbs to regulate fertility, the medicine woman must have experience in using them. In other words, she must have requested herbs to regulate her own fertility from a medicine woman herself. Once it works for her, she is then able to help other women. When a woman seeks help from the medicine woman she must bring a bunch of incense sticks and some gold paper to *fiv* (ask for help and agree to the service fee). This incense and gold paper will be burned to honor the medicine spirits that give her the knowledge and power to help women. The medicine woman must also be paid a certain fee. The fee for spacing children is minimal. In the case of abortion, however, the fee will be larger than for giving herbs to space children or to end fertility. Without this fee, the medicine woman will experience some ill health for handing out herbs to abort a baby.

> There are some Hmong who do not want children and there are Hmong medicines which can be given to them so that they won't have the children. When you go [to ask for help from a medicine woman] you must bring incense sticks and gold paper to burn for her spirits [the medicine spirits at the altar] and you have to pay her for the service. Then she will give you the medicine. This is to prevent her from getting sick. . . . The money must be paid to her. If you don't want the pregnancy then you must pay enough money so that it can prevent her from getting sick; having sore hands for giving out the medicine.

For terminating reproduction, both the woman and her husband must consult the medicine woman together. Both partners have to agree on the decision before the medicine woman can offer her services.

> If you want Hmong medicine to stop reproduction then both of you [couple] will have to agree and will have to go and *fiv* her before she is willing to give you anything. Normally *kws tshuaj* will ask you first if you want to have some more children in the future. If you want to then she won't do it.

Some herbs are fresh, and referred to as green herbs by the Hmong. Other herbs are in dried form. Fresh herbs can be leaves, stems and flowers, but dried herbs may be roots and bark mixed with leaves and dried in the sun before use or may sometimes be roots only. Some herbs can be grown as small shrubs in the backyard. However, most herbs are gathered in the forest. Usually, the herbs are boiled with chicken to make soup, but they can be boiled and drunk as tea. As mentioned, herbs for spacing children and stopping reproduction must be taken several times, but herbs for abortion need only be taken three times to be effective.

A medicine woman I interviewed mentioned two types of herbs that she grows in her garden. One herb is called *ncas liab*, and a second is named *paj kuab tub sab*. Both herbs are good for cleaning out the blood and for abortion. If a woman has difficulty conceiving because of the clotting of her blood, the herb is able to rid her of the bad blood only, and she may conceive afterwards. However, if the herb is taken during pregnancy, it can abort the baby. For abortion, the flower, leaf (mainly the tip of young leaves) and stem are selected to make chicken soup. Usually, three flowers and three tips are used. If there are no flowers (not in season), just the stems may be used.

Similarly, when a woman's menstruation does not flow properly or ceases, Hmong women resort to Hmong green herbs.

> When it does not flow properly then you use Hmong herbs to wash out the bad blood and the clotted blood. After this you will be back to normal. . . . If the bad blood remain inside the body this will make you have stomach pain.
>
> The Hmong have special herbs to use to renew that [clotted] blood so that your blood is new and you won't be pale.

Women say that the medicines are wild plants. Some herbs are in root form but may also be leaves or the stem of the plant.

Very often, however, women ask the medicine woman to prepare herbs for them. She prepares herbs for them to drink, usually over three nights one big cup or bowl for each night. Their menstruation will then flow properly.

> If the menses does not flow properly then you have to go and ask medicine from a *kws tshuaj* [medicine woman] to give medicine for you to drink to regulate your body so that you will have the menses again. You will have to take only two to three times before you will get better.

The medicine woman must be asked for assistance. During this process, fee is negotiated and agreed upon. If the treatment is not successful, no fee is paid. However, if the woman recovers, she must pay the agreed fee:

> If your menses is clotted you have to beg someone [medicine women] before they will give you any medicine. They will give you grown herbs and whatever they know they will use to help you. You will take the medicine and if it helps you then you will pay them the agreed amount.

CONCLUSIONS

The indigenous fertility regulation methods in Hmong culture reflect those of many parts of the world. This is clearly seen in a text by Newman (1985), which includes the prevalent practices of indigenous fertility regulation methods in Afghanistan, Colombia, Costa Rica, Egypt, Jamaica, Malaysia and Peru. Social researchers in this text have documented ways in which women have managed their fertility: contraceptives, emmenagogues, abortifacients, and fertility enhancers, among others.

For example, the Hmong practice of sexual abstinence in the period immediately following menstruation as a way to avoid conception has been documented in different parts of the world.[13] As Hansen (1975), in his writing about the "ethnophysiology of fertility" (Nichter and Nichter, 1996b: 10) of people of the Polynesian island of Rapa (1975: 53) notes:

> The uterus is conceived to be a mechanical organ which opens and closes. Remaining tightly closed most of the time, it opens for several days each month to allow the stale blood to run out. . . . Just as blood cannot escape a closed uterus, semen cannot enter it, so there is no possibility of conception during the greater part of the cycle. Conception could occur during menstruation but ideas that menstrual flow is contaminating lead them to avoid intercourse at this time. However, the uterus remains open for a few days after menstruating, and this is the time when, in Rapan eyes, conception occurs.

Rapan ideas, as presented by Hansen, may not be far removed from the perceptions of the Hmong, who also recognize the uterus as a dam that opens and closes at a particular time of the month.[14] Hmong women also believe that menstruation and the period that follows are the times when the uterus is open. Therefore, if sexual intercourse takes place, pregnancy will be the outcome. Because of this, women refrain from having sex with their husbands for a period of 20 days after menstruation.

Like women in less developed countries, Hmong women who use modern methods of fertility regulation also experience their so-called "side effects." But what is interesting is women's increased fear of modern contraception as a result of the rumors about these side effects. This is what Kunstadter and colleagues (1987) have found among the Hmong in northern Thailand. These rumors undermine the effectiveness of family planning programs in many parts of the world, and efforts have been undertaken to find ways to eradicate them (Nichter and Nichter, 1996b). But as Nichter and Nichter (1996b: 75) have pointed out, "Rumors about contraceptive methods would not appeal to the public if they did not resonate with some already existing tacit knowledge about the body—knowledge embedded in and reproduced through popular health practices and discourse about health." The Nichters' argument applies neatly to the Hmong perceptions about the body and their beliefs about health. The following examples may illustrate this point.

The fear that a condom may slip into vagina is common among Hmong women. This is similar to what Taylor (1990) has found among women in Rwanda. Despite the AIDS epidemic in Rwanda, women are reluctant to have their partners use them. They expressed the fear that the condom might remain lodged in the vagina after intercourse. According to Taylor, Rwandans "perceive risk in a manner which is consistent with their views concerning the social construction of the moral person. Of prime importance in this process is the body's perceived aptitude to engage in meaningful exchange and fertile sexuality." To Rwandan women, placing a condom between a woman and a man imposes a "blockage" against the flow of their secretions. For a man, the blockage means turning the semen back upon himself. For women, the fear is a risk of "becoming a blockage being" if a condom remains lodged inside their vagina after sexual intercourse. Sobo (1993) has found a similar notion of blockage/flow among women in Jamaica. Condoms, to Jamaican women, are an unrealiable and dangerous method, because they can "burst or slip off, often lodging inside women . . . and causing illness" (p. 61).[15] The Rwandan and Jamaican theories of bodily blockage/flow may be similar to Hmong women's perceptions about condoms.

Fears of the side effects of modern contraceptive methods, including loss of appetite, pain in the body and irregular menstruation, reflect interesting beliefs among women worldwide. Good (1980: 147), in her work with Iranian women, has stated that the fear of and complaints about side effects of contraceptive methods, particularly the pill, result from their impact on bodily functions. Good referred to this as "the disorders of womanhood," as all social classes of women in provincial Iran had complaints of, for example, heart distress, heart palpitations, weak nerves and aches and pains. Heart distress in particular, in Good's view, is "associated with *being female*—with pregnancy, with sexual intercourse, with contraception, with childbirth and raising children, and with being a wife" (p. 151). Although Hmong women do not articulate this idiom of distress as Good has described it, it is clear that Hmong women are also under pressure to reproduce. In Symond's study (1996) of Hmong women in northern Thailand, women complained that contraceptive pills or injections made them feel weak, with a poor appetite, and unable to work in the fields. More importantly, women claimed "to feel depressed and to be afflicted with what is known as *nyuab siab*, a difficult liver" (p. 118). Symonds pointed out that Hmong women well knew that if they refused to produce more children for the lineage, their husbands might take in junior wives. Thus, "It may be that the effects of social pressure to produce children, and subsequent feelings of depression, manifest themselves in the form of liver distress, the physical organ that provides an idiom for the expression of emotion in Hmong culture."

The notion that women have particular characteristics that make them susceptible to certain modern contraception methods brings up an interesting point. In her work with Iranian women, Good (1980) found that the women also believe that each person has a characteristic temperament, which is affected by climate and geographical location. Accordingly, "susceptibility to various disorders, to food categories which are illness-provoking, to chills, frights, or emotional upset varies according to one's temperament." And susceptibility to modern contraceptive methods, in Iranian women's eyes, is no exception. Therefore, some women may find that certain contraceptive methods are not suitable for certain women. This theory also applies to Hmong women, who believe that some modern fertility regulation methods only suit women of a certain nature. Because a woman does not know how she will react until she has tried a particular method, many women do not wish to conduct this experiment by risking their bodies and their health. This makes many women unwilling to initiate modern contraceptive methods to regulate their fertility.

Hmong women believe that women must be over age 40 before herbal medicines can be effective. Nichter and Nichter (1996b) and Bledsoe et al. (1994) have also noted that contraceptive methods are weighted differently at different points in the reproductive life span and in relation to both a woman's reproductive and productive capacity. In the Hmong culture, this is partly related to the need to produce many children, as I have discussed throughout this book. However, it is perhaps necessary to reiterate here that children in Hmong culture are important for the perpetuation of Hmong lineage, which in turn is essential for the survival of Hmong society.[16] As we have seen, Hmong women are reluctant to use any form of birth control even though they have knowledge of emmenagogues (or abortifacients). This is because, as Symonds (1996: 121) has noted,

> A women who desires to control her own reproduction through the use of birth control is socially discouraged from doing so, through the influence of a pervasive cultural discourse which suggests that in so doing she would also be upsetting the state of cosmological equilibrium that must be maintained through the continued and prolific reproduction of her husband's (and, in effect, her own) lineage.[17]

After having produced several children, women may not be under as much pressure as when they were young.[18] Since most Hmong women are married when they are quite young, by the time they are over age 40 they may have already given birth to several children. They have shown society that they have produced children for the continuation of Hmong society. Hence, Hmong women's belief is logical in the context of Hmong culture.

Abortion has been one among a continuum of fertility regulation options for many women in many parts of the world, but it does produce some ambiguities.[19] According to Hadley (1996: 30), "Abortion is probably the oldest, most common and universal method by which women have controlled their fertility, long before the law regulated it. Women determined to end their pregnancies have always known a wide variety of ways to do so. Until relatively recently it has certainly not attracted the shame or stigma which clings to it today." Hadley (1996: 162) has also stated that there is a "culture of shame" attached to abortion that causes it to be viewed differently than birth control. Because of this, abortion has tended to be seen as a moral issue and condemned by people in most parts of the world (Luker, 1984).

To some extent Hmong women also condemn those who abort their babies, but this condemnation largely depends on what groups these women belong to. It is interesting that Hmong women believe that certain groups of women, including older women and women who have had several children, have a right to abort their babies. The explanation for this belief also covers the use of herbal medicines to regulate fertility in older women who have produced several children for the continuation of the Hmong lineage and Hmong society. These women are seen as having the privilege of terminating their pregnancies if they do not wish to have more children. Those who are still young and have not produced "enough" children do not have this privilege. If they abort their babies, they are condemned by the society.

From this study, it became clear that, first, Hmong women do wish to regulate their fertility. However, society has placed a great deal of pressure on them to continue producing children. In a culture that values having many children, contraception is not easily accepted since it stops women from having children, which upsets the cosmological balance of society. Secondly, among those who have tried to regulate their fertility, a preference has been shown for indigeneous methods—particularly herbal medicines—over modern contraceptive methods. This preference has implications for those developing family planning programs for the Hmong.

What then can be done? Perhaps what is needed is, as Nichter and Nichter (1996b: 97) point out, "a cultural reading of the body and attentive listening to the voices of potential consumers." In these terms, this chapter has done just that. As Good (1980: 155) has suggested, "it may contribute toward the development of family planning programs that are sensitive to the cultural concerns of the population to be served."

NOTES

1. See later section on modern methods of fertility regulation, particularly sterilization. See also Chapter 15 on motherhood in a new country and women's concerns about having too many children in their new homeland.

2. See also Chapter 9 in this volume for further details about infant feeding practices.

3. See Chapter 6 for more details about confinement beliefs and practices in Hmong culture.

4. See Newman (1985) for details about indigeneous fertility regulation methods in many parts of the world.

5. See also Chapter 14 for further details about menstruation in Hmong society.

6. The notion of "bringing down" a delayed period has been reported in Mexico (Shedlin, 1982); Iran (Good, 1980); Afghanistan (Hunte, 1985); Colombia (Browner, 1980, 1985); Jamaica (Brody, 1981, 1985); Malaysia (Ngin, 1985); Ecuador (Scrimshaw, 1985); and the Philippines (Nichter and Vuckovic, 1994). According to Shedlin, women in Mexico do not see the bringing down of a delayed period as an abortion, and they speak about it freely.

7. See, for example, Newman (1972, 1985); Winikoff (1987); Hull (1991); Jacobson (1991); Eschen and Whittaker (1993); Nichter and Nichter (1996b); Jennaway (1996); and Whittaker (1996).

8. See also Chapter 2 for more details about sexuality in Hmong culture.

9. Whereas in Sri Lanka, for example, women only complain about weakness and the inability to do heavy work as the main side effects of sterilization (Nichter and Nichter, 1996b).

10. See also a case of soul loss in the introductory chapter. See also Bliatout (1988) on the fear of an operation among Hmong in the United States.

11. Laderman (1987) notes that women who do not want an "inconvenient" pregnancy try to get rid of the fetus by performing hot massage on their abdomen, which brings hot blood to the area. This makes their wombs uncomfortably hot and, hence, the fetus eventually falls out.

12. Although nearly all Hmong women believe that herbal medicines are effective in regulating their fertility, some women have also experienced side effects similar to those associated with Western birth control. One woman related: "When I was in Thailand, and after I had my third child I thought I didn't want to have children too close together. Someone had Hmong herbs for use as contraception so that the children would be spaced out. So I bought three packets and used them all. But after that I had a lot of back and stomach pain so I didn't take them anymore."

13. For example, the Indian subcontinent (Nichter and Nichter, 1996a; Gould, 1975; Mandelbaum, 1970); the Philippines (Rubel et al., 1975; Laing, 1984); Yucatan (Jordan, 1989); Peru (Maynard-Tucker, 1989); and Afghanistan (Hunte, 1985).

14. McGilvray (1982: 52) points out that for Batticaloa Tamils in Sri Lanka, the uterus is commonly seen as a flower and fecundity a time when it is in bloom.

15. According to Jamaican women, only doctors can remove condoms from their vaginas once they get stuck inside. This is also a common belief among Hmong women, and it is associated with inconvenience and fear of going into the hospital. The theory of blockage/flow is also discussed in great detail in Taylor's later publication (1992).

16. See also Kunstadter et al. (1987) and Symonds (1996) for discussions of the value of children in Hmong society and the reasons why Hmong women continue to produce more children for their husbands' lineage.

17. See also Chapter 11 in this volume for more details on the rebirth of souls and miscarriage in Hmong culture.

18. However, Symonds found that even women who have produced many children and believe their families are complete are still under pressure not to practice birth control of any kind. She mentioned that when she spoke to Hmong women in the presence of their mothers-in-law, the women would say that they did not use contraception. However, when they were alone they would admit that they were trying to use one method or another.

19. See, for example, Burnight and Leoprapai (1977); Riddle (1992, 1997); Hadley (1996); Johnson et al. (1996); Renne (1996); Rigdon (1996); Sobo (1996); and Lane et al. (1998). Riddle's book (1992) provides readers with a comprehensive historical account of abortion from the ancient world to the Renaissance.

Chapter 14

Blood Magic: Menstruation and Menopause

> Women, Women.... Well! if you don't have menses then you will not be able to have children, but if you have your menses then you will be able to have children.
>
> Hmong informant

> As earthly life is bounded by birth and death, so is the possibility of this life bounded by menarche and menopause
>
> (Delaney, 1988: 91)

INTRODUCTION

Menstruation is a universal physiological process in the lives of all women. But perceptions, meanings and practices related to it are not. As Buckley and Gottlieb (1988: 3) have stated: "While menstruation itself has at least a degree of biological regularity, its symbolic voicings and valences are strikingly variable, both cross-culturally and within single cultures." Menstruation, as such, is viewed and treated differently in different cultures. In most, menstruation is seen as being related to procreation; it gives women the power to conceive babies. But at the same time, menstruation is seen as "potentially polluting substances" (Delaney, 1988: 80) that can cause harm to others, particularly men. Because of this belief, "taboos"[1] exist in many cultures. Very often, these taboos impose restrictions on women's lives in order to safeguard others.

Menopause is a common aspect of life for women, but it is also a sociocultural event. The physical changes of menopause are only one part of a woman's life experiences. They are interwoven with the woman's social status, sexual role, personal circumstances, life history and state of health.[2] In her paper "Myth and the Menopause," Kaufert (1982: 144) stated that:

> Like childbirth and menstruation, there are two levels of reality to menopause. One is the actual physical changes that occur in a woman . . . all women who survive and have intact ovaries pass through the menopause. "Passage through the menopause" is also an event occurring within a socio-cultural context. It is this—the cultural dimension of the menopause—which forms the second level of its reality.

Kaufert has said that a woman who belongs to a culture that perceives the menopause as symptom-free will not experience menopausal symptoms related to physical changes in midlife, such as hot flashes and depression. These women will pass through the menopause without difficulty.

In this chapter, the experience of Hmong women is used as a paradigm to analyze cultural interpretations of menstruation and menopause. I will first discuss Hmong women's view of menstruation and its impact on their lives. The chapter then examines Hmong women's interpretations and experiences of menopause.

MENSTRUATION: BEING A WOMAN

> Menstruation! People who are ignorant would say that it is a dirty thing, but it is the most important thing for you. If you don't have that you are not able to have children. If you don't have that you will not look healthy and it makes you look anemic and unhealthy. If you have it you have no problems at all.

The Hmong recognize that menstruation is an essential part of being a woman. In this culture, being a woman means that one menstruates. The term commonly used by the Hmong to mean menstruation is *ua poj niam*, which literally means, "being a woman."

> To be a woman, you must have menstruation. If you are a woman it must come. If you are a woman you must have menstruation.

Menarche marks the beginning of womanhood among the Hmong. This is referred to as *nto nkauj*, which means that women have finished their childhood and reached womanhood or motherhood. It is believed that when a young girl begins to menstruate, she is capable of producing children.[3]

> People would say that you are at womanhood that is why you have menses. They say that you are *nto nkauj,* become a woman and you can become a mother.

Another woman related:

> When the girl starts to have menses it means that she has reached a motherhood. . . . Because when she has this she will be married and will be able to bear children. It means that you have the ability to conceive or bear children.

The Hmong have no elaborate "rite of passage" to mark the commencement of menarche, as is found in other cultures.[4] Women are only reminded that they are no longer young children and must be more cautious with men, because if they have sexual intercourse they may become pregnant. They are also told how to keep themselves clean and to pay particular attention to several rules observed in Hmong culture. This will be discussed in a later section.

MENSTRUATION AND HEALTH

Menstruation, at one level, is seen as "bad" blood that must be expelled from the body. Menstruation is believed to change the blood within the body. The circulation of "bad" blood enables the renewal of the blood, which in turn makes a woman healthy. Thus, Hmong women believe that a woman whose menstruation ceases for any reason will be unhealthy; she may become pale, skinny and eventually die.

> When you have your menses it is good. If you don't have it then you are like a person who is very unhealthy. Because you don't have your menses you are very pale and look like a person who is always sick.

The clotting of menstrual blood is seen as extremely dangerous to a woman's health. One woman told us about her relatives and acquaintances who died from the clots of their menstruation.

> If you don't have the blood you will become skinny and then you will die. . . . There are three people that I know who have died from blood clots. They became extremely skinny and their face was not normal; it became very yellow. They had no strength at all and became smaller and smaller and then died. Our [relative]'s first wife died of blood clots. My brother's

> eldest daughter had that and died too. The [X] family's aunt died of that too. I saw them with my own eyes.

MENSTRUATION, PREGNANCY AND THE BABY

At another level, menstruation is seen as closely associated with procreation, since women without menstruation are unable to produce children.

> Having the menses is good. If you don't have the menses then it means that your menses has dried up. If your menses has dried up that means that you will not bleed and then you will not be able to have children.

When discussing the relationship between menstruation and pregnancy, women offer two thoughts. First, menstruation "makes the baby." This is why women stop menstruating when they become pregnant.

> People say that when you have no more menses it means that it has become the baby and that is why you don't have any menses . . . until you give birth to the baby and after one month you will see it again for one time, then no more. When the next baby is going to be conceived then you will see the menses again.

Women use the metaphor of a dam for a fish to live in as the need for menstruation for the sake of the baby.

> I think that when you are pregnant, it will stay inside and not come out at all. . . . I think that when you conceive a baby your blood and water will make a dam for the baby; like a dam would be for the fish. When the baby is born then it will come out with the baby.

Second, women say that when menstruation stops it is used internally to feed the baby inside their womb.[5]

> Some women say that that is where the baby is going to grow from and that's why it stops and that menses becomes the baby's food. It may be like that because when you get pregnant you don't have that any more.

GOOD MENSES AND BAD MENSES: HEALTH AND FERTILITY

Hmong women make distinctions between good menses and bad menses. The color of the menstruation is used as an indication of good or bad blood. It is believed that good menstruation must be bright red. If it is dark it means bad blood. Bright blood will make the woman healthy.

In contrast, dark blood will make the woman pale and skinny; the indication of bad health.

> If you have menses which is no good, like it is not bright, then this means that there is a problem with your body and that is why you are pale.

The flow of blood is also used to identify good or bad menstruation. A moderate flow is believed to be best for any woman. A combination of light flow and dark color indicates bad health. A heavy flow is, however, believed to be the result of being "hit" by spirits.[6]

> For myself, if the blood comes a little bit at a time and black then it is no good. If your blood is no good then it will make you unhealthy. If that blood is very bright and good then it finishes quicker and you don't feel tired, only feel stronger.

The humoral quality of menstruation is also an identification of good or bad menses and is closely related to fertility. This humoral quality is based on the hot/cold dichotomy, as found in the Chinese medical system. It is believed that cold menstruation contributes to infertility.[7]

> It may be that your menses is very cold. If the menses is very cold then you can't have children. If the menses is warm and also the blood is bright that is when you can have children.

Good menstruation means successful conception. Good menstruation does not cause health problems, such as back and abdominal pains. Because of this, women who have good menses have a tendency to conceive easily. The color, the flow and the humoral quality of menstruation are also indications of the ability to conceive. When asked under what circumstances women may conceive, a common answer given is:

> If your body is healthy and that your menses flows properly, that your menses is bright and that is how you can have them [children]. But if your menses is not flowing properly then you will not be able to conceive.

Regularity of the period is also believed to be an indication of the ability to conceive.

> For good conception, the blood must be bright in color. Also for those women who have irregular period they will have children very far apart; they will find it hard to conceive.

When women talk about infertility, they very often indicate poor color and an inadequate flow of menstruation as the main causes.

> Periods vary from one person to person. It depends if they have always had only a little or a lot. If they have a little then they will have a little. . . . But [Y]'s wife told me that the reason why she can't conceive is because she has only a very small amount of period each time.

MENSTRUATION: SHAMEFUL MATTERS

Despite the fact that menstruation is good for women's health and important for procreation, most women also consider it "shameful" and "embarrassing." This is reflected in the interviews I conducted to ask the women about menstruation. The following conversation illustrates this point.

Pranee: I would like to ask you about menstruation, is this okay?

Neng: What do you want to know about it?

Pranee: Well, anything that you can tell me, I think it is related to having a baby.

Neng: Is it? We are to talk about your body having that dirty thing! Yes, you can, but what do you want to talk. . . . With the Hmong, it is the most embarrassing thing to talk about. . . . Yes, I am telling the truth, I became a shameful person because of my menstruation; it flowed too much.

She then asked me why I wanted to talk about the "shameful" thing. Another woman made a similar remark:

> I think it is a shameful thing, but you have to have it for you to have children. If you say it is a likable thing, no, it is not. I don't like it.

Because women no longer need to worry about the stain on their *tiab Hmong* (Hmong skirt), which causes great embarrassment, women feel somewhat relaxed about having no more menses. Some said:

> With the menses, Hmong in the villages have no underwear and no napkins so wherever they sat they will leave a mark. This is very embarrassing. Whenever the menses is due then you will worry a lot and feel scared that it will show. So when you don't have any more menses, you don't need to worry about it anymore.

Hmong women see menstruation as "dirty," and when other people can see a stain on their skirts or pants or the blood running down their legs, it causes considerable "embarrassment."

> I think that it is a dirty thing. For me I think why a woman has to have such an unhygienic thing like this. That is what I think. It is embarrassing, don't you think so? Ooh! I am really embarrassed about it and will not let anyone know that I am menstruating.

Similarly, another woman remarked:

> I think that because it is unclean, it is unhygienic. In Laos there are lots of people and if you can't keep it clean it stains your clothes and you feel embarrassed towards other people like the men around you and your children and family. You will feel that they can see you.

It must be noted that in Laos, most Hmong women did not have access to sanitary pads as in Australia. Women did not have anything to wear to prevent the running down of menstrual flow. In addition, the scarcity of materials prevented women from using anything to wipe off their blood. Most often, women had to let the blood run down their legs.

When their menstruation is apparent, women are criticized for not being able to hide their "embarrassment," even among other women.

> Even your peers would say, "Why isn't she embarrassed, why does she do it and everyone can see it?" Women as you are still saying this and what about the men if they see this they will stay away.

If men see women with menstrual marks on their clothes, they also talk about it. This is particularly true of young men. However, women also mentioned that despite their criticism, men will not choose a woman for marriage who is not menstruating, because they know that these women will have difficulty conceiving.

> Men! If they see women having that, some younger ones will talk about it. But, like I said before, if you don't have it then no one will want to marry you.

MENSTRUATION AND RESTRICTIONS

While menstruating, Hmong women do not have to take precautions with their diet, except for avoiding icy cold water and ice. Women believe that drinking icy cold water will cause the blood to clot and lead to health problems. This precaution is particularly observed after a long day of hard work in the field.[8]

> When you have menses you should not eat ice. If you eat it then your body will not be able to rid of the blood. When you eat the cold thing into your body it will make the blood clot and make you sick; pain in the stomach and you get all sort of sickness and this is no good for you.

The Hmong do not have many behavioral restrictions during the menstruating period. Women say they can perform their usual tasks and have contact with others in the community. However, there are restrictions of which women are well aware. These include not crossing over rivers, not washing their body or their menstrually stained clothes in rivers or dams and not throwing the water used to wash their menstrual blood in rivers. It is believed that these activities will offend nature spirits, who will become angry and strike them. This, in turn, may lead to miscarriage and infertility.[9]

> When you have your menses you should not go to wash these clothing in a river. When you have just grown up you do not know this so when you have your first menses you are very embarrassed about it so you go to wash your clothing in a river which is man-made and you must not throw the dirty water back into the river. If you wash your clothes and throw the water back into the river the spirit can hit you and this will cause you to be sick. If you wash you must wash it and throw it into the soil. If you throw it into the river it will make you sick and when you get married it will cause you to not have any children and it is very hard to fix. You may conceive but it is only after a long time of healing for you to conceive.

While menstruating, Hmong women totally avoid sexual intercourse. Their main reason is that "men do not like it because it is dirty." Women are too embarrassed to let their husbands see their menstrual blood, and therefore try to stay away from them. Most men understand this behavior and will not insist on sexual intercourse during this period.

> When you have menses you can't have sex with your husband because when it is like that it is very dirty. . . . For us, we don't like it because when you have that [menses] you are very embarrassed so you don't even sleep near your man.

Another woman said:

> When I have my menses I don't sleep with my husband because men don't like it. It is just dirty so men don't like it.

MENSTRUATION AND MENOPAUSE: THE LINK

Because menopause means that there will be no more menses, reaching menopause was seen by the women interviewed as being polluted no longer, but instead being clean. Women look forward to this stage in which they will no longer be seen as polluted and dirty. All Hmong women who have reached menopause say that they feel very relieved. They also believe that the cessation of menstruation makes them become "clean like men." One older woman told us about her embarrassment and bad experience with menstruation. She said that she sought herbal medicines to terminate her menstruation, which she succeeded in doing.

And now, she is "clean like the men."

> For me, I had bad menses and I hated it so much that is why I resorted to looking for medicines to get rid of it. I took medicines and so I am very clean like the men now. . . . I hate it so much that when it was gone I felt great. I was happy that I didn't have that anymore. I don't have to be embarrassed to other people anymore.

Those who have not reached menopause have ambivalent feelings about menstruation. On the one hand, it is essential for their procreation. On the other hand, however, having it causes uncomfortable feelings. At worst, if it does not come it may mean death.

> Being a woman, that is very dirty and if you don't have it then you may be afraid of dying and if you do have it, it is an uncomfortable thing to have. . . . The elderly say that if it just stops by itself then it may be a clot inside your body and that is why it can't flow and this can kill you. . . . So it is unclean but if you don't have it you may die too, and also it means that you can't have children.

THE MEANING OF MENOPAUSE

In the Hmong language there is no equivalent word for menopause. The concept of menopause is understood as *tsis coj khaub ncaws lawm,* which literally means "no more menstruation." In general, menopause is associated with *pog laus,* the terminology used for an old lady, an older person or a grandmother, and it is seen as a natural part of "growing old." Women's interpretations of menopause are presented in the following sections.

No More Children: No More Menstruation

Menopause is interpreted as the consequence of the transition from fertility to infertility. Hmong women perceive that women reach menopause only when they are no longer fertile; they have borne all of their children. The following conversation illustrates this point:

Pranee: How old is a woman when her menstruation stops completely?

Mai: After you have all of your children. . . . I don't know how old, it depends on the person. Some will have only seven or eight children and then their children will be finished and have no more, but some others will have over ten children before they finish their children, and that is when you have no more menstruation.

However, most Hmong women believe that in a lifetime a fertile woman may become pregnant up to 13 or 14 times. Hmong women also believe that early menarche means early menopause. According to the Hmong, if you have your first menses as early as about age ten or twelve, it will finish early. Even if you are not very old, it will stop. But if your menses start at the age of fourteen or fifteen, you will still have your menses when you are quite old. It is noted that all postmenopausal women in this study became menopausal relatively young, when they had just passed their forties (mean age, 43 years).

Menopause: No More Children

Women, once married, are expected to bear many children. Having borne her first child, a Hmong woman has fulfilled her most important role for the family since she has been able to provide continuity for the patrilineage. Most Hmong women believe that they must have at least as many children as their mother or mother-in-law.[10] Children are the assets of the family, particularly males. Children are necessary for one's well-being, not only in this life but also in the afterlife. If a woman does not bear children, there will be no one to look after her in old age. More importantly, if she does not have sons, there will be no one to care for the family altar and feed the ancestors, among whom she will be included when she dies. This makes having children a vital part of life for Hmong women.

These concerns cause some women to regret being no longer able to bear children. However, the majority of Hmong women have already borne many, and believe that menopause is a positive aspect of their lives.

Pranee: Do you think no more menses is a good thing or a bad thing?

Dia: It is a good thing.

Pranee: In what sense do you say it is a good thing?

Dia: It is good in that I will have no more children. . . . I am getting old and very tired of looking after children and if I don't have anymore, then it does not matter.

When I brought up the importance of bearing children among the Hmong and asked the women if it would worry them once they were no longer menstruating, their answers were much like this explanation.

Menopause as a Change of Role and Status

Hmong girls and adolescents do not have equal social or familial status with Hmong boys and men. However, their status changes when they marry and are able to bear a child. The birth of the first child brings a Hmong woman prestige.[11] Women gain respect and status from all of

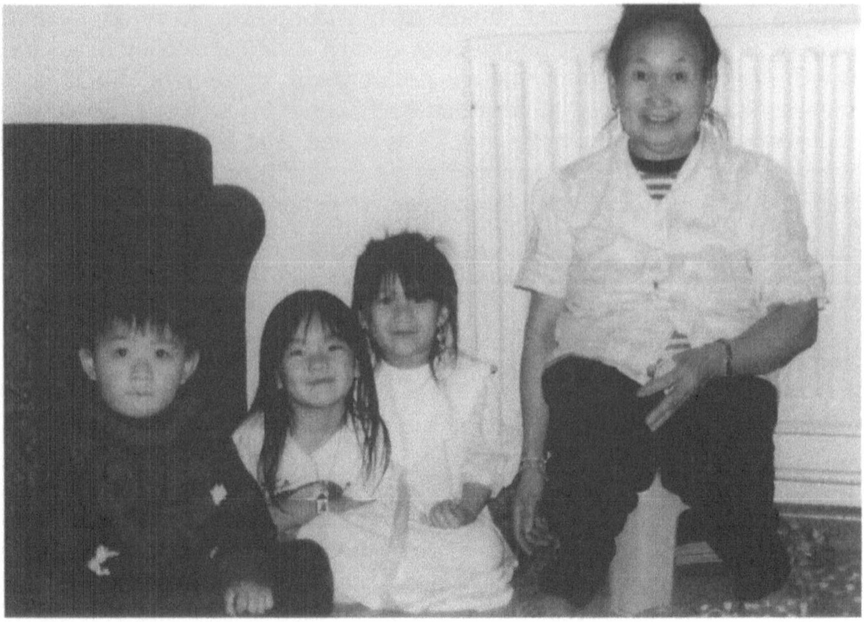

Photo 14.1 A Hmong grandmother with her grandchildren at home.

the community when they produce children. Once she becomes old, the woman's status changes again. Older women are referred to as *cov txwj laus* (respected elders) and are addressed as *pog laus* (grandmother) by all. Since menopause is associated with old age, postmenopausal women are, therefore, respected and have a higher status than when they were young.

Once women reach menopause, their role shifts from childbearing to childrearing; from caring for their own children to looking after their grandchildren (Photo 14.1). Women in the study said that their life with children did not end with menopause. By the time Hmong women reach menopause, their daughters or daughters-in-law have already reached the childbearing stage. The older women help rear and look after their grandchildren, since their daughters or daughters-in-law are engaging in childbearing and other domestic activities or working in the field.

> Older women are not bearing more children. At that time your children will be older and you can just relax, but if they have some children then you help them with their children.

Menopause and Aging

Women associate menopause with aging; when a woman has reached menopause, she is old.

> Now I think that I am old and that I will have no more children. I have had many children and that is why it is finished and that is why I don't have any more menses.

The majority of Hmong women do not see aging as problematic. By that time their children will have all grown up. They do not need to be as concerned about the survival and well-being of their children as they had when the children were younger.

> I am not too worried about getting old. By that time my children would have all grown up and I don't need to be worried about being poor, if it would be enough food to feed them, or if it would be enough clothes to keep them warm, that sort of things.

The Hmong have a strong belief in the Confucian values of filial piety. Adult children have a duty to look after and take good care of their aged parents. Among the Hmong, this duty extends even to the period after the death of their parents. Male children continue to feed and worship their deceased parents to ensure their reincarnation.[12]

However, some Hmong women worry about being old because they associate old age with the near-death stage. This means that they will not be with their children and grandchildren very long.

> I am worried that I am getting old and I may not live long any more because when you get old then you will die, that is what I think about.

THE EXPERIENCE OF MENOPAUSE

Postmenopausal women in the study were asked if any physical changes occurred after the cessation of menstruation. Interestingly, the women could not remember any physical changes after they became menopausal. However, all women recalled that their menstruation had become irregular and, in particular, lighter during the last year of their reproductive life. There were no reports of hot flashes, flushes or night sweating among these menopausal women. They said that nothing had changed physically.

> I have no effect from not having the menses. I still have good appetite but maybe I am old, that is why it is hard for me to put on weight but my appetite is the same and my health is the same.

And,

> I have not had any bad health since it stopped. I am today the same as I was before, no problems.

A number of women were surprised to learn that many Australian women experience some ill health when they become menopausal. Their interpretation of this information was that Australian women must not observe traditional restrictions after childbirth, as Hmong women do.[13] Hmong women, in common with women from other cultures in East and Southeast Asia, observe particular confinement practices during the first month after giving birth. These confinement practices, the Hmong believe, protect women and will keep them from having any ill health in old age. Therefore, any symptoms of ill health that occur from middle age onward are interpreted as resulting from not following the traditional confinement practices during childbearing years.

Women were also asked if they had experienced any emotional change or difficulty after menopause. Again, women said that they had not. Common answers were: "There is nothing, I am very comfortable and very happy." And "I am happy with my life, my children and my grandchildren. Nothing like that (emotional difficulty) has happened to me."

I also asked the women whether their health in general changed after menopause. Women found it rather amusing that I asked such a question. Some made remarks like:

> This is a natural part of growing old and when it stops because you are old then there should not be anything wrong with your health.

Another one remarked:

> When you are old and you just don't have it any more your health will still be the same as before, there is nothing wrong with not having any more menstruation because you are old.

The same question was asked of premenopausal women. Most women believed that the cessation of menstruation would not make them unhealthy. It would, however, have an effect on their "strength."

> When you do not menstruate, when you are about forty-five or so, you are old and can't do many things. You won't be as strong as before so you can't do too many things.

Women also believed that once menstruation ceased a woman may gradually become blind. This was considered to be associated with old age.

> They say that if you don't have that [menstruation] it makes you go blind. I can't thread the needle any more. That is what happens, it is a sign of getting older. When you get older you have no more blood so that you can't see as well as before.

CONCLUSIONS

In many societies, menstruation is perceived as "pollution"[14] because it is associated with dirt, mess and the uncleanliness of menstrual blood (Britton, 1996). This uncleanliness is seen as similar to other "dirt" (like saliva and semen) that crosses a body boundary. Thus, menstruation is a symbolic "matter out of place" (Douglas, 1966). As such, it becomes a "pollutant" that can be dangerous to social order. Because of this, rules, more widely known as "taboos," exist to protect human beings from the danger of women's menstruation. Menstruating women are usually "excluded" from normal activities such as cooking and looking for food.[15] They are also not allowed to have contact with their men for fear of contaminating or killing them.[16]

However, as Buckley and Gottlieb (1988), have pointed out, not all cultures have menstrual taboos. In some cultures, a belief also exists that menstruation is both polluting and purifying. Kuper (1947: 107) pointed out long ago that: "in certain situations . . . menstrual blood is not destructive, but is considered a life symbol or rather a life force." The notion that menstrual blood turns to nourish the fetus during pregnancy illustrates this point. In Sri Lanka, there is a belief that although menstrual blood is extremely polluted, the blood that goes to the baby is beneficial (McGilvray, 1982). If we use Douglas's interpretation to explain this, we may see that menstrual blood, like certain other bodily substances, only becomes polluting when it leaves the natural bounds of the body. This interpretation jibes with Hmong women's explanation of menstrual blood; that it makes and feeds the fetus during pregnancy. This, perhaps explains why menstruation is not seen as "polluted," as it is in many other cultures.

Menstruation, however, causes considerable embarrassment and discomfort among women. In the old days, women felt embarrassed because materials were scarce and there was nothing to help them hide their bleeding. It was considered dirty because the clothes they wore every day became dirty. The scarcity of clean running water because of their living situation contributed to this notion of "dirtiness" in the Hmong world view.

In Hmong culture, unlike many other cultures, there is no belief that menstrual blood may harm men. There are, however, "rules" that impose restrictions on menstruating women. Most are related to women's fertility; that is, they serve to ensure that women will be able to produce children. This can be seen from the beliefs that a menstruating woman should not consume "cold" food, since it will make her blood congeal and cause ill health; and that menstruating women should not cross a river or wash their menstrual blood in a river, as the spirits may trace them through the smell of the blood and cause miscarriage and fertility.

In this sense, as Gottlieb (1988: 74) has pointed out, menstruation can be seen as "a symbol of fertility, or life," rather than a polluting substance.

Menopause is seen as a natural part of life that any *pog laus* has to experience; it is part of growing old. By the time women become menopausal, they have borne all of their children, and their children have grown up. They have therefore done their duty, the duty of motherhood being to ensure the continuity of the family lineage by giving birth to sons, or to daughters who bring in sons-in-law. Once women reach this stage, they are more respected and become a "grandmother" to all. Women at this stage do not have to deal with the monthly business of menstruation. They no longer feel shameful about having menstruation and do not have to worry about being embarrassed by it. Women are able to feel more relaxed once their menstruation ceases. It is not surprising, then, that most of the Hmong women interviewed welcomed the menopause.

Why did Hmong women in this study appear to have no problems with menopause, as women do in most Western societies? I wish to discuss the two aspects of the Hmong world view that answer this question.

The Positive Attitude Toward Menopause

Brown has remarked (1982) that in traditional societies, the change in a woman's life in middle age appears to be positive. In most of these societies, a young woman is restricted and her life consists of "subservience and toil." Once she is middle-aged, she has more authority and leisure. Three major changes take place in the lives of middle-aged women in traditional societies. First, they are freed from many of the restrictions imposed on them when younger, such as menstrual restrictions. Second, they have authority over some younger kin, including making important decisions for them. Third, they are eligible for a special status that allows them to have more freedom, releasing them from confinement to the household. All of these changes improve the status of middle-aged women. It is these improvements to their lives that makes the meaning of menopause positive.

Bart's theory (1969) on the influence of status on women's experiences of menopause drew similar conclusions. Bart pointed out that as women age, their increased social status protects them from the negative effects of menopause. This is commonly found in traditional societies where kinship is practiced. According to Bart, six cultural characteristics act to protect middle-aged women. These are: "strong ties to family of origin and kin, extended family system, the residence patterns keeping one close to the family of orientation, strong mother-child relationship reciprocal in later life, institutionalised grandmother role and institutionalised mother-in-law role" (Bart, 1969: 14). Although the Hmong are a patrilineal and patrilocal society, when a woman moves into her husband's home after marriage, it does not reduce her strong ties with her natal kin. There are extended family networks, and several generations reside together in one household.[17] The Hmong also have strong mother-child reciprocal relationships. An aged mother is looked after and taken good care of by her adult children. When her sons are married, daughters-in-law are brought into her house. It is then her duty to teach and train her daughters-in-law to be good wives and mothers. Once she becomes a grandmother, her role changes from bearing her children to rearing grandchildren, and she is respected by all.[18]

According to Kaufert (1982), older women have more power and prestige in some traditional societies. However, women gain their power and prestige only when they are able to bear and raise children. Women without children—either because they are infertile or their children do not survive—face economic and social deprivation. The menopause ends their hope of becoming pregnant and having children. Women in these situations may perceive menopause as negative and do not welcome it. This study showed that Hmong women had gained all their power and prestige by fulfilling the important requirements of reproduction: bearing many children and having children survive to carry on their lineage.

Barnett's study, conducted in a small Peruvian town (1988), found that most postmenopausal women were relatively satisfied with their menopausal situation. Barnett determined that their satisfaction was linked to sociocultural beliefs such as the cultural recognition of adulthood, which is only granted to women and men over forty, the end of the daily and direct responsibility of caring for their children, and the satisfaction of filling their role of grandmother. Barnett also suggests that the internal rewards that accompany a woman's sense of accomplishment in her own principal role are equally important and are significant in determining the woman's perceptions of menopause. The present study indicates that at menopause Hmong women believe they have fulfilled their roles as Hmong mothers and, therefore, menopause is seen as a stage in which to reap the rewards for having done so.

The Experience of Menopause

Although menopause is inevitable for all women, physiological and emotional symptoms are not universally the same (Voda, 1993). Women in some cultures experience menopausal symptoms more than in others and, in some cultures, experience them not at all (Kaufert, 1982). Flint (1974), for example, has found that very few Indian women of the Rajput caste in the states of Rajasthan and Himachal Pradesh have problems with their menopause other than changes of the menstrual cycle. Flint reported that "there were no depressions, dizziness, no incapacitation nor any of the symptoms associated with what we call the menopausal syndrome" (Flint, 1975: 162). Similar to Flint, Beyene (1986, 1989) has reported the absence of any menopausal symptoms in Mayan women.

According to Flint (1975), the absence of menopausal symptoms among Indian women can be explained by the "reward" gained by women when they reach menopause and can no longer bear children. At menopause a woman is allowed to partake of activities that are "forbidden" during childbearing years. For example, the Rajput women have to live in "Purdah" (veiled and secluded) until their menopause, when they are no longer considered to be polluted. More importantly, their status is much more elevated than before menopause. Flint added that most women in the United States suffer severe menopausal symptoms, since menopause is a time of "punishment." At the time these women reach menopause, their children will have left home, leaving the women with an "empty nest" syndrome. Their husbands may also suffer a male climacteric and may be out looking for younger women to prove their virility. In addition, women in the United States do not gain status in old age. The life of Hmong women, however, fits very well with Flint's theory of "reward and punishment," and this may help to explain the absence of symptoms among them.

Beyene (1989) proposed a "biocultural analysis" to explain the absence and presence of menopausal symptoms. She put forward three hypotheses for the absence of symptoms in Mayan women. First, it may result from the women's positive attitudes toward menopause. When childbearing is over, a woman can be free. Second, the low nutritional status of Mayan women may lead to early onset of menopause and asymptomatology. Beyene found that Mayan women were already postmenopausal in their mid-forties, when most women in industrial nations are just entering the menopause. Hmong women in this study reached menopause at their mid-forties, approximately. Like Mayan women, their nutritional status is low. Their living situations in Laos were relatively poor because of their geographic location and the war. Even after being placed in refugee camps in Thailand and resettled in Australia, their situation did not improve a great deal. Finally, Beyene suggested that interference with normal reproductive function through the use of contraceptive drugs and interventions to prevent pregnancy, common among Western women, may cause menopausal symptoms among Western women. The majority of Hmong women interviewed did not use any Western birth control drugs or devices until they came to refugee camps in Thailand or settled in Australia.[19] Traditionally, Hmong women keep bearing children until menopause, with little interference with reproductive function. Beyene's three hypotheses may indeed explain the absence of menopausal symptoms among Hmong women in this study.

At present, it appears that the Hmong women in Melbourne continue to perceive menopause in a positive light and experience few so-called menopausal symptoms. However, the longer most Hmong women live here, the greater the process of adaptation to living in a Western environment will be. They are faced with many changes, and these changes may have consequences for the way in which the menopause is perceived and experienced. Because of the availability of Western health care and the relative unavailability of traditional herbal medicines and healers in Australia, Hmong women now seek help from mainstream health services when they experience ill health of any kind. This inevitably puts women in midlife into contact with current medical interpretations of menopause. Roberts (1985) has pointed out that once a woman reaches forty years of age, doctors tend to bring the menopause into all their discussions of her health. The question to be asked here is: Will Hmong women be encouraged to interpret menopause as a medically oriented event and thus experience menopausal symptoms in the way many Australian women do? Although evidence from previous studies that have examined women's lives in rapidly changing societies has indicated this may be the case,[20] it remains to be seen what will happen to Hmong women now living in Australia.

NOTES

1. This does not mean that all societies see menstruation as polluted and dangerous to others. Hence, "taboos" as such may not exist. Buckley and Gottlieb (1988: 7) have argued this in their critical analysis of theories of menstrual symbolism. They have pointed out that what is commonly found is a wide range of "rules for conduct regarding menstruation that bespeak quite different, even opposite, purposes and meanings."

2. See also Davis, 1986; Beyene, 1986; Barnett, 1988; Kaufert, 1982; and Chirawatkul, 1992, 1993.

3. Weideger (1977: 148) has said that "menarche is the sign and symbol of womanhood. It is the index of female sexuality as well as the potential for reproduction." See also McGilvray (1982) on the perceptions of menarche in Sri Lanka, and Britton (1996) on women's experience of menarche in England.

4. In many cultures, a rite of passage is performed to mark the beginning of their menstruation. According to Britton (1996: 652), "This rite of passage ritual is usually presented to the young women through a clear framework of meanings and practices." See McGilvray (1982) for elaborate rites as an example of rituals to mark the importance of menarche in Sri Lanka.

5. Good (1980: 150) has pointed out a similar belief among women in Iran. Although menstrual blood is considered pollution, the pollutant quality of the blood is seen as an essential element in reproduction. Women believe that menstrual blood turns into food for the baby during pregnancy. See also McGilvray (1982) for a similar belief among Sri Lankan women. Women in his study believed that menstruation blood stops during pregnancy because the blood goes

to nourish the baby. Delaney's (1988) study in Turkey pointed to the same belief among Turkish women.

6. See also Chapter 11 in this volume about the association between being struck by spirits and the loss of pregnancy.

7. See also Chapter 11 in this volume about hot and cold womb and its relation to infertility.

8. Several women, however, mentioned that they can drink cold water during menstruation. However, women who are likely to experience abdominal pain while menstruating will try to avoid it. As one said, "Some people say that they have no pain in the stomach or anywhere else they can drink it. For the ones that are at a higher risk of having stomach pain don't. . . . The ones that don't drink are the ones that have strong pain. Every time they have their menses they will lie down and at the end of it they will be very skinny. These are the ones that will not drink cold water."

9. See also Chapter 11 in this volume.

10. See Chapter 11 in this volume, Symonds (1991, 1996) and Kunstadter et al. (1987) for similar beliefs and practices among the Hmong in northern Thailand.

11. After giving birth to her first child, a Hmong woman becomes "Pao's mother." She is no longer addressed as "my younger daughter" by her parents, nor as "woman of Vang Jia Lee" by others. See also Chapter 2 in this volume and Symonds (1991, 1996).

12. See also Yang (1992) and Symonds (1991, 1996).

13. See also Chapter 6 in this volume, Symonds (1991, 1996) and Kunstadter et al. (1987) on Hmong confinement beliefs and practices.

14. See, for example, Good (1980), Furth and Chen (1992), Rozario (1992), Prendergast (1994) and Thuren (1994). Good (1980: 149) has pointed out that in Iran "menstrual blood (and the blood of childbirth) is not only physically polluting to the body, but is also ritually polluting. Menstrual blood is one of 10 or 12 categories of *nejasat*, items which are ritually unclean, including feces, urine, and the sweat of sexual exertion."

15. Britton (1996) points out that the seclusion of menstruating women has often been presented in negative terms. But feminist anthropologists have pointed to the positive functions of women's seclusion or exclusion. See Rosaldo (1974), Patterson (1986), Gottlieb (1988), Martin (1987) and Sobo (1993), for example. According to Rosaldo (1974: 38), "Pollution beliefs can provide grounds for solidarity among women." Menstrual huts for women's seclusion, for example, can also be sanctuaries for women. Patterson (1986: 490) reported that most women of Mogmog Island in the Pacific atoll of Ulithi actually enjoy the break from their normal routines and "spend the time happily talking or weaving." Their seclusion place, "women's house," serves as a community center for them.

16. See, for example, Sobo (1993) for her writing about menstruation in Jamaica. Sobo points out that women who wish to secure their men's love and money will use their menstrual blood in cooking as a way to "tie" the men to themselves. Therefore, women's intent to "tie" men is "central to menstruating women's 'unclean' state" (p. 116).

17. See also Chapter 1 in this volume, Symonds (1991, 1996), Kunstadter et al. (1987), Yang (1993) and Cooper et al. (1996).

18. See Chapter 2 in this volume about the relationship between a daughter-in-law and a mother-in-law.
19. See Chapter 13 in this volume. See also Symonds (1991, 1996) and Kunstadter et al. (1987) for fertility regulation in Hmong villages in northern Thailand.
20. See Flint and Samil (1990), Lock (1991), Chirawatkul (1992) and Chirawatkul and Manderson (1994).

Chapter 15

Conclusion: Motherhood in a New Country

> Motherhood—unmentioned in the histories of conquest and serfdom, wars and treaties, exploration and imperialism—has a history, it has an ideology, it is more fundamental than tribalism or nationalism.
>
> (Rich, 1992:34)

> If in Laos then I don't know, I may have about ten children, it could happen, because in Laos you need to have many children to be able to help you make the living on the farm. In this country, if you have many children, now it is ok, but when they grow older they will go to school and they will need to study and they will need money. I don't think that I will be able to provide for everyone if I have too many children.... Yes, it is the difficulty in raising up children here.
>
> Hmong informant

We have seen that women and reproduction play a significant role in Hmong society. Without women, children will not be produced, which will threaten the Hmong society at large. Becoming a mother is perceived by the society as an essential part of womanhood, and women are socialized to perceive this. But how do they view this concept when they are no longer in Laos? Migration has changed many things in Hmong lives. Although there is evidence that the Hmong always resist change wherever they live, from China to Southeast Asia and now in Western countries like Australia (Cooper et al., 1995; Quincy, 1995), we have also seen that the Hmong have had to change their ways to some extent in a new land. Are the concepts and practices of motherhood likely to change in a new environment? This chapter will examine this question.

MOTHERHOOD: ONLY FOR THE LUCKY ONES

Motherhood is seen as a positive part of life for women, since children look after them in old age and carry out essential rituals to send their souls back to heaven to be reborn.

> I think it is better to have children. For the Hmong, if you have children and when you get old, when you cannot support yourself, then your children can support you. So they will look after you in old age.

Only lucky women are able to become mothers. As one woman summarizes: "According to Hmong tradition then I must have more luck than those who cannot have children." In addition, women's fortune and luck in having children is granted by *Txoov Kab Yeeb* and is inscribed on papers they were given to bring to earth when they were born (their mandate of life).[1] Women see this as a gift to them.

> They say that having many children because heaven has given you the ability to do so. So it is a gift that the heaven has given you.

Hmong women realize that conceiving, giving birth and raising children are not easy tasks for them. However, the rewards gained mean security in old age.

> It is a hard work to do but you also feel that you must have at least one or two children so that when you get older you do not envy other people who have children. If you don't have any at all then when you get older and you see other old people have children to love them, cook for them and look after them and that is when you start to envy them. But talking about when you give birth to children and bring them up it is very difficult for you. But when you get old it must be better for you.

Becoming a mother and having children also means that they will not be too lonely in old age, since there will be many grandchildren around. One woman who had become a grandmother offered the following remarks:

> You have children and their children are with you and this makes you feel less lonely. You may not have young children anymore but your sons and

> daughters-in-law will have children and you look after their children while they go to work or go to school. The children may make a lot of noise but it won't make you worried at all. If you stay by yourself, or just the couple by themselves, how are you going to live day by day?

What, then, are the consequences for "unlucky" women who are not able to have a baby?[2] As one woman summarized them:

> The ones that cannot bear children their husbands will not love them and the relatives will not treat them well either. They say that because they can't have children so their husbands should marry another woman and so later on in their life they will not be a respectable people.

As illustrated throughout this book, Hmong women greatly value their children. This is reflected in their child rearing practices.[3] (See Photo 15.1.) I was struck by comments made by many women during the interviews when they said that in whatever they did in connection with raising children, it was important not to make "the child sorry." Although the women's explanations were related to child health, I believe that they showed their love and care for their children as well. For example, whatever ritual parents have performed for one child will be performed for all the other children. This is to show the children that they are all loved and cared for by the parents.

> With my family we choose to do it [*hu plig*; a soul-calling ceremony] for all of them. When you do one then you have to do for the rest of the children. If you don't do that then the children will say that you love one but don't love another. So the baby will bother you by becoming sick often even when they are not sick because they feel sorry.

THE HEALTH CONSEQUENCES OF BEING A MOTHER

A common perception of Hmong women is that motherhood has negative consequences for their health. Motherhood may give them many rewards, but it also has an impact on their health. Women believe that the stresses and strains of conceiving, carrying pregnancy to term and giving birth to children causes their own health to deteriorate. The more children they bear, the poorer their health will become.

> Talking about being a mother, I think that my health before having children is much better because when you haven't got any children you do not feel the stress and strains on your body. After you have children you feel these stress and strains. The more you have the worse the stress and strains on your body.

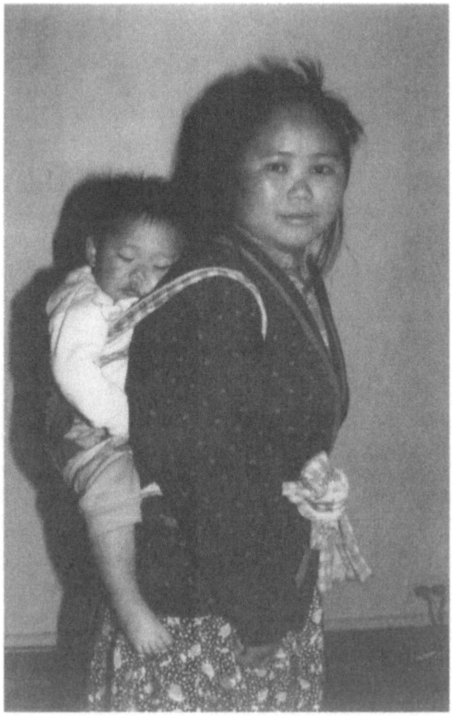

Photo 15.1 A mother carrying her young child on her back.

Despite the fact that in Hmong culture women practice the 30-day confinement rest after giving birth,[4] they believe that they cannot completely rest because they still have to perform certain chores in their household. In addition, although there are many prohibitions during the confinement period which they must observe in order not to cause ill health in old age, they may sometimes ignore them unintentionally.

> When you have children during your confinement period you do not take a good rest and you might do that sort of thing which you should not do during the confinement. So when you are older you get sick. Even if you take a good rest you still have to do the house chores like cooking when there is no one to do it for you, you have to do it yourself. This contributes to that.

Women talk about ill health they have experienced as something which they cannot do anything about. Hence, they simply treat it as part of their lives.

> With this health problem I don't know what to do about it so I just leave it alone. It is not a constant thing; I mean it just comes and goes with the

> change of weather. Some days when it rains I can feel that but when it changes to a sunny day I don't feel that much.

Because of this belief, it is not surprising to see that some Hmong women wish to regulate their fertility[5] or stop reproduction completely. When younger women were asked how many children they wished to have, they usually replied, three or four—if they had the choice. Some women mentioned that even if they still lived in Laos, where they had to rely on many children for survival, they would want to stop having so many.

> If I can do then I will not want any more children because if you have too many it is a very hard work. If I can control myself to not fall pregnant then I do not want anymore, but if I can't then I will have to have them. Even if I still live in Laos I would still say the same thing.

Nevertheless, some women still want to have as many children as they can, to follow the Hmong tradition. Some women also believe that they have been accepted in Australia only as refugees, and that if they are no longer allowed to stay in the new country, they may have to return to Laos. If they have to return to live in their own tradition, they will need many children to fulfill their needs and for survival. Hence, these mothers feel that they may as well conceive while they are still capable of it.

> Why do I want many children! It is because there are never enough children. Traditionally there are a lot of roles [tasks] to do so if you don't have enough children then the jobs won't be done. The children will have to help with the housework. And if we are not allowed to stay in this country and go back to Laos, we will definitely need the extra help for survival on the farm. . . . If the country [Laos] is back to normal, with no more war, and they said that that is your country and you must go back then we must go.

Women also talk about the emotional side of motherhood. Anxiety over rearing children, particularly the first child, is a common experience of many women. Will they become ill? Will they recover? Will they survive? These are common anxieties that women continuously experience.

> You worry about the baby getting sick. When you have your first baby it will have the most sickness of all. With the Hmong, the first one is always getting sick and you will have to always *ua neeb* or *hu plig* almost all the time. You have one done and they say it is because of something else and you have to fix that too. You do it for two or three days then the baby will be sick again and you have to repeat the whole cycle again until the child grows a bit older. The ones after that first are not sick that often. . . . Hmong are always like that; the first one gets sick most often.

SEX PREFERENCES: TRADITIONAL AND CURRENT

When outsiders ask men what sex they would prefer a child to be, the answer is usually "boys." Boys are favored far more than girls, since boys carry on the clan name, carry out important rituals and feed their ancestors—tasks prohibited to women. This, however, does not mean that Hmong girls have no value. On the contrary, they are assets of the family as well.[6] When the same question is posed to a mother, we see that to her, both boys and girls are equally important.

> Boys and girls, I would like to have them in equal numbers. It is better. If you have more boys and fewer girls then you would want to have more of the girls. . . . If you have equal number of girls and boys, it is good because there is a lot of help amongst them. . . . The Hmong traditionally practice that when the girls get married they leave and do not come back [to live with you]. The boys even if they get married they still live with the parents; this is why we call the girls "girl visitors" and the boys "the boys at home." This is the tradition with the Hmong people. But if you have equal numbers of both, this would be much better.

One woman had already had seven children including both boys and girls, but she wished to have one more child before ending her fertility. She said:

> Whether a boy or a girl it will be good as long as I have one more. If it is a boy or a girl, it doesn't matter much.

She was asked her reason for her lack of a preference for either sex for her last child. The following is her explanation:

> Traditionally boys are preferred because the boys will look after you, carry on the *dab qhuas* to the next generation. The girls, if they stay with you until old then that is not a good thing so when they get a bit older they will marry into another family. Therefore, if you have only a few boys then you will be very sad with having too many girls because they will leave you. So people will prefer to have more boys. But sometimes it can't be helped. So if you have a boy or a girl then it would not matter.

As illustrated, the reasons women wish to have boys or girls are somewhat different from traditional expectations.[7] Sentimental value is an important factor in their preferences for one sex or the other, and women certainly want to have daughters as well as sons. But to have too many daughters means losing them when the girls grow up. In Laos, the daughters may be married out to men in different villages, sometimes too far away for the girls to pay frequent visits. Women's concern about their loss when their daughters are married out is a serious matter.[8]

MOTHERS IN THE NEW COUNTRY

Being a mother in a new country produces several uncertainties in many Hmong women. In despite of living in a new country, most Hmong women still wish to see children carry on their traditions, but they also realize that this may not be possible in the future.

Although traditionally children look after aged parents, women are not so certain that they will be taken care of by their children in their new homeland. This causes considerable anxiety among them.

> In this country, I don't know if I can manage my children. I am still doubtful if they will support me when they grow up. I am still very worried about this. . . . In my country I would not be worried about this. But being here the children take on the Western culture. I mean like when they go to school they go to learn the Western culture and I am very worried that they would not carry on our tradition. But then it depends on the children so you must try your best to teach them when they come home.

Many Hmong women continue to have children in their new homeland. Although some do this because they believe they have not yet had enough children, others do so because they fear that some of their children may not follow their traditions. One woman talked about having several children:

> I don't know about the future but I think that I should have a few children so if one does not love me then the other one will. But I don't know about this in this country whether when they grow up they will love me or not. If they follow the Hmong tradition then if one does not love their parents then the other one will still love them.

Some women, however, are not so certain about the value of having many children. This is mainly related to their living situation in Australia, where people in most households are unemployed and have to rely on Social Security benefits. Having too many children may mean poverty for the family.

> I don't know about this in this country. But in Laos the ones with lots of children, they say that, it means lots of family member. This is greatly valued because the bigger the family the better the chance of survival since they are able to grow and harvest food. But I don't know about this in this country. I think it can be valuable, but sometimes I think that you will become poorer.

Migration has therefore had an impact on the way Hmong women see motherhood. There is considerable uncertainty about the process of becoming a mother and raising children in the new country. Most obvious is the women's apprehension about the future generations changing traditions.

FINAL WORDS

> When our generation has died out then the next may not follow our customs anymore. There is no one to teach them and the customs will be lost. I am worried that they will be disappearing. . . . I have had my turn, so it is up to them what they want to do so long as I don't know about it [after her death], it does not matter.

This book has illustrated that the Hmong in Australia, and Hmong women in particular, have tried to maintain the Hmong way despite living in a Western society. They have resisted assimilation into a host culture, as their ancestors did in China and Southeast Asia. In some ways, they have succeeded. But they are also influenced in many ways by the new rules in their new country. They have adopted tactics, covertly and overtly, so that their culture can survive, but at the same time they do not wish to break the rules of their new homeland. In this way they believe they may live in harmony with other Australians. Because of this adaptation, the older generations are now worrying that their culture may disappear. How long they can maintain the Hmong way and whether they will remain as they have always been remain to be seen. But I hope that they will continue the many practices of their culture that can set good examples to follow for those of us in the West.

NOTES

1. See Chapter 1 in this volume concerning *Txoov Kab Yeeb* and fertility in Hmong cosmology.
2. See also Chapter 11 on the cultural construct of infertility in Hmong society.
3. See Chapters 8 and 9 on child rearing and infant feeding practices among Hmong women.
4. See Chapter 6 on Hmong confinement practices.
5. See Chapter 14, Kunstadter et al. (1987) and Symonds (1991, 1996) on fertility regulation among Hmong women.
6. See Chapter 2 and Symonds (1996) on the brideprice that young Hmong women will bring into the family.
7. See also Kunstadter et al. (1987) on the perceptions of the value of girls among Hmong parents in the north of Thailand.
8. See also Chapter 2 on marriage and Savina (1930) on his account of the sadness of Hmong mothers when their daughters are married out.

References

Adler, S. R., 1995. "Refugee Stress and Folk Belief: Hmong Sudden Deaths." *Social Science and Medicine* 40 (12): 1623–1629.

Appell, L.W.R. 1988. "Menstruation Among the Rungus of Borneo: An Unmarked Category." In *Blood Magic: The Anthropology of Menstruation*, edited by T. Buckley and A. Gottlieb, 94–112. Berkeley: University of California Press.

Barnett, E. A., 1988. "*La Edad Critica*: The Positive Experience of Menopause in a Small Peruvian Town." In *Women and Health: Cross-Cultural Perspectives*, edited by P. Whelan, 40–54. Granby, MA: Bergin & Garvey.

Bart, P., 1969. "Why Women's Status Changes in Middle Age." *Sociological Symposium* 3 (Fall): 1–18.

Baumslag, N., and D. L. Michels. 1995. *Milk, Money, and Madness: The Culture and Politics of Breastfeeding*. Westport, CT: Bergin & Garvey.

Becker, G., and R. D. Nachtigall. 1994. "Born to be a Mother: The Cultural Construction of Risk in Infertility Treatment in the U.S." *Social Science and Medicine* 39 (4): 507–518.

Beyene, Y., 1986. "Cultural Significance and Physiological Manifestations of Menopause: A Biocultural Analysis." *Culture, Medicine and Psychiatry* 10 (1): 47–71.

Beyene, Y., 1989. *From Menarche to Menopause: Reproductive Lives of Peasant Women in Two Cultures*. Albany, NY: State University of New York Press.

Bledsoe, C. A., A. Hill, U. D'Alessandro, and P. Langerick. 1994. "Constructing Natural Fertility: The Use of Western Contraceptive Technologies in Rural Gambia." *Population and Development Review* 20 (1): 81–113.

Bliatout, B. T., 1982. *Hmong Sudden Unexpected Nocturnal Death Syndrome: A Cultural Study*. Portland, OR: Sparkle Publishing Enterprises.

Bliatout, B. T., 1986. "Guidelines for Mental Health Professionals to Help Hmong Clients Seek Traditional Healing Treatment." In *The Hmong in Transition*, edited by G. L. Hendricks, B. T. Downing, and A. S. Deinard, 349–364. New York: The Center for Migration Studies.

Bliatout, B. T., 1988. "Hmong Attitudes towards Surgery: How It Affects Patient Prognosis." *Migration World* 16 (1): 25–28.

Bliatout, B. T., 1991. "Hmong Healing Practitioners." *Hmong Forum* 2: 58–66.

Britton, C. J. 1996. "Learning About 'The Curse': An Anthropological Perspective on Experiences of Menstruation." *Women's Studies International Forum* 19 (6): 645–653.

Borg, S., and J. Lasker. 1982. *When Pregnancy Fails*. London: Routledge.

Brody, E. B., 1981. *Sex, Contraception, and Motherhood in Jamaica*. Cambridge, MA: Harvard University Press.

Brody, E. B., 1985. "Every Day Knowledge of Jamaican Women." In *Women's Medicine: A Cross-Cultural Study of Indigenous Fertility Regulation*, edited by L. F. Newman, 161–177. New Brunswick, NJ: Rutgers University Press.

Brown, J. K. 1982. "Cross-Cultural Perspectives on Middle Aged Women." *Current Anthropology* 23 (2): 143–154.

Brown, P. J., M. C. Inhorn, and D. J. Smith. 1996. "Disease, Ecology and Human Behavior." In *Medical Anthropology: Contemporary Theory and Method*, rev. ed., edited by C. F. Sargent and T. M. Johnson, 183–218. Westport, CT: Praeger.

Browner, C. H., 1980. "The Management of Early Pregnancy: Folk Concepts of Fertility Control." *Social Science and Medicine* 14b (1): 25–32.

Browner, C. H. 1985. "Traditional Techniques for Diagnosis, Treatment, and Control of Pregnancy in Cali, Colombia." In *Women's Medicine: A Cross-Cultural Study of Indigenous Fertility Regulation*, edited by L. F. Newman, 99–123. New Brunswick, NJ: Rutgers University Press.

Buckley T., and A. Gottlieb, eds. 1988. *Blood Magic: The Anthropology of Menstruation*. Berkeley, University of California Press.

Burnight, R. G., and B. Leoprapai. 1977. "Attitudes of Rural Thai Women towards Induced Abortion." *Journal of Biosocial Science* 9: 61–72.

Camey, X. C., C. G. Barrios, X. R. Guerrero, R. M. Nunez-Urquiza, D. G. Hernandez, and A. L. Glass. 1996. "Traditional Birth Attendants in Mexico: Advantages and Inadequacies of Care for Normal Deliveries." *Social Science and Medicine* 43 (2): 199–207.

Carter, H. 1998. "Postnatal Sex Can Kill." *The Herald Son*, October 2, p. 23.

Castle, S. E., 1994. "The (Re)Negotiation of Illness Diagnoses and Responsibility for Child Death in Rural Mali." *Medical Anthropology Quarterly* 8 (3): 314–335.

Cecil, R. 1994. " 'I Wouldn't Have Minded a Wee One Running About': Miscarriage and the Family." *Social Science and Medicine* 10 (10): 1415–1422.

Cecil, R., ed. 1996a. *The Anthropology of Pregnancy Loss: Comparative Studies in Miscarriage, Stillbirth and Neonatal Death*. Oxford: Berg.

Cecil, R., ed. 1996b. "Introduction: An Insignificant Event? Literary and Anthropological Perspectives on Pregnancy Loss." In *The Anthropology of Preg-*

nancy Loss: Comparative Studies in Miscarriage, Stillbirth and Neonatal Death, edited by R. Cecil, 1–14. Oxford: Berg.

Cecil, R., and J. C. Leslie. 1993. "Early Miscarriage: Preliminary Results from a Study in Northern Ireland." *Journal of Reproductive and Infant Psychology* 11 (2): 89–95.

Cerquone, J. 1986. *Refugees from Laos: In Harm's Way*. Washington, D.C.: American Council for Nationalities Service.

Chalmers, B., and D. Meyer. 1992a. "A Cross-Cultural View of the Psychosocial Management of Miscarriage." *Journal of Psychosomatic Obstetrics and Gynaecology* 13 (3): 163–176.

Chalmers, B., and D. Meyer. 1992b. "A Cross-Cultural View of the Emotional Experience of Miscarriage." *Journal of Psychosomatic Obstetrics and Gynaecology* 13 (3): 177–186.

Chan, S., 1994. *Hmong Means Free: Life in Laos and America*. Philadelphia, PA: Temple University Press.

Cheung, N. F. 1997. "Chinese Zuo Yuezi (Sitting in for the First Month of the Postnatal Period) in Scotland." *Midwifery* 13 (2): 55–65.

Chindasri, N., 1976. *The Religion of the Hmong Njua*. Bangkok: The Siam Society.

Chindasri, N., 1983. "Hmong Shamanism." In *Highlanders of Thailand,* edited by J. McKinnon and W. Bhruksasri, 187–193. Kuala Lumpur: Oxford University Press.

Chirawatkul, S., 1992. *The Social Construction of Menopause in Northeastern Thailand*. Paper presented at the Fourth Tropical Health and Nutrition Conference, The University of Brisbane, Brisbane, Australia.

Chirawatkul, S., 1993. *Sud Lyad, Sud Luuk: The Social Construction of Menopause in Northeast Thailand*. Doctoral dissertation, Tropical Health Program, University of Queensland, Queensland, Australia.

Chirawatkul, S., and L. Manderson. 1994. "Perceptions of Menopause in Northeast Thailand: Contested Meaning and Practice." *Social Science and Medicine* 39 (11): 1545–1554.

Chu, C. 1996. "Tso Yyueh-Tzu (Sitting the Month) in Contemporary Taiwan." In *Maternity and Reproductive Health in Asian Societies,* edited by P. L. Rice and L. Manderson, 191–204. Amsterdam: Harwood Academic Publishers.

Chu, C. M., 1993. *Reproductive Health Beliefs and Practices of Chinese and Australian Women*. Taipei: Population Studies Center, National Taiwan University.

Chu, C. M-Y. 1980. "Menstrual Beliefs and Practices of Chinese Women." *Journal of the Folklore Institute* 17 (1): 38–55.

Conquergood, D., P. Thao, and X. Thao. 1989. *I Am a Shaman: A Hmong Life Story with Ethnographic Commentary*. Southeast Asian Refugee Studies Occasional Paper Number 8. Minneapolis: Center for Urban and Regional Affairs, University of Minnesota.

Conton, L. 1985. "Social, Economic and Ecological Parameters of Infant Feeding in Usino, Papua New Guinea." In *Infant Care and Feeding in the South Pacific,* edited by L. B. Marshall, 97–119. New York: Gordon and Breach.

Cooper, R., 1983. "Sexual Inequality among the Hmong Highlanders of Thailand." In *The Highlanders of Thailand,* edited by J. McKinnon and W. Bhruksasri, 174–186. Kuala Lumphur: Oxford University Press.

Cooper, R. M., and J. Lumley. 1996. "Mothers' Knowledge of the Risk Factors and Anxiety about SIDS." *Journal of Paediatrics and Child Health* 32 (4): 310–315.

Cooper, R., N. Tapp, G. Y. Lee, and G. Schworer-Kohl. 1995. *The Hmong*. Bangkok: ArtAsia Press.

Cosminsky, S., 1982. "Childbirth and Change: A Guatemalan Study." In *Ethnography of Fertility and Birth*, edited by C. P. MacCormack, 205–229. London: Academic Press.

Croghan, R., 1990. "First-Time Mothers' Accounts of Inequality in the Division of Labour." *Feminism and Psychology* 1: 221–246.

Datan, N., A. Antonovsky, and B. Moaz. 1981. *A Time to Reap: The Middle Age of Women in Five Israeli Subcultures*. Baltimore: Johns Hopkins University Press.

Davies, D. P., 1985. "Cot Death in Hong Kong: A Rare Problem?" *Lancet* 2: 1346–1349.

Davis, D. L., 1986. "The Meaning of Menopause in a Newfoundland Fishing Village." *Culture, Medicine and Psychiatry* 10 (1): 73–94.

DeFrain, J., 1991. "Learning About Grief from Normal Families: SIDS, Stillbirth, and Miscarriages." *Journal of Marital and Family Therapy* 17 (3): 215–232.

Delaney, C., 1988. "Mortal Flow: Menstruation in Turkish Village Society." In *Blood Magic: The Anthropology of Menstruation*, edited by T. Buckley and A. Gottlieb, 75–93. Berkeley: University of California Press.

Dettwyler, K. A., 1987. "Breastfeeding and Weaning in Mali: Cultural Context and Hard Data." *Social Science and Medicine* 24 (8): 633–644.

de Zoysa, I., D. Carson, R. Feachem, B. Kirkwood, E. Lindsay-Smith, and R. Loewenson. 1984. "Perceptions of Childhood Diarrhoea and Its Treatment in Rural Zimbabwe." *Social Science and Medicine* 19 (7): 727–734.

Dobson, S. M., 1988. "Transcultural Health Visiting: Caring in a Multi-Cultural Society." *Recent Advances in Nursing* 20: 61–80.

Donato, M., 1988. Letter published in *Bitter-sweet . . . Hellogoodbye*, section 1, edited by J. M. Lamb. Belleville, IL: Charis Communications.

Donnelly, N. D., 1994. *Changing Lives of Refugee Hmong Women*. Seattle: University of Washington Press.

Douglas, M., 1966. *Purity and Danger: An Analysis of Concepts of Pollution and Taboo*. London: Routledge and Kegan Paul.

Douglas, M., 1970. *Natural Symbols*. New York: Pantheon Books.

Early, E. A., 1993. "Fertility and Fate: Medical Practices among Baladi Women of Cairo." In *Everyday Life in the Muslim Middle East*, edited by D. L. Bowen and E. A. Early, 102–108. Bloomington: Indiana University Press.

Ebin, V., 1982. "Interpretations of Infertility: The Aowin People of South-West Ghana." In *Ethnography of Fertility and Birth*, edited by C. P. MacCormack, 141–159. London: Academic Press.

Edwards, L. E., C. J. Rautio, and E. Y. Hakanson. 1987. "Pregnancy in Hmong Refugee Women." *Minnesota Medicine* 70: 633–655.

Ehrenreich, B., and D. English. 1978. *For Her Own Good: 150 Years of the Experts' Advice to Women*. New York: Anchor.

Eichinger Ferro-Luzzi, G., 1974. "Food Avoidances during the Puerperium and Lactation in Tamilnad." *Ecology of Food and Nutrition* 3: 7–15.

Eschen, A., and M. Whittaker. 1993. "Family Planning: A Base to Build on for Women's Reproductive Health Services." In *The Health of Women: A Global*

Perspective, edited by M. Koblinsky, J. Timyan, and J. Gay, 105–131. Boulder, CO: Westview Press.

Fadiman, A. 1997. *The Spirit Catches You and You Fall Down: A Hmong Child, Her American Doctors, and the Collision of Two Cultures*. New York: Farrar, Straus and Giroux.

Faller, H. D. 1985. "Perinatal Needs of Immigrant Hmong Women: Surveys of Women and Health Care Providers." *Public Health Reports* 100 (3): 340–343.

Faller, H. S. 1992. "Hmong Women: Characteristics and Birth Outcomes." *Birth* 19 (3): 144–150.

Farooqi, S., I. J. Perry, and D. G. Beevers. 1993. "Ethnic Differences in Infant-Rearing Practices and Their Possible Relationship to the Incidence of Sudden Infant Death Syndrome (SIDS)." *Paediatrics and Perinatal Epidemiology* 7 (9): 245–252.

Feldman-Savelsberg, P. 1994. "Plundered Kitchens and Empty Wombs: Fear of Infertility in the Cameroonian Grassfields." *Social Science and Medicine* 39 (4): 463–474.

Fernandez, E. L., and G. M. Guthrie. 1984. "Belief Systems and Breast Feeding among Filipino Urban Poor." *Social Science and Medicine* 19 (9): 991–995.

Fernandez, M. E. L., and B. M. Popkin. 1988. "Prelacteal Feeding Patterns in the Philippines." *Ecology of Food and Nutrition* 21: 303–314.

Fishman, C., R. Evans, and E. Jenks. 1988. "Warm Bodies, Cool Milk: Conflicts in Post Partum Food Choice for Indochinese Women in California." *Social Science and Medicine* 26 (11): 1125–1132.

Flint, M. 1974. "Menarche and Menopause of Rajput Women." Doctoral dissertation, Department of Anthropology, City University of New York, New York.

Flint, M. 1975. "The Menopause: Reward or Punishment." *Psychosomatic Medicine* 16: 161–163.

Flint, M., and R. S. Samil. 1990. "Cultural and Subcultural Meanings of the Menopause." *Annals of the New York Academy of Sciences* 592 (13): 134–148.

Fuller, N., and B. Jordan. 1981. "Maya Women and the End of the Birthing Period: Postpartum Massage-and-Binding in Yucatan, Mexico." *Medical Anthropology* (Winter): 35–50.

Furth, C., and C. Shu-Yueh. 1992. "Chinese Medicine and the Anthropology of Menstruation in Contemporary Taiwan." *Medical Anthropology Quarterly* 6 (1): 27–48.

Gantley, M., D. P. Davies, and A. Murcott. 1993. "Sudden Infant Death Syndrome: Links with Infant Care Practices." *British Medical Journal* 306 (6864): 16–20.

Geddes, W. R. 1976. *Migrants of the Mountains: The Cultural Ecology of the Blue Miao (Hmong Njua) of Thailand*. Oxford: Oxford University Press.

Gethin, A., and B. Macgregor. 1998. "Cry Baby, Cry." *Melbourne's Baby* (July): 8–9.

Goldfarb, M. 1982. *Fighters, Refugees, Immigrants: A Story of the Hmong*. Minneapolis, MN: Carolrhoda Books.

Goldsmith, J. 1990. *Childbirth Wisdom from the World's Oldest Societies*. Brookline, MA: East West Health Books.

Good, M-J. D. 1980. "Of Blood and Babies: The Relationship of Popular Islamic Physiology to Fertility." *Social Science and Medicine* 14B: 147–156.

Gottlieb, A. 1988. "Menstrual Cosmology among the Beng of Ivory Coast." In *Blood Magic: The Anthropology of Menstruation*, edited by T. Buckley and A. Gottlieb, 55–74. Berkeley: University of California Press.

Gould, K. 1975. "Sexual Practices and Reproduction Decisions." *Journal of the Christian Medical Association of India* 4: 547–550.

Gove, S., and G. Pelto. 1994. "Focused Ethnographic Studies in the Programme for the Control of Acute Respiratory Infections of the World Health Organization." *Medical Anthropology* 15:409–424.

Grace, J., 1998. "The Treatment of Infants and Young Children Suffering Respiratory Tract Infection and Diarrhoeal Disease in a Rural Community in Southeast Indonesia." *Social Science and Medicine* 46 (10): 1291–1302.

Green, E. C., A. Jurg, and A. Djedje. 1994. "The Snake in the Stomach: Child Diarrhea in Central Mozambique." *Medical Anthropology Quarterly* 8 (1): 4–24.

Greer, G., 1984. *Sex and Destiny: The Politics of Human Fertility*. London: Secker and Warburg.

Gunnlaugsson, G., and J. Einarsdottir. 1993. "Colostrum and Ideas About Bad Milk: A Case Study from Guinea-Bissau." *Social Science and Medicine* 36 (3): 283–288.

Hadley, J., 1996. *Abortion: Between Freedom and Neccessity*. London: Virago.

Hamilton-Merrit, J., 1993. *Tragic Mountains: The Hmong, the Americans, and the Secret Wars for Laos, 1942–1992*. Bloomington: Indiana University Press.

Hang, D., 1986. "*Tam Tuab Neeg*: Connecting the Generations." In *The Hmong World* I, edited by B. Johns and D. Strecker, 33–41. New Haven, CT: Yale Southeast Asia Studies.

Hansen, F. A., 1975. *Meaning in Culture*. London: Routledge and Kegan Paul.

Harding, M. E., 1973. *Women's Mysteries*. New York: Bantam Books.

Hart, D. V., R. J. Coughlin, and P. Anumanrajadhon. 1965. *Southeast Asian Birth Customs: Three Studies in Human Reproduction*. New Haven, CT: Human Relations Area File.

Helsel, D., D. B. Petitti, and P. Kunstadter. 1992. "Pregnancy among the Hmong: Birthweight, Age, and Parity." *American Journal of Public Health* 82 (10): 1361–1364.

Hey, V., 1989. "A Feminist Exploration." In *Hidden Loss: Miscarriage and Ectopic Pregnancy*, edited by V. Hey, C. Itzin, L. Saunders, and M. Speakman, 51–72. London: The Woman's Press.

Hmong Australia Society Inc., 1998. *A Report of Hmong Member in Victoria, 1998*. Melbourne: Hmong Australia Society Inc.

Hoff, W., and N. Maseko. 1986. "Nurses and Traditional Healers Join Hands." *World Health Forum* 7 (2): 412–426.

Hogel, J., and A. Prins. 1991. *Prospects for Collaborating with Traditional Healers in Africa*. Arlington, VA: Management Sciences for Health (PRITECH Project).

Hollingsworth, A. O., L. P. Brown, and D. A. Brooten. 1984. "The Refugee and Childbearing: What to Expect?" *Research in Nursing* 4 (November): 45–58.

Holm, J., and J. Bowker. 1994. *Rites of Passage*. London: Pinter Publishers.

Homans, H., 1982. "Pregnancy and Birth as Rites of Passage for Two Goups of Women in Britain." In *Ethnography of Fertility and Birth*, edited by C. P. MacCormack, 231–268. London: Academic Press.

Howell, R. R., F. H. Moriss, and L. K. Pickering. 1986. *Human Milk in Infant Nutrition and Health*. Springfield, IL: Charles C Thomas.

Hull, T. 1991. *Government and Society in Southeast Asian Family Planning Programs: The Cases of Indonesia, Vietnam and the Philippines*. Paper presented at the 1991 Annual Meeting of the Population Association of America. Canberra: Department of Politics and Social Change, Australian National University.

Hull, V., and M. Simpson. 1985. "Breastfeeding, Child Health and Child Spacing." In *Breastfeeding Child Health and Child Spacing: Cross-Cultural Perspectives*, edited by V. Hull and M. Simpson, 1–10. London: Croom Helm.

Hunte, P. A., 1985. "Indigenous Methods of Fertility Regulation in Afghanistan." In *Women's Medicine: A Cross-Cultural Study of Indigenous Fertility Regulation*, edited by L. F. Newman, 43–75. New Brunswick, NJ: Rutgers University Press.

Inhorn, M. C., 1994a. *Quest for Conception: Gender, Infertility, and Egyptian Medical Traditions*. Philadelphia: University of Pennsylvania Press.

Inhorn, M. C., 1994b. "Interpreting Infertility: Medical Anthropological Perspectives." *Social Science and Medicine* 39 (4): 459–461.

Inhorn, M. C., 1994c. "Kabsa (A. K. A. Mushahara) and Threatened Fertility in Egypt." *Social Science and Medicine* 39 (4): 487–505.

Inhorn, M. C., 1996. *Infertility and Patriarchy: The Cultural Politics of Gender and Family Life in Egypt*. Philadelpia: University of Pennsylvania Press.

Jacobson, J. L., 1991. *Women's Reproductive Health: The Silence Emergency*. Washington, D.C.: Worldwatch Institute.

Jambunathan, J., and S. Stewart. 1995. "Hmong Women in Wisconsin: What Are Their Concerns in Pregnancy and Childbirth?" *Birth* 22 (4): 204–210.

Jeffery, P., R. Jeffery, and A. Lyon. 1988. *Labour Pains and Labour Power: Women and Childbearing in India*. London: Zed Books.

Jelliffe, D. B., and E. E. P. Jelliffe. 1978. *Human Milk in the Modern World*. Oxford: Oxford University Press.

Jenkins, C. L., and P. F. Heywood. 1985. "Ethnopediatrics and Fertility among the Amele of Lowland Papua New Guinea." In *Breastfeeding Child Health and Child Spacing: Cross-Cultural Perspectives*, edited by V. Hull and M. Simpson, 11–34. London: Croom Helm.

Jennaway, M., 1996. "Of Blood and Foetuses: Female Fertility and Women's Reproductive Health in a North Balinese Village." In *Maternity and Reproductive Health in Asian Societies*, edited by P. L. Rice and L. Manderson, 37–59. Amsterdam: Harwood Academic Press.

Johnson, B. R., M. Horga, and L. Andronache. 1996. "Women's Perspectives on Abortion in Romania." *Social Science and Medicine* 42 (4): 521–530.

Johnson, C., and S. Yang. 1992. *Myths, Legends and Folk Tales from the Hmong of Laos*. St. Paul: Linguistics Department, Macalester College.

Jordan, B., 1978. *Birth in Four Cultures: A Cross-Cultural Investigation of Childbirth in Yucatan, Holland, Sweden, and the United States*. Vermont: Eden Press.

Jordan, B., 1989. "Cosmopolitan Obstetrics: Some Insights from the Training of Traditional Midwives." *Social Science and Medicine* 28 (9): 925–944.

Julian, R., 1994. "When the Rain Is White." Paper presented at the Women as Migrants Conference, The University of Melbourne, Melbourne, Australia.

Kase, N., 1974. "Estrogens and the Menopause." *Journal of the American Medical Association* 227 (3): 318–319.

Kaufert, P., and P. Gilbert. 1986. "Women, Menopause, and Medicalization." *Culture, Medicine and Psychiatry* 10 (1): 7–21.

Kaufert, P. A., 1982. "Myth and the Menopause." *Sociology of Health and Illness* 4 (2): 141–166.

Kay, M. A., ed. 1982. *Anthropology of Human Birth*. Philadelphia, PA: F.A. Davis Company.

Kendal, L., 1987. "Cold Wombs in Balmy Honolulu: Ethnogynecology among Korean Immigrants." *Social Science and Medicine* 25 (4): 367–376.

King, J., and A. Ashworth. 1987. "Historical Review of the Changing Pattern of Infant Feeding in Developing Countries: The Cases of Malaysia, the Caribbean, Nigeria and Zaire." *Social Science and Medicine* 25 (12): 1307–1320.

Kitzinger, S., 1978. *Women as Mothers*. London: Fontana Books.

Kitzinger, S., 1982. "The Social Context of Birth: Some Comparisons between Childbirth in Jamaica and Britain." In *Ethnography of Fertility and Birth*, edited by C. P. MacCormack, 181–203. London: Academic Press.

Klein, R. D., 1989. "The Making of This Book." In *Infertility: Women Speak About Their Experiences of Reproductive Medicine*, edited by R. D. Klein, 1–7. London: Pandora.

Kleinman, A. 1992. "Local Worlds of Suffering: An Interpersonal Focus for Ethnographies of Illness Experience." *Qualitative Health Research* 2: 127–134.

Kocturk, T., and R. Zetterstrom. 1989. "The Promotion of Breastfeeding and Maternal Attitudes." *Acta Paediatrics Scandinevea* 78 (6): 817–823.

Kunstadter, P. 1994. *Determinants and Consequences of Hmong Age at Marriage in Sacramento*. Paper presented at the 10th Annual Southeast Asia Education Fair, Sacramento, California, March.

Kunstadter, P., C. Kesmanee, and P. Pothi-art. 1987. *Hmong and Karen Health and Family Planning: Cultural and Other Factors Affecting Use of Modern Health and Family Planning Services by Hilltribes in Northern Thailand*. Bangkok: Family Health Division, Department of Health.

Kuper, H. 1947. *An African Aristocracy: Rank among the Swazi*. London: Oxford University Press for the International African Institute.

Laderman, C. 1983. *Wives and Midwives: Childbirth and Nutrition in Rural Malaysia*. Berkeley: University of California Press.

Laderman, C. 1987. "Destructive Heat and Cooling Prayer: Malay Humoralism in Pregnancy, Childbirth and Postpartum Period." *Social Science and Medicine* 25 (4): 357–367.

LaFontaine, J. S. 1972. "Ritualization of Women's Life-Crises in Bugisu." In *The Interpretation of Ritual, Essays in Honour of A. I. Richards*, edited by J. S. LaFontaine, 159–186. London: Tavistock.

Laing, J. 1984. "Natural Family Planning in the Philippines." *Studies in Family Planning* 15 (2): 49–61.

Lane, S. D., J. M. Jok, and M. T. El-Mouelhy. 1998. "Buying Safety: The Economics

of Reproductive Risk and Abortion in Egypt." *Social Science and Medicine* 47 (8): 1089–1099.
Layne, L. L. 1990. "Motherhood Lost: Cultural Dimensions of Miscarriage and Stillbirth in America." *Women & Health* 16 (3/4): 69–98.
Layne, L. L. 1997. "Breaking the Silence: An Agenda for a Feminist Discourse of Pregnancy Loss." *Feminist Studies* 23 (2): 289–315.
Lazarus, E. S., 1990. "Falling Through the Cracks: Contradictions and Barriers to Care in a Prenatal Clinic." *Medical Anthropology* 12:269–287.
Lazarus, E. S. 1994. "What Do Women Want?: Issues of Choice, Control, and Class in Pregnancy and Childbirth." *Medical Anthropology Quarterly* 8 (1): 25–46.
Lee, G. Y. 1981. "The Effects of Development Measures on the Socio-Economy of the White Hmong." Ph.D. thesis, Department of Anthropology, The University of Sydney, Sydney, Australia.
Lee, G. Y. 1986. "Minority Politics in Thailand: A Hmong Perspective." Hmong homepage (http://www.stolaf.edu/people/cdr/hmong/hmong-au/thaihmg.htm) .
Lee, G. Y. 1999. "The Hmong." In *The Australian People: An Encyclopedia of the Nation, Its People and Their Origin*, 2nd ed., edited by J. Jupp. Canberra: Angus and Robertson.
Lee, G. Y., and W. A. Smalley. 1991. "Perspectives on Pahawh Hmong Writing." Southeast Asian Refugee Studies Newsletter, Spring, 8–9.
Lee, N. N. Y., Y. F. Chan, D. P. Davies, E. Lau, and D. C. P. Yip. 1989. "Sudden Infant Death in Hong Kong: Confirmation of Low Incidence." *British Medical Journal* 298: 721.
Lefkarites, M. P. 1992. "The Sociocultural Implications of Modernizing Childbirth among Greek Women on the Island of Rhodes." *Medical Anthropology* 13: 385–412.
Lemoine, J. 1983. *Showing the Way*. Translated by K. White. Bangkok: Pandora Press.
Lemoine, J. 1986. "Shamanism in the Context of Hmong Resettlement." In *The Hmong in Transition*, edited by G. L. Hendricks, B. T. Downing, and A. S. Deinard, 337–348. New York: The Center for Migration Studies.
Letherby, G. 1993. "The Meanings of Miscarriage." *Women's Studies International Forum* 16 (2): 165–180.
Littlewood, J. 1996. "Stillbirth and Neonatal Death." In *Conception, Pregnancy and Birth*, edited by C. A. Niven and A. Walker, 148–158. Oxford: Butterworth and Heinemann.
Livo, N. J., and D. Cha. 1991. *Folk Stories of the Hmong: Peoples of Laos, Thailand, and Vietnam*. Englewood: Libraries Unlimited.
Lock, M. 1982. "Models and Practice in Medicine: Menopause as Syndrome or Life Transition?" *Culture, Medicine and Psychiatry* 6 (3): 261–280.
Lock, M. 1991. "Contested Meanings of the Menopause." *The Lancet* 337 (8752): 1270–1272.
Lock, M., and N. Scheper-Hughes. 1990. "A Critical-Interpretive Approach in Medical Anthropology: Rituals and Routines of Discipline and Dissent." In *Medical Anthropology: A Handbook of Theory and Method*, edited by T. M. Johnson and C. F. Sargent, 47–62. New York: Greenwood Press.

Lovell, A. 1983. "Some Questions of Identity: Late Miscarriage, Stillbirth and Perinatal Loss." *Social Science and Medicine* 17 (11): 755–761.

Luker, K. 1984. *Abortion and the Politics of Motherhood.* Berkeley: University of California Press.

Lusetich, R. 1994. "Cultures Clash as Nomads Confront US Medical Law." *The Australian*, December 10, p. 5.

McClain, C. S., 1975. "Ethno-Obstetrics in Ajijic." *Anthropological Quarterly* 48: 38–56.

McClain, C. S. 1982. "Toward a Comparative Framework for the Study of Childbirth: A Review of the Literature." In *Anthropology of Human Birth*, edited by M. A. Kay, 25–59. Philadelphia: F. A. Davis Company.

McClain, C. S., ed. 1991. *Women as Healers: Cross Cultural Perspectives.* New Brunswick NJ: Rutgers University Press.

MacCormack, C. P., ed. 1982. *Ethnography of Fertility and Birth.* London: Academic Press.

MacCormack, C. P. 1982. "Biological, Cultural and Social Adaptation in Human Fertility and Birth: A Synthesis." In *Ethnography of Fertility and Birth*, edited by C. P. MacCormack, 1–23. London: Academic Press.

McGilvray, D. 1982. "Sexual Power and Fertility in Sri Lanka: Batticaloa Tamils and Moors." In *Ethnography of Fertility and Birth*, edited by C. P. MacCormack, 25–74. London: Academic Press.

McKenna, J. J. 1998. *SIDS, Infant Sleeping Arrangements and Culture: What Are the Connections?* Public lecture given at Kensington Campus, the University of New South Wales, August 5.

McKenna, J. J., and S. Mosko. 1993. "Evolution and Infant Sleep: An Experimental Study of Infant Parent Co-Sleeping and Its Implications for SIDS." *Acta Paediatrics* Supplement 389 (9): 31–36.

Maclean, U. 1971. *Magical Medicine.* Harmondsworth: Penguin Books.

McNamer, M. 1986. "Musical Change and Change in Music: Implications for Hmong Identity." In *The Hmong World 1*, edited by B. Johns and D. Strecker, 137–163. New Haven, CT: Yale Southeast Asia Studies.

McNee, A., N. Khan, S. Dawson, J. Gunsalam, V. L. Tallo, L. Manderson, and I. Riley. 1995. "Responding to Cough: Boholano Illness Classification and Resort to Care in Response to Childhood ARI." *Social Science and Medicine* 40 (9): 1279–1289.

Madden, M. E. 1994. "The Variety of Emotional Reactions to Miscarriage." *Women & Health* 21 (2/3): 85–104.

Mandelbaum, D. 1970. *Human Fertility in India.* Berkeley: University of California Press.

Manderson, L. 1981. "Roasting, Smoking and Dieting in Response to Birth: Malay Confinement in Cross-Cultural Perspectives." *Social Science and Medicine* 15B: 509–520.

Manderson, L. 1982. "Bottle Feeding and Ideology in Colonial Malaya: The Production of Change." *International Journal of Health Service* 12 (4): 597–616.

Manderson, L., and M. Mathews. 1981. "Vietnamese Behavioral and Dietary Precautions During Pregnancy." *Ecology of Food and Nutrition* 11: 1–8.

Martin, E. 1987. *The Woman in the Body: A Cultural Analysis of Reproduction.* Boston: Beacon Press.

Mathews M., and L. Manderson. 1980. "Infant Feeding Practices and Lactation Diets amongst Vietnamese Immigrants." *Australian Paediatrics Journal* 16: 263–266.

Mathews, M., and L. Manderson. 1981. "Vietnamese Behavioral and Dietary Precautions During Confinement." *Ecology of Food and Nutrition* 11: 9–16.

Mattison, W., L. Lo, and T. Scarseth. 1994. *Hmong Lives: From Laos to La Crosse.* La Crosse: The Pump House.

Maynard-Tucker, G. 1989. "Knowledge of Reproductive Physiology and Modern Contraceptives in Rural Peru." *Studies in Family Planning* 20 (4): 215–224.

Michaelson, K., ed. 1988. *Birth in America: Anthropological Perspective.* South Hadley, MA: Bergin & Garvey.

Minichiello V., R. Aroni, E. Timewell, and L. Alexander. 1995. *In-Depth Interviewing: Principles, Techniques, Analysis.* 2nd ed. Melbourne: Longman.

Mitchell, R. 1980. "Vietnamese Child-Rearing Practices." Unpublished paper. Department of Further Education, Language and Migrant Education Center, Melbourne, Australia.

Morse, J. M. 1984. "The Cultural Context of Infant Feeding in Fiji." *Ecology of Food and Nutrition* 14:287–296.

Morse, J. M. 1989. "Cultural Variation in the Behavioural Response to Parturition: Childbirth in Fiji." *Medical Anthropology* 12: 35–54.

Morse, J. M., ed. 1992. *Qualitative Health Research.* Newbury Park, CA: Sage Publications.

Morse, J. M., C. Jehle, and D. Gamble. 1990. "Initiating Breastfeeding: A World Survey of the Timing of Postpartum Breastfeeding." *International Journal of Nursing Studies* 27 (3): 303–313.

Mottin, J. 1980. *The History of the Hmong.* Bangkok: Odeon Store.

Moua, J. L. 1996. "The Uses of Herbal Medicine in Health Care Practices of Hmong Refugees, and Policy Implications in Merced County, California." Masters thesis, California State University, Stanislaus.

Mougne, C. 1978. "An Ethnography of Reproduction: Changing Patterns of Fertility in a Northern Thai Village." In *Nature and Man in South East Asia,* edited by P. A. Stott, 68–106. London: School of Oriental and African Studies, University of London.

Muecke, M. A. 1976. "Health Care Systems as Socializing Agents. Childbirth in North Thai and Western Ways." *Social Science and Medicine* 10: 377–383.

Mull, D. S. 1992. "Mother's Milk and Pseudoscientific Breastmilk Testing in Pakistan." *Social Science and Medicine* 34 (11): 1277–1290.

Murphy, P., and K. Chamberlin. 1994. The Hmong: A Basic Handbook for Health Care Professionals. Chico, CA: School of Nursing, CSU.

Neff, D. L. 1994. "The Social Construction of Infertility: The Case of the Matrilineal Nayars in South India." *Social Science and Medicine* 39 (4): 475–485.

Nelson, E. A. S. 1989. "Sudden Infant Death Syndrome and Child Care Practices." MD thesis, University of Otago, New Zealand.

Nelson, E. A. S. 1997. "Cross Cultural Child Care." Keynote paper presented at the 11th Australian SIDS Conference, Melbourne, June 20–22.

Newman, L. F. 1972. *Birth Control: An Anthropological View.* Module No. 27. Reading, Mass.: Addison-Wesley.

Newman, L. F., ed. 1985. *Women's Medicine: A Cross-Cultural Study of Indigenous Fertility Regulation*. New Brunswick, NJ: Rutgers University Press.

Ngin, C-S. 1985. "Indigenous Fertility Regulating Methods among Two Chinese Communities in Malaysia." In *Women's Medicine: A Cross-Cultural Study of Indigenous Fertility Regulation*, edited by L. F. Newman, 25–41. New Brunswick, NJ: Rutgers University Press.

Nichter, M. 1993. "Social Science Lessons from Diarrhea Research and Their Application to ARI." *Human Organization* 52(1): 53–67.

Nichter, M., and M. Nichter. 1994. "Acute Respiratory Illness: Popular Health Culture and Mother's Knowledge in the Philippines." *Medical Anthropology* 15: 353–375.

Nichter, M., and M. Nichter. 1996a. "Modern Methods of Fertility Regulation: When and for Whom Are They Appropriate?" In *Anthropology and International Health: Asian Case Studies*, edited by M. Nichter and M. Nichter, 71–108. Amsterdam: Gordon and Breach Publishers.

Nichter, M., and M. Nichter. 1996b. "Cultural Notions of Fertility in South Asia and Their Impact on Sri Lankan Family Planning Practices." In *Anthropology and International Health: Asian Case Studies*, edited by M. Nichter and M. Nichter, 3–33. Amsterdam: Gordon and Breach Publishers.

Nichter, M., and N. Vuckovic. 1994. "Agenda for an Anthropology of Pharmaceutical Practice." *Social Science and Medicine* 39(11): 1509–1525.

Niehof, A., 1988. "Traditional Medication at Pregnancy and Childbirth in Madura, Indonesia." In *The Context of Medicines in Developing Countries*, edited by S. van der Geest and S. R. Whyte, 235–252. Dordricht, Holland: Kluwer Academic Publishers.

Nyce, J. M., and W. H. Hollinshead. 1984. "Southeast Asian Refugees of Rhode Island: Reproductive Beliefs and Practices among the Hmong." *Rhode Island Medical Journal* 67: 361–366.

Oakley, A. 1979. *Becoming a Mother*. Oxford: Martin Robertson.

Oakley, A. 1986. *The Captured Womb: A History of the Medical Care of Pregnant Women*. New York: Basil Blackwell.

Oakley, A., A. McPherson, and H. Roberts. 1990. *Miscarriage*. Harmondsworth, G. B.: Penguin.

Obeyesekere, G. 1981. *Medusa's Hair: An Essay on Personal Symbols and Religious Experience*. Chicago: University of Chicago Press.

Oden, M. 1986. "Cot Deaths in Hong Kong." Letter, *Lancet* 8471 (I): 214.

Park, K-J-Y., and L. M. Peterson. 1991. "Beliefs, Practices, and Experiences of Korean Women in Relation to Childbirth." *Health Care for Women International* 12:261–269.

Patterson, C. 1986. "In the Far Pacific at the Birth of Nations." *National Geographic* 170 (4): 460–499.

Pearson, R. 1982. "Understanding the Vietnamese in Britain, Part III: Health Beliefs, Birth and Child Care." *Health Visitor* 55(10): 533–540.

Pillsbury, B. L. K. 1978. " 'Doing the Month': Confinement and Convalescence of Chinese Women after Childbirth." *Social Science and Medicine* 12: 11–22.

Potter, G. S., and A. Whiren. 1982. "Traditional Hmong Birth Customs: A Historical Study." In *The Hmong in the West: Observations and Reports*, edited by B. T. Downing and D. P. Olney, 48–62. Minneapolis: Southeast

Asian Refugee Studies Project, Center for Urban and Regional Affairs, University of Minnesota.

Prendergast, S. 1994. *This Is the Time to Grow Up: Girls' Experiences of Menstruation in School*. London: Family Planning Association.

Puddifoot, J. E., and M. P. Johnson. 1997. "The Legitimacy of Grieving: The Partner's Experience at Miscarriage." *Social Science and Medicine* 45 (6): 837–845.

Pyke, C. V., 1987. "Medicinal Ethnobotany of Hmong Refugees in Thailand." *Journal of Ethnobiology* 7(1): 13–26.

Quincy, K. 1995. *Hmong: History of a People*. Cheney, WA: Eastern Washington University Press.

Quine, L., and D. Rutter. 1996. "Birth Experiences." In *Conception, Pregnancy and Birth*, edited by C. A. Niven and A. Walker, 114–119. Oxford: Butterworth and Heinemann.

Raphael-Leff, J. 1991. *Psychological Processes of Childbearing*. London: Chapman and Hall.

Reinharz, S. 1988. "What Is Missing in Miscarriage?" *Journal of Community Psychology* 16 (January): 84–103.

Reissland, N., and R. Burghart. 1988. "The Quality of a Mother's Milk and the Health of Her Child: Beliefs and Practices of the Women of Mithila." *Social Science and Medicine* 27 (5): 461–469.

Renne, E. P. 1996. "The Pregnancy That Doesn't Stay: The Practice and Perception of Abortion by Ekiti Yoruba Women." *Social Science and Medicine* 42 (4): 483–494.

Rice, P. L. 1993. *My Forty Days: A Cross-Cultural Resource Book for Health Care Professionals in Birthing Services*. Melbourne: The Vietnamese Antenatal/Postnatal Support Project.

Rice, P. L. 1994. "When I Had My Baby Here!" In *Asian Mothers, Australian Birth*, edited by P. L. Rice, 117–132. Melbourne: Ausmed Publications.

Rice, P. L. 1995. "*Pog Laus, Tsis Coj Khaub Ncaws Lawm*: The Meaning of Menopause in Hmong Women." *Journal of Reproductive and Infant Psychology*, Special Issue on the Menopause 13 (2): 79–92.

Rice, P. L. 1997. "Giving Birth in a New Home: Childbirth Traditions and the Experience of Motherhood among Hmong Women from Laos." *Asian Studies Review* 20 (3): 133–148.

Rice, P. L. 1998. *Children! Children!: The Social Construction of Infertility among Hmong Women in Australia*. Paper presented at the Fourth National Hmong Conference, Denver, CO, April 16–18.

Rice, P. L., and L. Manderson, eds. 1996. *Maternity and Reproductive Health in Asian Societies*. Amsterdam: Harwood Academic Publishers.

Rice, P. L., and C. Naksook. 1998. "Childrearing and Cultural Beliefs and Practices among Thai Mothers in Victoria: Implications for the Sudden Infant Death Syndrome." *Journal of Paediatrics and Child Health* 34 (4): 302–306.

Rice, P. L., B. Ly, and J. Lumley. 1994. "Soul Loss and Childbirth: The Case of a Hmong Woman." *Medical Journal of Australia* 160 (9): 577–578.

Rice, P. L., C. Naksook, and L. Watson. 1999. "After Birth: Confinement Practices During Hospital Stay and upon Returning Home among Thai Women in Australia." *Midwifery* 15 (1): 47–57.

Rich, A. 1992. *Of Woman Born: Motherhood as Experience and Institution*. London: Virago Press.

Riddle, J. M. 1992. *Conception and Abortion from the Ancient World to the Renaissance*. Cambridge: Harvard University Press.

Riddle, J. M. 1997. *Eve's Herbs: A History of Contraceptive and Abortion in the West*. Cambridge: Harvard University Press.

Rigdon, S. M. 1996. "Abortion Law and Practice in China: An Overview with Comparisons to the United States." *Social Science and Medicine* 42 (4): 543–560.

Riordan, J. 1993. "The Cultural Context of Breastfeeding." In *Breastfeeding and Human Lactation*, edited by J. Riordan and K. G. Auerback, 27–48. Boston: Jones and Bartlett.

Roberts, H. 1985. *The Patient Patients: Women and Their Doctors*. London: Pandora Press.

Romalis, S. 1981. *Childbirth: Alternatives to Medical Control*. Austin: University of Texas Press.

Rosaldo, M. Z. 1974. "Women, Culture and Society: A Theoretical Overview." In *Women, Culture and Society*, edited by M. Z. Rosaldo and L. Lamphere, 17–42. Stanford, CA: Stanford University Press.

Rothman, B. K. 1984. "The Meaning of Choice in Reproductive Technology." In *Test-tube Women: What Future for Motherhood?*, edited by R. Arditi, R. D. Klein, and S. Minden, 23–33. Boston: Pandora Press.

Rothman, B. K. 1989. *Recreating Motherhood*. New York: W. W. Norton & Company.

Rothman, B. K. 1991. *In Labor: Women and Power in the Birthplace*. New York: W. W. Norton & Company.

Rozario, S. 1992. *Purity and Communal Boundaries: Women and Social Change in a Bangladeshi Village*. London: Zed Books.

Rubel, A., K. Weller-Fahy, and M. Trosdal. 1975. "Conception, Gestation and Delivery According to Some Mananabang of Cebu." *Philippine Quarterly of Culture and Society* 3: 131–145.

Sargent, C. 1982. "Solitary Confinement: Birth Practices among the Bariba of the People's Republic of Benin." In *Anthropology of Human Birth*, edited by M. A. Kay, 193–210. Philadelphia: F. A. Davis Company.

Savage, O. M. N. 1996. " 'Children of the Rope' and Other Aspects of Pregnancy Loss in Cameroon." In *The Anthropology of Pregnancy Loss: Comparative Studies in Miscarriage, Stillbirth and Neonatal Death*, edited by R. Cecil, 95–109. Oxford: Berg.

Savina, F. M. 1930. *Histoire des Miao*. Hong Kong: Imprimerie de la Société des Missions-Étrangeres.

Scheinberg, C. A. 1983. "Childbirth Interactions of Hmong Refugees in California with Health Providers: An Historical and Ethnographic Perspective." M.A. thesis, Department of Anthropology, California State University, Fullerton.

Scheper-Hughes, N. 1984. "Infant Mortality and Infant Care: Cultural and Economic Constraints on Nurturing in Northeast Brazil." *Social Science and Medicine* 19 (5): 535–546.

Scheper-Hughes, N. 1991. "Social Indifference to Child Death." *The Lancet* 337 (8750): 1144–1147.

Scheper-Hughes, N. 1992. *Death without Weeping: The Violence of Everyday Life in Brazil*. Berkeley: University of California Press.

Scott, G. M. 1986. "Migrants without Mountains: The Politics of Sociocultural Adjustment among the Lao Hmong Refugees in San Diego." Ph.D. diss., Department of Anthropology, University of California at San Diego, San Diego.

Scrimshaw, S. C. M. 1985. "Bringing the Period Down: Government and Squatter Settlement Confront Induced Abortion in Ecuador." In *Micro and Macro Levels of Analysis in Anthropology: Issues in Theory and Research*, edited by B. R. DeWalt and P. J. Pelto, 121–146. Boulder: Westview Press.

Sha, J. L. 1990. *Mothers of Thyme: Customs and Rituals of Infertility and Miscarriage*. Ann Arbor, MI: Lida Rose Press.

Shea, P. D., A. Riggio, and Y. Yang. 1995. *The Whispering Cloth: A Refugee's Story*. Honesdale, PA: Boyds Mills Press.

Shedlin, M. 1982. *Anthropology and Family Planning: Culturally Appropriate Intervention in a Mexican Community*. Ph.D. diss., Columbia University, New York.

Sich, D. 1981. "Traditional Concepts and Customs on Pregnancy, Birth and Post Partum Period in Rural Korea." *Social Science and Medicine* 15B: 65–69.

Simonds, W. 1988. "Confessions of Loss: Maternal Grief in True Story, 1920–1985." *Gender & Society* 2 (2): 149–171.

Small, R., P. L. Rice, J. Yelland, and J. Lumley. 1999. "Mothers in a New Country: The Role of Culture and Communication in Vietnamese, Turkish and Filipino Women's Experiences of Giving Birth in Australia." *Women & Health* 28 (3): 77–101.

Smalley, W. A., C. K. Vang, and G. Y. Yang. 1990. *Mother of Writing: The Origin and Development of a Hmong Messianic Script*. Chicago: University of Chicago Press.

Sobo, E. 1992. " 'Unclean Deeds': Menstrual Taboos and Binding 'Ties' in Rural Jamaica." In *Anthropological Approaches to the Study of Ethnomedicine*, edited by M. Nichter, 101–126. Amsterdam: Gordon and Breach Science Publishers.

Sobo, E. 1993. "Bodies, Kin, and Flow: Family Planning in Rural Jamaica." *Medical Anthropology Quarterly* 7 (1): 50–73.

Sobo, E. 1996. "Abortion Traditions in Rural Jamaica." *Social Science and Medicine* 42 (4): 495–508.

Steinberg, S. 1996. "Childbearing Research: A Transcultural Review. *Social Science and Medicine* 43 (12): 1765–1784.

Stone, D. 1998. "When the Shaman Pulls the String." *The Age Extra/Features*, October 31, p.5.

Symonds, P. V., 1991. "Cosmology and the Cycle of Life: Hmong Views of Birth, Death and Gender in a Mountain Village in Northern Thailand." Ph.D. diss., Department of Anthropology at Brown University, Providence, RI.

Symonds, P. V., 1996. "Journey to the Land of Light: Birth among Hmong Women." In *Maternity and Reproductive Health in Asian Societies*, edited by P. L. Rice and L. Manderson, 103–123. Amsterdam: Harwood Academic Press.

Tapp, N. 1985. "Categories of Change and Continuity among the Hmong." Ph.D. diss., Department of Anthropology, School of Oriental and African Studies, University of London.

Taylor, C., 1990. "Condoms and Cosmology: The 'Fractal' Person and Sexual Risk in Rwanda." *Social Science and Medicine* 31 (9): 1023–1028.

Taylor, C., 1992. "The Harp That Plays by Itself." In *Anthropological Approaches to the Study of Ethnomedicine*, edited by M. Nichter, 127–147. Amsterdam: Gordon and Breach Science Publishers.

Thao, P., X. Thao, and D. Conquergood, 1986. "I Am a Shaman." In *The Hmong World* 1, edited by B. Johns and D. Strecker, 164–193. New Haven, CT: Yale Southeast Asia Studies.

Thao, T. C. 1986. "Hmong Customs on Marriage, Divorce and the Rights of Married Women." In *The Hmong World* 1, edited by B. Johns and D. Strecker, 74–98. New Haven, CT: Yale Southeast Asia Studies.

Thao, X. 1984. "Southeast Asian Refugees of Rhode Island: The Hmong Perception of Illness." *Rhode Island Medical Journal* 67: 323–330.

Thao, X. 1986. "Hmong Perceptions of Illness and Traditional Ways of Healing." In *The Hmong in Transition*, edited by G. L. Hendricks, B. T. Downing, and A. S. Deinard, 365–378. New York: The Center for Migration Studies.

Thuren, B-M. 1994. "Opening Doors and Getting Rid of Shame: Experiences of First Menstruation in Valencia, Spain." *Women's Studies International Forum* 17 (2/3): 217–228.

Townsend, K., and P. L. Rice. 1996. "A Baby Is Born in Site 2 Camp: Pregnancy, Birth and Confinement among Cambodian Refugee Women." In *Maternity and Reproductive Health in Asian Societies*, edited by P. L. Rice and L. Manderson, 125–143. Amsterdam: Harwood Academic Publishers.

Townsend, J. M., and C. L. Carbone. 1980. "Menopausal Syndrome: Illness or Social Role—A Transcultural Analysis." *Culture, Medicine and Psychiatry* 4 (3): 229–248.

Trueba, H. T., L. Jacob, and E. Kirton. 1990. *Cultural Conflict and Adaptation: The Case of Hmong Children in American Society*. New York: Falmer Press.

Trueba, H. T., and Y. Zou. 1994. *Power in Education: The Case of Miao University Students and Its Significance for American Culture*. Washington, D.C.: Falmer Press.

van der Geest, S., and S. Whyte. 1989. "The Charm of Medicines: Metaphors and Metonyms." *Medical Anthropology Quarterly* 3 (4): 345–367.

Van Esterik, P. 1985. "The Cultural Context of Breastfeeding in Rural Thailand." In *Breastfeeding Child Health and Child Spacing: Cross-Cultural Perspectives*, edited by V. Hull and M. Simpson, 139–161. London: Croom Helm.

Van Gennep, A. V. 1960. *The Rites of Passage*. Chicago: University of Chicago Press.

van Keep, P., and J. Kellerhals. 1975. "The Aging Woman. About the Influence of Some Social and Cultural Factors on the Change in Attitude and Behaviours That Occur after Menopause." *Acta Obstetrica Gynecology Scandinavia* (Suppl.) 51: 19–27.

Vang, C. K., G. Y. Yang, W. A. Smalley, M. Moua, and S. Yang. 1990. "The Life of Shong Lue Yang: Hmong 'Mother of Writing.'" Southeast Asian Refugee Studies Occasional Papers, No. 9. Center for Urban and Regional Affairs, University of Minnesota, Minneapolis.

Vang, L., and J. Lewis. 1990. *Grandmother's Path, Grandfather's Way: Oral Lore, Generation to Generation*. Rancho Cordova, CA: Lue Vang and Judy Lewis.

Vang, M. M., 1994. "Hmong Mothers and Daughters: Cultural Adjustment and Conflict." Master's thesis, California State University, Stanislaus.

Vangay, J. 1988. "Hmong Parents' Cultural Attitudes and the Sex-Ratio Imbalance of Hmong Merced High School Graduates." Master's thesis, California State University, Stanislaus.

Vincent Priya, J. 1992. *Birth Traditions and Modern Pregnancy Care*. Shaftesbury: Element.

Voda, A. 1993. Book Review. *Signs: Journal of Women in Culture and Society* (Winter): 447–451.

Vong-Ek, P. 1993. "How Popular Beliefs Influence Breastfeeding Practices in Northeast and Central Thailand." *Journal of Primary Health Care and Development* 6 (1): 61–76.

Vue, K., and C. Vue. 1995. *The Hmong People of Southeast Asia*. Melbourne: Victorian Co-oporative on Children's Services for Ethnic Groups.

Wang, J. A., 1998. "Health Care Behaviour of Hmong Refugees in Sydney." Master's thesis, Department of Geography, University of Sydney, Sydney, Australia.

Watson, L., A. Potter, R. Gallucci, and J. Lumley. 1998. "Is Baby Too Warm? The Use of Infant Clothing, Bedding and Home Heating in Victoria, Australia." *Early Human Development* 51: 93–107.

Weideger, P. 1977. *Menstruation and Menopause: The Physiology and Psychology, the Myth and the Reality*. Harmondsworth, Middlesex: Penguin Books.

Weise, H. J., 1976. "Maternal Nutrition and Traditional Food Behavior in Haiti." *Human Organization* 35 (2): 193–200.

Wembah-Rashid, J. A. R. 1996. "Explaining Pregnancy Loss in Matrilineal Southeast Tanzania." In *The Anthropology of Pregnancy Loss: Comparative Studies in Miscarriage, Stillbirth and Neonatal Death,* edited by R. Cecil, 75–93. Oxford: Berg.

Westermeyer, J. 1988. "Folk Medicine in Laos: A Comparison between Two Ethnic Groups." *Social Science and Medicine* 27 (8): 769–778.

Whiteford, L. M., and Gonzalez, L. 1995. "Stigma: The Hidden Burden of Infertility." *Social Science and Medicine* 40 (1): 27–36.

Whittaker, A. 1996. "White Blood and Falling Wombs: Ethnogynaecology in Northeast Thailand." In *Maternity and Reproductive Health in Asian Societies,* edited by P. L. Rice and L. Manderson, 207–225. Amsterdam: Harwood Academic Press.

Williamson, M. H. 1983. "Sex Relations and Gender Relations: Understanding Kwoma Conception." *Mankind* 14 (1): 13–23.

Wilson, C. S., 1973. "Food Taboos of Childbirth: The Malay Example." *Ecology of Food and Nutrition* 2: 267–274.

Wilson, P. 1966. *Female Forever*. New York: M. Evans.

Winikoff, B. 1987. "Family Planning and the Health of Women and Children." *Technology in Society* 9: 415–438.

Woollett, A., N. Dosanjh, P. Nicholson, H. Marshall, O. Djhanbakhch, and J. Hadlow. 1995. "The Ideas and Experiences of Pregnancy and Childbirth of Asian and Non-Asian Women in East London." *British Journal of Medical Psychiatry* 68: 65–84.

Woollett, A., and N. Dosanjh-Matwala. 1990. "Pregnancy and Antenatal Care: The Attitudes and Experiences of Asian Women." *Child: Care, Health and Development* 16: 63–78.

Woollett, A., and P. Nicholson. 1998. "The Social Construction of Motherhood and Fatherhood." In *Current Issues in Infancy and Parenthood*, edited by C. A. Niven and A. Walker, 1–14. Oxford: Butterworth Heinemann.

World Health Organization, 1988. *World Health Organization: A Brief Summary of Its Work.* Australian Canberra: Government Publishing Service.

Yang, D. 1992. "The Hmong: Enduring Traditions." In *Minority Cultures of Laos: Kammu, Lua', Lahu, Hmong, and Iu-Mien*, edited by J. Lewis, 249–326. Rancho Cordova, CA: Southeast Asia Community Resource Center.

Yang, D. 1993. *Hmong at the Turning Point*. Minneapolis MN: WorldBridge Associates.

Yelland, J., S. Gifford, and M. Macintyre. 1994. "Explanatory Models About Maternal and Infant Health and Sudden Infant Death Syndrome among Asian-Born Mothers." In *Asian Mothers, Australian Birth*, edited by P. L. Rice, 175–190. Melbourne: Ausmed Publications.

Yelland, J., R. Small, J. Lumley, P. L. Rice, V. Cotronei, and R. Warren. 1998. "Support, Sensitivity, Satisfaction: Filipino, Turkish and Vietnamese Women's Experiences of Postnatal Hospital Stay." *Midwifery* 14 (3): 144–154.

Yoddumnern-Attig, B., O. Pituckmahaket, and U. Kanungsukkasem. 1993. "The Main Types and Steps of Sampling." In *Qualitative Methods for Population and Health Research*, edited by B. Yoddumnern-Attig, G. A. Attig, W. Boonchalaksi, K. Richter, and A. Soonthorndhada, 91–100. Salaya, Thailand: Institute for Population and Social Research, Mahidol University at Salaya.

Index

About the Author

PRANEE LIAMPUTTONG RICE is Senior Lecturer in the School of Public Health, La Trobe University, Melbourne, Australia. She has published several books and papers including *Maternity and Reproductive Health in Asian Societies* (with Lenore Manderson, editors, 1996), *Living in a New Country: Understanding Migrants' Health* (editor, 1999) and *Qualitative Research Methods: A Health Focus* (with Douglas Ezzy, 1999).

www.ingramcontent.com/pod-product-compliance
Ingram Content Group UK Ltd.
Pitfield, Milton Keynes, MK11 3LW, UK
UKHW041131071026
15587UKWH00009B/410

9 780897 896795